SAUNDERS SOLUTIONS IN
**VETERINARY PRACTICE**

SMALL ANIMAL
# EXOTIC PET MEDICINE

*Commissioning Editor:* Robert Edwards
*Development Editor:* Ewan Halley
*Project Manager:* Priya Dauntess
*Designer/Design Direction:* Charles Gray
*Illustrator:* Merlyn Harvey

# SAUNDERS SOLUTIONS IN VETERINARY PRACTICE

## SMALL ANIMAL
# EXOTIC PET MEDICINE

Series Editor: Fred Nind BVM&S, MRCVS

## Lesa Longley

MA BVM&S DZooMed (Mammalian) MRCVS
RCVS Recognised Specialist in Zoo & Wildlife Medicine
College of Medicine & Veterinary Medicine
University of Edinburgh
UK

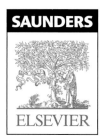

SAUNDERS

ELSEVIER

Edinburgh   London   New York   Oxford   Philadelphia   St Louis   Sydney   Toronto   2010

**SAUNDERS**
ELSEVIER

First published 2010

ISBN: 978-0-7020-2985-1

**British Library Cataloguing in Publication Data**
A catalogue record for this book is available from the British Library

**Library of Congress Cataloging in Publication Data**
A catalog record for this book is available from the Library of Congress

**Notice**

Knowledge and best practice in this field are constantly changing. As new research and experience broaden our knowledge, changes in practice, treatment and drug therapy may become necessary or appropriate. Readers are advised to check the most current information provided (i) on procedures featured or (ii) by the manufacturer of each product to be administered, to verify the recommended dose or formula, the method and duration of administration, and contraindications. It is the responsibility of the practitioner, relying on their own experience and knowledge of the patient, to make diagnoses, to determine dosages and the best treatment for each individual patient, and to take all appropriate safety precautions. To the fullest extent of the law, neither the Publisher nor the Authors assume any liability for any injury and/or damage to persons or property arising out or related to any use of the material contained in this book.

*The Publisher*

**ELSEVIER**
your source for books,
journals and multimedia
in the health sciences

**www.elsevierhealth.com**

Working together to grow
libraries in developing countries

www.elsevier.com | www.bookaid.org | www.sabre.org

ELSEVIER    BOOK AID
International    Sabre Foundation

The
publisher's
policy is to use
**paper manufactured
from sustainable forests**

Printed in China

# Contents

# Acknowledgements

I would like to thank friends and family who have encouraged me along my journey to becoming an exotics clinician, and to those veterinary surgeons and clients that have assisted me on the way. In particular my appreciation goes to Dermod Malley – for his inspiration, teaching, and friendship.

Thank you all for your support.

Lesa Longley

# Introduction

*Saunders Solutions in Veterinary Practice* series is a new range of veterinary textbooks which will grow into a mini-library over the next few years, covering all the main disciplines of companion animal practice.

Readers should realize that it is not the authors' intention to cover all that is known about each topic. As such the books in the *Solutions Series* are not standard reference works. Instead they are intended to provide practical information on the more frequently encountered conditions in an easily accessible form based on real-life case studies. They cover that range of cases that fall between the boringly routine and the referral. The books will help practitioners with a particular interest in a topic or those preparing for a specialist qualification. The cases are arranged by presenting sign rather than by the underlying pathology, as this is how veterinary surgeons will see them in practice.

Each case also includes descriptions of underlying pathology and details of the nursing required, both in the veterinary clinic and at home. It is hoped that the books will also, therefore, be of interest to veterinary students in the later parts of their course and to veterinary nurses.

Continuing professional development (CPD) is mandatory for many veterinarians and a recommended practice for others. The *Saunders Series* will provide a CPD resource which can be accessed economically, shared with colleagues and used anywhere. It will also provide busy veterinary practitioners with quick access to authoritative information on the diagnosis and treatment of interesting and challenging cases. The robust cover has been made resistant to some of the more gruesome contaminants found in a veterinary clinic because this is where we hope these books will be used.

Joyce Rodenhuis, Mary Seager and Robert Edwards were the inspiration for the Series and both the Series editor and the individual authors are grateful for their foresight in commissioning the series and their unfailing support and guidance during their production.

## SMALL ANIMAL EXOTIC PET MEDICINE

There is a tendency for practitioners to panic when presented with so called 'exotic' animals, and it can indeed feel challenging to be faced with a species that you have never encountered before. But do not despair. This book will help you. Specifically, it will reassure you that by going back to the basics of obtaining a good history, applying the skills of observation and clinical examination that you would use in a more familiar species and the judicious use of clinical aids are all that you need to reach a diagnosis in the vast majority of cases.

We also hope that the book will persuade you that an animal obtained by the owner for little or no money is not valueless to them and that many owners of 'exotic' pets will be just as willing to work hard and pay your fees to get a sick one back to health, as any cat or dog owner.

The warm glow of satisfaction when an 'exotic' case gets better is an experience to be savoured and the author and I hope that this book will help share it.

Fred Nind
Series Editor

# 1 The exotic pet consultation

## INTRODUCTION

Exotic pets are different from the more usual domestic pet, not just in their appearance but also in their husbandry requirements. While most owners know the basics of how to keep a dog or cat well fed, many novel/exotic pet owners can be misguided as to the dietary needs of their animal. Many exotic pet species – particularly reptiles – originate from tropical climes with very specific environmental requirements, and, when kept in more temperate regions, necessitate close attention to husbandry details in order to be maintained in good health. For this reason, it is imperative for the exotic pet veterinary practitioner to meticulously investigate the *husbandry* details of the animal. Many owners are closely bonded with their pets and willing to have extensive veterinary treatments if the animal becomes ill (Fig. 1.1). The *history* of the problem as noted by the owner should also be assessed comprehensively.

For many of these unusual pets, the *clinical examination* may be reduced compared with that of other species. Some, such as the Roborovsky hamster, may just be too small to assess in detail. Others, such as tortoises, may have a shell encasing the main body cavity, precluding palpation.

By attaining a sound knowledge of common problems in exotic pet species, the clinician should be able to quickly assess the patient for frequent pathologies. Often, the veterinary clinician identifies a disease process that is not directly related to the problem for which the animal was presented. On some occasions, the animal is presented for a routine health check – particularly with a new pet – and this is an ideal opportunity for the clinician to assess the animal and its living conditions for any potential factors that may predispose to disease in the future. This form of preventative healthcare is to be encouraged among clients – as prevention is eminently preferable to treatment – and many veterinary practices promote 'well-animal' checks of exotic species (Fig. 1.2).

## HISTORY TAKING

As there are many differences in husbandry requirements and predispositions for disease within taxonomic groups, suggested questions are listed in the introductory sections throughout the book.

In general, topics to cover include:
- Period of ownership
- Diet: what is offered by the owner and what is eaten by the animal, including any supplements
- Enclosure: size, structure, any supplemental heating and/or lighting, substrate
- Handling/training
- Breeding: behaviour and/or production
- Previous medical problems: minor issues may have previously been treated by the owner
- Current problem: date of onset, progression, whether intermittent or continuous
- Any other changes in the animal: thirst/appetite, urine/faecal output, behaviour
- In-contact animals: including any problems noted in them.

## CLINICAL EXAMINATION

Ideally, adapt the normal small animal examination to these pets. The author adopts the approach of starting with the head and working caudally, although it is equally feasible to assess by body system.

It is important to note that many of these animals will not be accustomed to handling, and the procedure will be stressful. Prepare all equipment before restraining the animal – including any equipment necessary for laboratory sampling – to minimize the period of handling.

Perform a general physical examination to obtain an indication of the health of the individual. This will be especially important if further investigation or treatment is required, e.g. anaesthesia or surgery, that may be

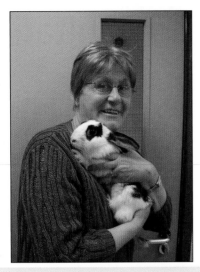

Figure 1.1 Many owners are closely bonded with their pets, and willing to have extensive veterinary treatments if the animal becomes ill.

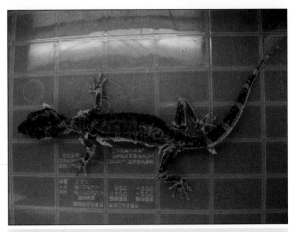

Figure 1.3 A thorough clinical examination should be performed even in small animals such as this leopard gecko (*Eublepharis macularius*). Care should be taken not to overly stress debilitated animals such as this emaciated specimen.

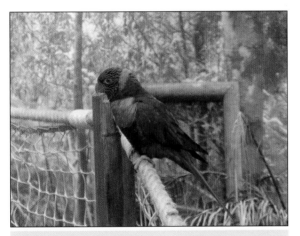

Figure 1.2 'Well-animal' veterinary health checks are particularly useful for birds such as this rainbow lorikeet (*Trichoglossus haematodus*), since many birds hide signs of illness until pathology is severe.

metabolically stressful and potentially fatal in an extremely unwell animal.

This should be followed by a more intensive assessment of the problem(s) noted during history taking. This may lead the clinician to examine other parts of the animal in more detail. For example, an ocular problem in a gecko may be associated with retained skin (Fig. 1.3) and the rest of the integument should be assessed to determine if dysecdysis has resulted in other problems

such as missing digits (after constrictive lesions caused by retained skin compromise the circulation).

## FORMATION OF DIFFERENTIAL DIAGNOSES

Although not always a clear-cut part of the consultation with the client, the veterinary clinician should formulate a list of possible differential diagnoses for the presenting signs. During the consultation, this may be a brief list of common problems that may be further investigated, although a more in-depth list will be appropriate for animals that are shown not to have these diagnoses. This list will enable the clinician to design a plan and discuss reasoning for investigations and potential treatments.

## INVESTIGATIONS

Each case will require specific investigations. As alluded to above, some laboratory samples may be taken during the initial examination. For example, swabs may be taken from lesions for microscopic and bacteriological assessment.

At other times, it will be necessary to use chemical restraint on the patient in order to investigate further. For example, many exotic pets require sedation or anaesthesia prior to phlebotomy or radiography. These requirements will vary greatly between species, e.g. many reptiles can be blood sampled and imaged conscious, while birds generally need to be anaesthetized.

Although minor superficial procedures may sometimes be performed under analgesia and local anaesthesia, all species require general anaesthesia for more invasive surgery.

## DISCUSSION WITH OWNER

The risks of chemical restraint and any procedures to be performed should be discussed with the owner so that they may give informed consent. These risks will vary between species and between animals. The use of off-label drugs should also be discussed, as few drugs are licensed for use in exotic species.

Often, exotic pets are prey species and hide signs of illness – or show only very subtle signs – until they are extremely ill. The owner should not be given unrealistic hopes for the recovery of their pet. However, as the clinician becomes more experienced, they should be able to identify those cases that are likely to respond to treatment.

The owner should be given a clear indication of the prognosis for the animal, along with an accurate estimation of the fees likely to be incurred in the processes of investigation and treatment. Most exotic pets are not insured and many conditions require extensive investigation to reach a diagnosis and for some – particularly reptiles – treatment may be prolonged and therefore expensive.

In some cases, the owner may not be willing or able to afford further investigation and expensive treatment. In these instances, the clinician should be able to provide good husbandry advice for the animal and potentially medication based on likely common conditions. Where an animal is suffering but treatment is not possible, the clinician should impress upon the client the need for animal welfare, and persuade them to permit euthanasia of the pet.

# SECTION 1

# MAMMALS

# 2 Mammals – an introduction

Small mammals are commonly kept as pets. Various species may be presented to the veterinary clinician, often with diverse husbandry requirements and disease predispositions. Presenting signs may be subtle and vague. This chapter will aim to discuss some basic biology and husbandry for these species, as well as providing the clinician with an outline on basic techniques to assess and treat the animals. The ensuing chapters will demonstrate approaches to an assortment of cases.

## TAXONOMY

Taxonomic classification of mammals commonly seen as pets is given in Table 2.1.

## BIOLOGY

This is a brief synopsis for common pet species. Further information may be found in Table 2.2, specific case reports later in the text or in references listed in the Further reading section.

### Leporidae (rabbit)

Rabbits are highly social, and should be kept with a companion (preferably both neutered). They dig burrows in the wild. An exercise area should be provided. Wood shavings and hay or straw are commonly used as substrates. Outdoor hutches should be secure. Indoor rabbits can be litter-trained; care should be taken to ensure cables and houseplants are protected from chewing. Chewable toys can be offered, e.g. cardboard boxes. Scent is an important sense to rabbits. As a prey species, fear elicits either immobility or a flight response. Thumping of the hindlegs is an alarm call.

This species is herbivorous, adapted to a low-quality, high-fibre diet – eating grass and weeds in the wild. Captive animals should be fed similarly, usually on a diet of good quality meadow hay supplemented with leafy green vegetables and wild plants such as dandelions. Concentrate mixes should be avoided, particularly 'muesli'-type mixes where selective feeding is possible. Water is usually provided in a sipper bottle, as the dewlap may get wet and skin infection could result if a bowl is used.

The dental formula is: incisors 2/1, canines 0/0, premolars 3/2, molars 3/3. All teeth are continuously growing (hypsodontic, with open roots). Rabbits cannot vomit. Gastrointestinal transit time is rapid in these hindgut fermenters, with bacterial fermentation in the caecum. Indigestible fibre stimulates gastrointestinal motility. The colon separates fibrous from non-fibrous particles; the former are excreted as hard faecal pellets. Soft mucus-covered caecal pellets are expelled separately and eaten (caecotrophy), allowing absorption of nutrients and bacterial fermentation products, as well as digestion of previously undigested food.

Rabbits should be vaccinated against myxomatosis and viral haemorrhagic disease.

### Sciuridae (chipmunk, prairie dog)

**Chipmunks** are omnivorous, eating seeds, buds, leaves and flowers in the wild. Captive animals are fed a commercial mix supplemented with fresh or dried fruit, vegetables and occasional nuts. These little rodents are escape artists, and their enclosure needs to be secure. Cage furniture should include branches, ropes and drainpipes. They can be housed singly, in pairs, or as a harem (with one male to two or three females). The testes descend in mature males during the breeding season (January–September).

**Prairie dogs** are social animals. They should be provided with tunnels and deep bedding (such as wood shavings or paper) for digging. Prairie dogs are herbivores, and hindgut/caecal fermenters. They can be fed on rodent food and grass hay, with fresh greens as a

**Table 2.1** Taxonomic classification of mammals commonly seen as pets

| Order | Suborder | Family | Subfamily | Species |
|---|---|---|---|---|
| Lagomorpha | – | Leporidae | – | Rabbit (*Oryctolagus cuniculus*) |
| Rodentia | Sciurognathi | Sciuridae (squirrel-like rodents) | – | Siberian chipmunk (*Tamias sibiricus*)<br>Prairie dog (*Cynomys ludovicianus*) |
| | | Muridae (mouse-like rodents) | Murinae | Mouse (*Mus musculus*)<br>Rat (*Rattus norvegicus*) |
| | | | Cricetinae<br>Gerbillinae | Hamster (e.g. golden hamster, *Mesocricetus auratus*)<br>Gerbil (e.g. Mongolian gerbil, *Meriones unguiculatus*) |
| | Hystricognathi (cavy-like rodents) | Caviidae<br>Chinchillidae<br>Octodontidae | –<br>–<br>– | Guinea pig (*Cavia porcellus*)<br>Chinchilla (*Chinchilla laniger*)<br>Degu (*Octodon degus*) |
| Insectivora | – | Erinaceidae | Erinaceinae | African pygmy hedgehog (*Atelerix albiventris*) |
| Diprotodontia (in the Marsupialia) | – | Petauridae | – | Sugar glider (*Petaurus breviceps*) |
| Carnivora | – | Mustelidae | Mustelinae | Ferret (*Mustela putorius furo*) |
| Primates | Haplorhini | Callitrichidae<br>Cebidae | –<br>– | Common marmoset (*Callithrix jacchus*)<br>Common squirrel monkey (*Simia sciureus*) |

treat. Obesity is common in pet prairie dogs. Water is provided in a sipper bottle. Males have an open inguinal canal (as in guinea pigs), and the testes may be retracted intra-abdominally.

## Muridae (mouse, rat, hamster, gerbil)

These species also exhibit coprophagy; they cannot vomit. The dental formula for this group is: incisors 1/1, canines 0/0, premolars 0/0, molars 3/3. The incisors are hypsodontic, while the molars are brachyodontic (permanently rooted).

**Mice** are omnivorous or herbivorous. Pet animals are usually fed a commercial rodent diet supplemented with a small amount of fresh food, fruit and vegetables. They are housed in either a wire cage with a solid plastic bottom, or a plastic enclosure with a mesh roof. Sawdust or wood shavings are utilized as substrate, with shredded newspaper or commercial rodent bedding in the nest box. Cardboard boxes and paper to tear, drainpipes and wheels are useful enrichment. Cage hygiene is important.

**Rats** have a similar diet and housing requirement to mice. Fur yellowing is normal in aged animals.

**Hamsters** have large cheek pouches for food storage. They are omnivorous and hoard food. Commercial hamster mixes are available for captive animals. They have bilateral pigmented sebaceous glands on their flanks; these are used for territorial marking and mating behaviour. Common species kept as pets include Syrian (*Mesocricetus auratus*), Chinese (*Cricetulus griseus*) and Russian (e.g. Roborovski, *Phodopus roborovskii*) hamsters. These animals are escape artists, and enclosures should be secure. They are usually housed in wire cages or plastic enclosures with tunnels. Paper or hay should be provided in the nest box. Exercise wheels are used at night.

**Gerbils** have a large ventral scent gland on the mid-abdomen, used for territorial marking. The gland is more pronounced in young males. Urine is very concentrated in this desert adapted species. Commercial rodent mix can be supplemented with fresh fruit and vegetables, hay, and occasional treats of raisins. Gerbils are highly social and should be maintained in a group (ideally same sex), usually in a glass or plastic tank. The 'gerbillarium' should have a deep (15 cm) substrate of sawdust, wood shavings or peat and hay. Sand should be avoided, as rostral abrasions are common.

**Table 2.2** Biology of selected mammals commonly kept as pets

| Species | Longevity | Average weight | Sexual maturity | Sexing | Gestation | Litter size | Weaning age | Rectal temperature (°C) | Heart rate (/min) | Respiratory rate (/min) |
|---|---|---|---|---|---|---|---|---|---|---|
| Rabbit | 5–10 years | 1–10 kg (depends on breed) | 4–8 months (F before M) | M: greater ano-genital distance, round preputial opening F: elliptical vulval opening | 28–32 days | 4–12 | 6 weeks | 38.5–40.0 | 180–300 | 30–60 |
| Chipmunk | 4–6 years (<12 years reported) | 72–120 g | – | M: longer ano-genital distance, obvious prepuce | 31–32 days | 3–5 | 42 days | – | – | 75 |
| Prairie dog | 10 years | 0.5–2.2 kg (M>F) | 2–3 years | M: scrotal sac easily visible, longer ano-genital distance | 30–35 days | 2–10 (average 5) | 6 weeks | 35.3–39.0 | 83–318 | – |
| Mouse | 1.5–2.5 years | 20–40 g | 6–7 weeks | M: longer ano-genital distance F: separate vaginal and urethral orifices | 19–21 days | 6–12 | 21 days | 37.5 | 500–600 | 100–250 |
| Rat | 2.5–3.5 years | 225–500 g (M larger) | 6–8 weeks | M: testicles usually visible in juveniles F: separate vaginal and urethral orifices | 20–22 days | 6–16 | 21 days | 38 | 260–450 | 70–150 |
| Hamster | 1–3 years (depending on species) | Syrian 85–150 g Chinese 27–35 g Russian 30–50 g | 6–8 weeks (7–14 weeks for Chinese) | M: longer ano-genital distance F: separate vaginal and urethral orifices | Syrian: 15–18 days Chinese: 21 days Russian: 18 days | Syrian: 5–9 Chinese: 4–5 Russian: 4 | Syrian: 21–28 days Chinese: 21 days Russian: 16–18 days | 37.6 | 280–412 | 33–135 |
| Gerbil | 3–4 years | 70–120 g | 10–12 weeks | M: longer ano-genital distance F: separate vaginal and urethral orifices | 24–26 days (27–48 days if lactating) | 3–7 | 20–26 days | 37–38.5 | 300–400 | 90–140 |
| Guinea pig | 4–8 years | F: 750 g–1 kg M: 1–1.2 kg | F: 4–6 weeks M: 9–10 weeks | M: protrude penis by pressing either side of genital opening F: shallow vaginal groove between urethra and anus | 59–72 days | 1–6 | 3 weeks | 37.2–39.5 | 190–300 | 90–150 |

**Table 2.2** Biology of selected mammals commonly kept as pets *continued*

| Species | Longevity | Average weight | Sexual maturity | Sexing | Gestation | Litter size | Weaning age | Rectal temperature (°C) | Heart rate (/min) | Respiratory rate (/min) |
|---|---|---|---|---|---|---|---|---|---|---|
| Chinchilla | 8–10 years | 400–600 g (F larger) | 6–9 months | M: longer ano-genital distance than F, testes in inguinal canal (no true scrotum) F: cone-shaped urogenital papilla (with urethra) similar appearance to prepuce, vaginal closure membrane | 111 days | 1–6 | 6 weeks | 37–38 | 100–150 | 45–80 |
| Degu | 7 years | 170–300 g | 6 months | M: intra-abdominal testes, greater ano-genital distance | 90 days | 1–10 | 4 weeks | 37.9 | – | – |
| African pygmy hedgehog | 3–5 years (<10 years in captivity) | F: 250–400 g M: 500–600 g | 2 months | M: prepuce on mid-abdomen, testes in para-anal recess (can palpate in reproductively active M) F: urogenital opening few mm cranial to anus | 34–37 days | 1–7 (average 3) | 4–6 weeks | 36.1–37.2 | – | – |
| Sugar glider | 12–14 years (captivity) | 95–160 g (M larger) | F: 8–12 months M: 12–14 months | M: mid-ventral pedunculated scrotum and bifurcated penis F: pouch (contains two teats) | 16 days (before fetus in pouch) | 1–2 | 70 days (leave pouch), independent at 16 weeks | 32 (body temperature) | – | – |
| Ferret | 5–15 years (usually <10 years) | M: 1–2 kg F: 500–900 g | 8–12 months | M: testicles in scrotum in breeding season (December– July), longer ano-genital distance with obvious prepuce | 42 days | 7–14 | 6 weeks | 37.8–40.0 | 200–400 | 33–36 |
| Common marmoset | 15–20 years | 350–400 g | M: 15–24 months F: 14–24 months | M: greater ano-genital distance, testes in scrotum | 130–150 days | 1–4 (average 2) | 2–3 months | 39–40 | 200–350 | 50–70 |

M, male; F, female.

## Caviidae (guinea pig)

Guinea pigs have sebaceous glands over the dorsum, rump and perineal areas. As with other Hystricognathi, they have large tympanic bullae. Digestion is mainly by caecal fermentation. They should be fed a diet of hay, fresh vegetables, and some commercial mix. Guinea pigs have a daily requirement for vitamin C, approximately 30 mg/kg per day (higher levels are required during pregnancy, lactation and illness). The dental formula for hystricognaths is: incisors 1/1, canines 0/0, premolars 1/1, molars 3/3. All teeth are continuously growing (hypsodont).

They are usually housed in a hutch with a large run area. They are a sociable species and usually kept in single-sex groups (castrated if male to reduce aggression), pairs or harems. At least one hide area should be provided per guinea pig. The flooring should be smooth, with a substrate of wood shavings or shredded paper.

Male guinea pigs have large seminiferous vesicles. A vaginal membrane is present in females, except during oestrus and parturition. Both sexes have a pair of inguinal nipples.

## Chinchillidae (chinchilla)

Chinchillas have very dense fur, with up to 90 hairs per follicle. They are hindgut fermenters. They should be fed mainly hay with a small amount of commercial pellets; fruit and green vegetables can be given as occasional treats.

This species is usually housed in pairs, single-sex groups or a harem (one male with up to five females). Enclosures should be multilevel to permit horizontal and vertical activity. The enclosure is usually composed of wire mesh (15 × 15 mm) with wooden shelves and nest box. Dust baths should be provided for 10 minutes daily. Originating from the Andes, chinchillas are adapted to low humidity and cooler temperatures.

## Octodontidae (degu)

Degus are native to Chile, and susceptible to heat stress (in environmental temperatures greater than 30°C). They are used in sleep biology and jet-lag studies, but very few medical data are published on this species. Degus are hindgut fermenters. Tail slip is common if they are incorrectly restrained.

The captive diet should be predominantly grass hay, with rodent mix and a small amount of fresh greens. Degus are sociable and kept in pairs or groups. Their enclosure is similar to that for chinchillas, although they should be provided with bedding for digging and storing food. They will use an exercise wheel, and may use a dust bath.

## Erinaceidae (African pygmy hedgehog)

African pygmy hedgehogs (or four-toed hedgehogs) originate from equatorial and central Africa. They are nocturnal and solitary. Novel objects may result in 'anting' or 'anointing' behaviour, where the hedgehog hypersalivates to create a foam which it then spits onto itself. Animals may hiss or 'puff up' in defence. Unlike the European hedgehog (*Erinaceus europaeus*), they do not hibernate.

The dental formula for hedgehogs is: incisors 3/2, canines 1/1, premolars 3/2, molars 3/3. Wild hedgehogs are insectivorous and omnivorous, requiring a relatively high-protein and low-fat diet. Captive animals are fed cat food or insectivore diet, vegetables, insects and a vitamin/mineral supplement.

Their enclosure should have smooth walls, deep (10 cm) bedding and a hide box. The ambient temperature should be 24–30°C, often requiring some form of supplemental heating. The hedgehogs like to dig and use exercise wheels, and may swim or bathe in shallow water.

## Petauridae (sugar glider)

Sugar gliders are nocturnal and arboreal. The gliding membrane (patagium) stretches from the fifth digit of the forepaws to the ankles, and they can glide up to 50 m. For this reason, large areas should be made available for exercise. The enclosure should be a minimum of 2 m wide × 2 m long × 1.8 m high, with branches at either end to allow gliding. Supplemental heating is usually required to prevent the animals entering a state of torpor. They are sociable and kept in groups. Scent marking allows group members to recognize each other. Males develop a scent gland on their forehead, and have anal glands and scent glands on their chest; females have scent glands within their pouch but scent mark with urine.

In the wild, the diet of the sugar glider varies seasonally – being mainly gum/sap from eucalyptus or acacia trees during the winter, and mainly insects for the rest of the year. Sugar gliders have specialized incisors for gouging bark. Several 'recipes' have been developed for the sugar glider diet, usually a mix of insectivore/carnivore diet and Leadbeater's Mixture (a honey, protein, vitamin and mineral supplement mix). Sugar gliders should be fed in the evening.

As marsupials, sugar gliders have a common opening for the urinary and digestive tracts, the cloaca. Assessment of core body temperature via a cloacal probe is less reliable than rectal probes in other species.

## Mustelidae (ferret)

Some ferrets are kept as working animals (particularly in the UK) and others purely as pets. They are carnivorous, and are fed on either whole carcasses (e.g. pigeon or rabbit) or a commercial ferret diet. The gastrointestinal transit time is quite rapid, being approximately 3 hours.

The heart is relatively caudal (at the level of the sixth to eighth ribs). Ferrets should be vaccinated against canine distemper virus. Dental disease is common and the teeth should be brushed if possible.

Ferrets should be housed in an enclosure measuring at least 55 × 50 × 40 cm. The substrate is usually wood shavings. Most animals like to sleep in a towel or blanket, in a hammock or a box.

## Callitrichidae and Cebidae (common marmoset, squirrel monkey)

Non-human primates are rarely kept as pets, many species require a licence to be kept as such legally in the UK. Callitrichids (marmosets and tamarins) are the most common species seen. Zoonotic diseases should be considered when handling primates.

These species are omnivorous, but exact dietary requirements vary. Callitrichids eat a large proportion of fruit, but commercial kibble diets are available for most species. Besides the primate's daily requirement for vitamin C, New World primates (particularly callitrichids) require vitamin D3 so should be exposed to ultraviolet light (UV-B) to enable calcium and phosphorus metabolism. Where invertebrates are fed, these should be gut-loaded with calcium supplement.

## HISTORY

Some pertinent topics to discuss with owners during the initial consultation with an exotic pet mammal are listed in Box 2.1. Although the basic outline is very similar to that for other companion animals, it is noteworthy that greater emphasis is paid to husbandry conditions (including housing and diet). This is to gain an understanding of any factors that may predispose disease in the animal. Unfortunately husbandry-related disease is common in exotic pets.

Husbandry conditions can vary widely between species and owners. For example, some rabbits are housed indoors, while others are outdoors. Size of enclosure and any furniture present will have a significant bearing on the animal's activity and fitness. Inadequacies may potentially predispose to disease; for example, poor ventilation may be associated with a build-up of ammonia, respiratory irritation, and thus an increased risk of respiratory disease in rodents.

Unlike other companion animals, diets may also be extremely varied and the veterinary clinician should be cognizant of locally available proprietary brands and their suitability for the species in question. For most exotic pet mammals, it can be difficult to ascertain how much food is being eaten, and less observant owners

---

### BOX 2.1  SUGGESTED TOPICS TO COVER DURING HISTORY TAKING FOR SMALL MAMMALS

- Species (±breed)
- Age
- Gender
- Source, e.g. petshop, breeder
- Period in owner's possession (if this is relatively short, husbandry details from the previous carer may be important)
- Vaccination history (rabbits, ferrets)
- Reproductive history
- Other animals in household (or potential in-contact animals, e.g. wildlife)
- Housing: size, construction materials, location, substrate, cleaning regime
- Diet: what food is offered and what is eaten, water provision
- Previous medical history (including any treatments)
- Current problem: time period, outline of clinical signs noted by owner
- Current physiology: appetite, thirst, faecal and urine output (including number/size of faecal pellets, frequency/volume of urine, and description of both)
- Question owner further about the pet's current health: any other clinical signs of disease or changes in behaviour (these may be subtle)
- Companion animals in same enclosure/airspace/indirect contact: any health problems (current or previous).

may not notice reduced appetite in their pet for some time.

It is useful to ask the owner how habituated the pet is to handling, as this will affect how the animal reacts to restraint for clinical examination.

## CLINICAL EXAMINATION

### Handling/restraint

#### Rabbit

Rabbits can be nervous, particularly if not habituated to handling, and are susceptible to spinal fractures. They should therefore be handled gently but firmly. Most rabbits can be picked up with one hand under the thorax and the other under the abdomen or hindquarters. Fractious individuals can be picked up by the scruff and the body weight supported under the hindquarters. For medication of restless rabbits, it can be useful to wrap the patient in a towel (the 'burrito' wrap) with the head left exposed.

When restrained on a table, a hand covering the rabbit's eyes will reduce stimulus, and a hand over the lumbar region will reduce the risk of jumping and spinal trauma (Fig. 2.1a). To examine the ventral body surface, the rabbit is supported under the thorax and held vertically against the handler's chest, again supporting the lumbar region (Fig. 2.1b).

#### Chipmunk

Habituated animals may be cupped in your hands. Others may be restrained around their thoracic girdle. Some may require general anaesthesia with an inhalant agent to permit a full clinical examination.

#### Prairie dog

Tame individuals can be picked up by supporting the thorax and hindquarters. A towel may be used to assist restraint of other animals, to protect the handler from bites and scratches.

#### Mouse

Grasp the mouse at the base of the tail, and allow it to grip onto a cage bar or your clothing. Alternatively, the mouse may be grasped by the scruff of the neck.

#### Rat

Rats rarely bite. Hold the rat around the thoracic girdle; a thumb can be placed under one mandible to restrain the head. Support the abdomen in larger animals.

#### Hamster, gerbil, degu

Cup these small animals in your hands. Individuals not used to handling may be scruffed. Hamsters have ample skin over the back and shoulders, and a large pinch

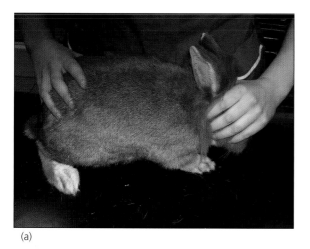

(a)

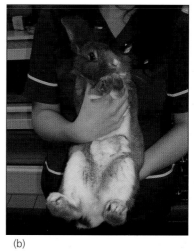

(b)

**Figure 2.1** Restraint of a rabbit (*Oryctolagus cuniculus*): (a) on the table for dorsal examination, and (b) for ventral examination.

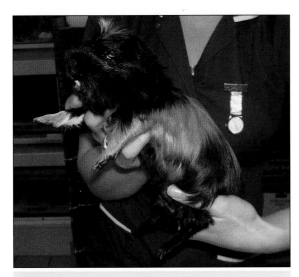

**Figure 2.2** Handling a guinea pig (*Cavia porcellus*).

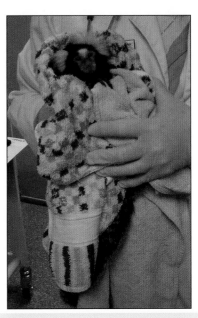

**Figure 2.3** Restraint of a common marmoset (*Callithrix jacchus*) using a towel.

should be taken to prevent the animal from turning its head. Degloving tail injuries may occur in gerbils and degus that are incorrectly handled.

### Guinea pig

This species may be flighty; initial capture is easiest performed by cornering the individual in a box or enclosure. Part of the clinical examination may be performed with the animal restrained on a table, with one hand over the head and the other over either the head or the thoracic girdle. When lifting guinea pigs, they should be supported under and/or around the thorax and under the abdomen (Fig. 2.2).

### Chinchilla

This species should be held around the shoulders to restrain. When lifting chinchillas, support the hind feet and/or grasp the tail base. Warn owners beforehand that 'fur slip' is possible (particularly if the animal is not habituated to handling or the veterinary practitioner is not experienced at such restraint).

### African pygmy hedgehog

African pygmy hedgehogs should be handled using protective gloves. The spines will at best be uncomfortable to handle, and at worst may inoculate the handler with bacterial or fungal isolates that result in a deep dermatitis. Although habituated pets may permit some examination, general anaesthesia with gaseous agents may be necessary to perform a full clinical assessment.

### Sugar glider

Sugar gliders are notoriously difficult to catch, and towels or small nets may be useful. Once captured, the animal can be restrained by taking hold of the skin on the scruff. If it cannot be securely restrained by hand, anaesthesia may be induced with gaseous agents to permit examination.

### Ferret

Most pet ferrets are well used to being handled. New pets may be more likely to bite, but most are just inquisitive. Grasp the animal around the thoracic girdle to restrain. It is not imperative to support the hindlegs, but animals may prefer support caudally on a table or arm during examination. Scruffing the animal will usually elicit a 'yawn' and the oral cavity can be assessed.

### Non-human primates

The species, size and demeanour of the primate will dictate whether conscious restraint for examination is possible. Small, less aggressive animals such as common marmosets may be handled using a towel (Fig. 2.3). Larger or less tractable non-human primates will often require sedation or anaesthesia before handling, with drugs administered either by injection (for sedatives or anaesthetics) while restrained in a net or using a squeeze cage, or in an induction chamber (for administration of gaseous anaesthetics to smaller individuals).

## Clinical examination (Box 2.2)

Initially observe the patient from a distance, including assessment of demeanour, locomotion, and respiratory pattern/noise. Check the transport container for evidence of urination or faeces. Then restrain the animal for examination from head to tail. This may be limited in small species or those susceptible to stress, when handling time should be minimized.

Check for oculo-nasal discharge; signs of oral discomfort (e.g. ptyalism); mucous membranes; dentition (only incisors are visible during conscious examination of rabbits and most rodents), use an otoscope or speculum to check cheek teeth in rabbits, guinea pigs and chinchillas (the author usually does this at the end of the clinical examination as it is relatively stressful for the animal); auscultate the thorax, palpate and auscultate the abdomen; look over and palpate the skin and feet (common conditions include pododermatitis and overgrown nails); and check the perineal region for soiling. Take the rectal temperature in larger species (rabbit, guinea pig, chinchilla, non-human primate and ferret). Assess the animal's body condition (e.g. using a point scale system) and always weigh on small digital scales; this is vital to monitor weight and for accurate drug dosing.

## INVESTIGATION

### Phlebotomy

Anaesthesia or sedation may be required to perform phlebotomy (Table 2.3) in many of these species. Restraint for jugular access in particular can be stressful. The risk of anaesthesia should be balanced against the potential gains of obtaining blood for analysis. In ill animals, anaesthesia is usually performed using inhalant agents such as isoflurane or sevoflurane.

Use an insulin syringe with a swaged-on needle for small veins to reduce the risk of collapsing the vein due to excessive suction. Venepuncture is difficult in guinea pigs, particularly the jugular vein, which is usually buried under a thick layer of fat.

In laboratory rodents, blood may be collected from the orbital venous plexus or via cardiac puncture. These routes are not recommended in pet species unless the animal is anaesthetized for euthanasia (e.g. to collect blood for investigation of a group problem).

Small mammals have approximately 7 ml of blood per 100 g of body weight. It is safe to sample 7–10% of this

---

### BOX 2.2  CHECKLIST FOR CLINICAL EXAMINATION

- Confirm species/breed and sex
- Weigh (using digital scales)
- Head: eyes, ears (use otoscope in larger species), nares, oral cavity (including otoscopic examination in rabbit, chinchilla, guinea pig and degu), observe and palpate for symmetry
- Thorax: auscultate lungs and heart, ± percuss (to assess for fluid presence) or compress thoracic cavity (to assess compliance)
- Abdomen:
  - Gastrointestinal tract: palpate, auscultate (herbivores), ± percuss (assess for tympany)
  - Urinary tract: palpate (e.g. for bladder stones)
  - Reproductive tract: palpate for pregnancy or abnormalities (e.g. uterine masses)
- External genitalia/reproductive system: discharges, swellings, wounds, mammary gland swelling/discharge
- Skin: palpate for masses, assess for lesions or discharges (e.g. alopecia, crusts, wounds), check feet for pododermatitis
- Musculoskeletal: observe locomotion, palpate and examine limbs
- Nervous system: observe demeanour, perform further neurological tests if warranted (e.g. if head tilt, facial asymmetry or ataxia present)
- Body temperature: routinely taken in larger species, but may be traumatic in conscious small rodents; rectal or aural thermometer.

---

from a healthy individual. Thus 0.5–0.7 ml of blood can be withdrawn from a 100 g animal. Ill animals will have less capacity for blood regeneration, and may already be anaemic; in these individuals, a smaller sample should be taken. Similarly, animals require time to regenerate blood constituents and large samples should not be repeated frequently (as a guide, a healthy mammal will take approximately 2 weeks to regenerate a 10% blood loss).

### Radiography

As usual, two orthogonal views should be taken when radiographing a body part. Most commonly, this is a lateral view (usually a right lateral by convention) and a

**Table 2.3** Preferred sites for phlebotomy in small mammals

| Site | Comment | Species |
|------|---------|---------|
| Lateral tail artery | Warm tail before access | Rat |
| Cephalic vein | Small volume only, easily accessible | Rabbits, prairie dog, rodents, African pygmy hedgehog |
| Lateral saphenous vein | Small vessel, mobile, but easily accessible | Any (but limited use in tiny species) |
| Jugular vein | Stressful, anaesthesia required in species other than the rabbit and some ferrets | Rabbit, prairie dog, guinea pig, chinchilla, ferret, African pygmy hedgehog |
| Anterior vena cava | Anaesthesia required | Rat, guinea pig, African pygmy hedgehog, ferret |
| Marginal auricular vein | Use a small syringe (may collapse the vein with excessive suction). Use 25 gauge needle. Reports exist of vascular damage and necrosis | Rabbit |
| Femoral vein | Anaesthesia required. Apply pressure for a few minutes afterwards to prevent haematoma formation | Rodents, sugar glider, non-human primates |
| Ventral coccygeal artery | Warm tail before access | Mouse, sugar glider |

ventro-dorsal (or dorso-ventral) view. Other views may be indicated at other times; for example, several skull radiographs are taken to assess dental disease. In some instances, the body part may be anatomically inaccessible to a true lateral view, such as the proximal hindlimb in small animals, and an oblique view is taken. It may also be useful to take oblique views to assess a particular area or elucidate a specific lesion.

It is usually possible to take more than one image of a small species on a single radiographic plate, providing collimation is good and scatter minimal. Owing to the small size of many patients, the entire body is often radiographed on one view. This is useful to give the practitioner an overview of the animal, but may not provide optimum settings for imaging individual body regions. The use of special films such as mammography or dental film may be indicated to provide higher resolution in imaging very small animals. Digital radiography will permit post-exposure alteration of the image.

## Sampling

Many samples can be collected from small mammals as in other pets for laboratory analysis.

*Urine* can be collected via cystocentesis or catheterization in larger species, or free-catch (e.g. natural voiding on an upside-down incontinence pad, or after gentle manual expression). Ultrasound-guided cystocentesis under anaesthesia is recommended in rodent species.

Endotracheal washes and bronchoalveolar lavage can be performed in many species under general anaesthesia. These will produce samples that can be analysed cytologically and bacteriologically.

Other samples that may be sent for *bacteriology* include swabs from infected wounds and abscesses. Often abscess capsular material yields better culture results than purulent material from the centre of the abscess, which may be sterile.

*Cytology* may be performed on fine needle aspirates (FNAs) from masses. In some cases, an incisional or excisional biopsy may be required to reach a diagnosis. Skin scrapes are useful for diagnosis of ectoparasites; anaesthesia may be necessary to perform the scraping.

## TREATMENT

### Basic procedures

#### Drug administration

The most basic of routes for administration of drugs, fluids or nutritional support is the *oral* route. Although references exist for medication in feed or drinking water, dosing is very variable with this technique and the author does not recommend it. Animals may drink less than expected if they dislike the taste of the medication (or like it too much and drink more), or their thirst may be affected by their illness. However, the in-feed or in-water route may be useful for medicating large groups of animals where it will not be possible to dose animals individually.

A more accurate technique is to dose using a syringe. The tip is placed into the side of the mouth (into the diastema in lagomorphs and rodents). Unfortunately, in unhabituated animals, this may be more stressful for both owner and animal.

*Subcutaneous* injections are often used to administer medication in small mammals. In most species, the scruff of the neck dorsally between the scapulae is commonly used. In guinea pigs, there is a thickened mantle of skin in this region, and it is advisable to use skin more caudally or laterally over the thorax. In sugar gliders, the patagium (or wing membrane) should be avoided as the blood supply – and therefore the absorption rate – is particularly slow in this region. In general, fluids administered subcutaneously are relatively slowly absorbed, but in some species this may be the only route accessible.

*Intramuscular* injections may be used for certain medications, including sedative or anaesthetic drugs where more rapid absorption is required. Muscle groups are small in these species, and the total volume injected should be small to avoid muscle damage (for example, a maximum of 0.1 ml at a single site in the quadriceps muscle of a hamster). The lumbar or quadriceps muscles are used routinely in most species. Patient size permitting, the author prefers to inject into the lumbar muscles in conscious animals, as muscle movement and damage is more likely during quadriceps injection.

The *intraperitoneal* route is commonly used for administration of fluids. The patient is restrained – preferably anaesthetized – in dorsal recumbency and slightly tilted to the left (so the bladder is less likely to be penetrated). A small needle is inserted at a 30–45° angle into the right caudal quadrant of the abdomen. If aspiration before injection reveals any fluid or other material, the needle is withdrawn and the procedure started again with a fresh needle and syringe. Absorption is relatively rapid with this route, and it is often used for administration of anaesthetic agents in research rodents.

It is relatively straightforward to insert and maintain an *intravenous* catheter in larger species such as rabbits (e.g. marginal auricular vein, cephalic vein, or lateral saphenous vein) and ferrets (e.g. cephalic or lateral saphenous vein), but intravenous access can be difficult in small mammals. The lateral tail vein may be accessed in larger rodents such as rats, but catheter placement is technically difficult. The intravenous route provides direct access to the circulation and is optimum for administration of fluids and medication to debilitated animals.

For animals where veins cannot be readily accessed, the *intraosseous* route is used. Commonly the proximal femur or tibia is used. Specialist intraosseous needles are available, but often prohibitively expensive for small mammal clients. An alternative is to use small hypodermic needles; sterile fine gauge orthopaedic wire may be inserted into the needle as a stylet to reduce the risk of the needle becoming blocked. Tape and/or suture material may be used to retain intraosseous needles in place.

> **CLINICAL TIP**
>
> - Fluids should always be warmed to body temperature before administration. Cool fluids will rapidly result in hypothermia in small animals.
> - Fluid therapy:
>   - The normal fluid requirement for a guinea pig is 100 ml/kg per day
>   - Remember to add losses due to dehydration/diarrhoea, etc.
>   - If possible, administer by continuous rate infusion (CRI); otherwise, divide the total volume into two or three treatments per day.

### Assist-feeding

Some animals benefit from *hand-feeding*, particularly if they have locomotor difficulty. This may be more readily accepted from a bonded owner than a veterinary nurse in a stressful hospital situation.

For patients more reluctant to feed, various convalescent diets are available for *syringe-feeding*. The diet should be selected based on the species, ensuring a close match to the animal's normal diet. For example, commercial herbivore or carnivore diets are available in powder form that can be mixed with water and administered orally via a syringe. Nutrition given in this way should be administered slowly to allow the patient to swallow.

If patients are unwilling or unable to take food directly from the oral cavity, a naso-oesophageal or oesophageal *feeding tube* may be placed. These tubes permit rapid administration of nutrition to the oesophagus and thence the stomach, which reduces handling time and stress to the patient.

> ### CLINICAL TIPS
>
> - Note that rabbits do not usually cough when a tube enters their trachea.
> - Radiography should be performed to check positioning of a naso-oesophageal tube.
> - Alternatively, an endoscope orally may be used to visualize the tube in the oesophagus (rather than in the trachea).

## Anaesthesia

### Pre-anaesthesia

Evaluate the patient as described above. This will include a detailed history and as thorough a clinical examination as is possible (this may be limited by the size of some small mammals).

If the patient is severely debilitated and/or has been chronically unwell, it may benefit from stabilization before anaesthesia is induced. Often this includes rehydration (orally or by injection), warming (e.g. in an incubator) and nutritional support (e.g. by assist-feeding).

### Pre-medication

Most small rodents are not pre-medicated if gaseous agents are to be used for induction of anaesthesia. However, in species such as guinea pigs and chinchillas, pre-medication may be useful to reduce stress (Table 2.4).

### Inhalation agents

Most volatile anaesthetic agents may be used in small mammals. Isoflurane or sevoflurane are used for preference, as they are rapidly excreted and therefore recovery is rapid. Sevoflurane is less irritant to the respiratory passages and less likely to result in discomfort or breath-holding. Sevoflurane is administered to effect and usually requires higher concentrations than isoflurane (Table 2.5).

**Table 2.4** Commonly used pre-medicants in small mammals

| Drug | Dose (mg/kg) | Route | Species |
|---|---|---|---|
| Acepromazine + butorphanol | 1.7 + 1.7 | PO | Sugar glider (sedation and analgesia) |
| Acepromazine | 0.25–1.0 | IM/SC/IV | Rabbit |
| | 0.5–1.0 | IM | Prairie dog, mouse, rat, hamster, guinea pig, chinchilla |
| | 0.1–0.5 | SC/IM | Ferret |
| | 0.5–1.0 | PO/SC/IM | Non-human primates |
| Fentanyl/fluanisone (Hypnorm®, Janssen) | 0.2–0.5 ml/kg | IM | Rabbit |
| | 0.5–1.0 ml/kg | IM/IP | Gerbil |
| | 0.3 ml/kg | IM | Ferret |
| | 0.3 ml/kg | SC/IM | Non-human primates |
| Ketamine | 5–20 | IM | Non-human primates |
| Medetomidine | 0.1–0.5 | IM/SC | Rabbit |
| | 0.5 | IM | Prairie dog |
| | 0.1 | SC | Mouse, rat, hamster, gerbil, guinea pig |
| | 0.08–0.20 | SC/IM | Ferret |
| | 0.2 | IM | African pygmy hedgehog |
| Midazolam | 0.5–2.0 | IM/IV/IP | Rabbit |
| | 1.0–2.0 | IM | Rodents |
| | 0.3–1.0 | SC/IM | Ferret |
| | 0.1–0.5 | IM/IV | Non-human primates |

IM, intramuscular; IP, intraperitoneal; IV, intravenous; PO, perioral; SC, subcutaneous.

**Table 2.5** Isoflurane use in small mammals

| Drug | Concentration (%) | | Species |
| --- | --- | --- | --- |
| | Induction | Maintenance | |
| Isoflurane | 3–5 (after pre-medication) | 1.5–1.75 | Rabbit |
| | 4–5 | 1.75–2.5 | Prairie dog |
| | 2–5 | 0.25–4.0 | Rodents |
| | 5 | 2–3 | Ferret |
| | 5 | 1–3 | Sugar glider |
| | 3–5 | 0.5–3 | African pygmy hedgehog |
| | 4 | 0–3 | Non-human primates |

**Table 2.6** Commonly used injectable anaesthetic protocols in small mammals

| Drug | Dose (mg/kg) | Route | Species |
| --- | --- | --- | --- |
| Acepromazine + ketamine | 0.4–0.5 + 40–50 | IM | Prairie dog |
| | 0.5–0.75 + 40 | IM | Chinchilla |
| Medetomidine + ketamine | 0.5 + 10–20 | IM | Prairie dog |
| | 1.0 + 50–75 | IM/IP | Mouse |
| | 0.5 + 75 | IM/IP | Rat |
| | 0.5 + 40 | IM/IP | Guinea pig |
| | 0.06 + 5.0 | IM/IP | Chinchilla |
| | 0.08 + 5.00 | IM | Ferret |
| | 0.1 + 5.0 | IM | African pygmy hedgehog |
| | 0.1 + 10.0–15.0 | IM | Non-human primates (light anaesthesia) |
| Medetomidine + ketamine + butorphanol | 0.1 + 5.0 + 0.5 | IM | Rabbit |
| | 0.08 + 5.00 + 0.10 | IM | Ferret |
| Fentanyl/ fluanisone, followed by midazolam | 0.2–0.3 ml/kg + 0.5–2.0 | IM + IV | Rabbit |
| Fentanyl/ fluanisone, followed by diazepam | 0.4 ml/kg + 5 | IP | Mouse |
| | 0.4 ml/kg + 2.5 | IP | Rat |
| | 1 ml/kg + 2.5 | IM | Guinea pig |

Many species are induced in a chamber, particularly the small rodents. Larger animals such as ferrets may be restrained while a facemask is applied, but this may be stressful. The main advantage of induction using a mask is easier monitoring of the patient. Maintenance of anaesthesia in small mammals is usually with volatile agents. In small species, a closely fitting facemask is applied. Where possible, the animal is intubated.

Oxygen should always be provided to anaesthetized patients, even in animals where an injectable anaesthetic regime has been used to induce anaesthesia and no volatile agent is required.

### Injectable agents

These are not commonly used solely, but are useful in conjunction with gaseous agents. Injectable agents are especially useful for prolonged or painful procedures, as an agent with analgesic properties can be included in the protocol (Table 2.6). These regimes are also used where provision of gaseous agents may be impaired, for example during dental procedures. Oxygen should always be provided where possible.

### Monitoring anaesthesia

As with other animals, body systems should be monitored throughout anaesthesia.

The respiratory system can be assessed using a stethoscope (bell or, in larger animals, oesophageal). The chest and/or anaesthetic reservoir bag are observed for movement. Capnography is useful, although care should be taken not to increase resistance in the anaesthetic circuit for small animals by using an in-line sampler.

The cardiovascular system is usually monitored by palpating a pulse (e.g. the femoral artery in most species, and also the central auricular artery in rabbits), and a stethoscope (as above). An electrocardiogram (ECG) and pulse oximeter (e.g. on the ear or tongue) may be useful.

A rectal (or aural in larger species) thermometer is used to assess body temperature. This is vital in smaller animals, as they are at an increased risk of hypothermia during anaesthesia.

Several reflexes can be checked to assess depth of anaesthesia. These include the toe or tail pinch, corneal reflex, palpebral reflex (unreliable in rabbits), and jaw tone. Muscular reactions to any surgical stimuli should also be monitored.

### Peri-anaesthetic care

Heat loss should be minimized by several methods, including: supplemental heating (e.g. a hot-air blanket, heat pad or hot water bottle), minimal surgical clip, reduced wetting of the patient during preparation, and insulation (e.g. using bubble-wrap). The animal can be recovered in an incubator after the procedure. Care should be taken to avoid over-heating, and body temperature should be monitored until the patient is recovered from anaesthesia.

Many animals benefit from fluids at the time of anaesthesia, particularly when injectable anaesthetic agents have been utilized that may affect renal function. After recovery, the animal's food and water intake, and urine and faecal output should be monitored. If food and water intake are reduced, assist-feeding and rehydration therapy should be administered. Prokinetics should be given if faecal output is reduced. Pain will prolong recovery, and analgesia should be administered if a painful procedure has been performed.

## Surgery

In order to minimize surgical time, all equipment should be readied before the procedure. As mentioned above, care should be taken not to cool the animal by excessive use of surgical preparation fluids.

Tissues should be handled gently, particularly the gastrointestinal tract in herbivores that are susceptible to ileus. Attention should be paid to haemostasis, as an apparently small volume of blood may be a significant volume to the small patient.

Owing to their propensity for self-trauma, skin wounds in small mammals are usually closed using absorbable suture material in an intradermal pattern. If a pattern with exposed knots is required (e.g. to relieve skin tension), consideration should be given to the use of some sort of protection to prevent trauma – such as a buster collar on rabbits, or a bandage covering the wound (although this too may be chewed).

## EUTHANASIA

This is usually achieved by overdosing anaesthesia. Use the intravenous route if you can gain access, for example the marginal auricular vein in rabbits. For most small species anaesthesia is induced with a volatile anaesthetic agent as outlined above, followed by intracardiac pentobarbitone.

# 3 Post-spay complications in a rabbit

**INITIAL PRESENTATION**

Inappetence and lethargy after ovariohysterectomy in a rabbit.

## INTRODUCTION

Surgical procedures involving the abdominal cavity of rabbits are historically associated with many potential complications, including wound breakdown and gastrointestinal ileus (Box 3.1). While the benefits of ovariohysterectomy (spaying) (Box 3.2) in the general population far outweigh these risks, they should nonetheless be discussed with clients before the procedure is performed on their pet. This case outlines the strong interplay between medical therapy and nursing care, and surgical treatment of complications after spaying in one individual.

**CASE PRESENTING SIGNS**

A 10-month-old female English rabbit (*Oryctolagus cuniculus*) was presented with inappetance, lethargy, and reduced faecal output 3 days after ovariohysterectomy.

## HUSBANDRY

The rabbit was obtained from a local rescue centre 2 months prior to being presented for neutering. The patient's sibling was obtained and spayed at the same time (with no problems noted). The rabbits were fed on a diet of hay, commercial extruded concentrate pellets for rabbits, and mixed fresh vegetables. They had been housed indoors initially, but had access to the owners' garden after being vaccinated against myxomatosis and viral haemorrhagic disease.

## CASE HISTORY

The ovariohysterectomy was routine, using poliglecaprone 25 (Monocryl®, Ethicon, Livingstone, UK) suture material for ligatures, polydioxanone (PDS®, Ethicon) for the muscle layer, and poliglecaprone 25 for the subcutaneous and intradermal layers. The rabbit was overweight (body condition score 3/5), with excessive intra-abdominal fat, making the procedure technically more difficult. (Dietary advice was given to the owner at discharge, advising a reduction in the quantity of concentrate pellets being offered.) She was discharged 2 days after surgery, by which point she was eating and passing normal faeces, and the wound had a normal appearance. Analgesia was continued (meloxicam at 0.3 mg/kg PO q24hr, off-label use) for 3 days.

A day later (3 days after surgery), the rabbit represented at the clinic (Box 3.3). She had not eaten and had been quiet at home. Faecal output was reduced and the rabbit appeared to have abdominal discomfort.

## CLINICAL EXAMINATION

The rabbit's weight had reduced slightly (from 2.93 kg pre-surgery to 2.6 kg 3 days after surgery). Auscultation of the abdomen showed reduced gut sounds on the left-hand side, and a large mass was palpated in the caudal abdomen. The rabbit was reluctant to move, but did not appear to have locomotor dysfunction (Box 3.3). A moderate tachypnoea was present (respiratory rate 100 breaths/minute, normal range 32–60).

## BOX 3.1 POTENTIAL COMPLICATIONS AFTER ABDOMINAL SURGERY IN RABBITS

- Wound dehiscence, e.g. after self-trauma or excessive activity, resulting in herniation if linea alba closure dehisces
- Seroma formation
- Haemorrhage – with haematoma formation or bruising
- Infection: of wound, peritonitis
- Gastrointestinal ileus (particularly if gastrointestinal tract is handled roughly or excessively)
- Adhesions
- Reaction to suture material (particularly if catgut is utilized)
- Hepatic lipidosis (associated with fasting of obese individuals during the procedure and recovery period).

## BOX 3.2 REASONS FOR SPAYING FEMALE RABBITS

- Prevent unwanted pregnancies (permitting neutered does to live with uncastrated bucks)
- Prevent pseudopregnancy
- Reduce territorial aggression
- Reduce incidence of or treat uterine neoplasia (commonly adenocarcinoma)
- Prevent or treat other uterine pathologies such as pyometra, uterine aneurysm and hydrometra.

## BOX 3.3 SIGNS OF PAIN IN RABBITS

Clinical signs of pain are usually vague in rabbits, often being a subtle change from normal behaviour. Normal grooming ceases and some individuals show aggression. Signs may include reluctance to move, anorexia and changes in physiological parameters (heart rate, respiratory rate and body temperature). Abdominal pain may be evidenced by a crouched posture and tooth grinding. Some rabbits may be restless, intermittently jumping and circling. Those with urinary tract pain may show signs of dysuria.

## DIFFERENTIAL DIAGNOSES

The differentials for *reduced appetite and faecal output* were:
- Gastrointestinal ileus post-surgery, associated with rough handling of intra-abdominal organs
- Pain/discomfort after surgery
- Peritonitis (infectious or sterile)
- Wound infection
- Other gastrointestinal disease: including infection, intussusception, foreign body (uncommon)
- Metabolic dysfunction, e.g. hepatic lipidosis
- Wound dehiscence, possibly with herniation of abdominal contents. (Remember that the linea alba may be compromised with or without loss of integrity of the skin wound.)

## CASE WORK-UP

### Trial with supportive care

Gastrointestinal ileus is extremely common after a stressor such as surgery. Prevention is preferable to cure, and it is advisable to administer prokinetics and assist feed rabbits after surgery until appetite and faecal output return to normal (as was done in this case). Re-instigation or continuance of prokinetics, assist feeding, and fluid therapy (see Nursing aspects box below) are indicated in a rabbit with reduced appetite and/or faecal output. An improvement should be seen within 24–48 hours. In the case of this patient, fluids were administered intravenously (Fig. 3.1).

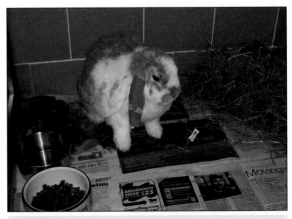

**Figure 3.1** Rabbit receiving intravenous fluids. The catheter is placed in the marginal auricular vein.

## Blood analysis

Since this rabbit did not respond to supportive care, a blood sample was taken from the jugular vein (conscious) for a health check (Box 3.4, Fig. 3.2). Haematology and biochemistry results were unremarkable.

The following procedures were then completed under sedation with fentanyl/fluanisone (0.3 ml/kg IM Hypnorm®, VetPharma Ltd, Leeds, UK).

## Abdominal radiography

Lateral and ventro-dorsal views were taken of the abdomen (Fig. 3.3). These showed some gas building up in the gastrointestinal tract, particularly the caecum – supporting the diagnosis of hypomotility.

## Abdominal ultrasound

Flocculant free fluid was present within the peritoneal cavity. This was aspirated, and an in-house Romanowsky stain demonstrated many inflammatory cells (neutrophils and lymphocytes), some erythrocytes, but no bacteria (ruling out the differential of infected peritonitis). Creatinine in the fluid was 326 µmol/l, suggesting that some urine may be present (normal creatinine levels in blood are 44.2–229 µmol/l, and this rabbit's blood value had been 166 µmol/l). The left renal pelvis and ureter were dilated. Attempts to follow the left ureter caudally were not successfull beyond a mass-like structure.

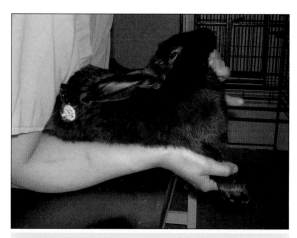

**Figure 3.2** Positioning for jugular phlebotomy in a rabbit. The rabbit is restrained similarly to a cat, with the neck extended. This position will affect the rabbit's breathing (mis-aligning the trachea from the nasal passages), and should not be maintained for prolonged periods.

---

### BOX 3.4   PHLEBOTOMY SITES IN RABBITS

- Jugular vein
- Marginal auricular vein
- Lateral saphenous vein
- Cephalic vein.

---

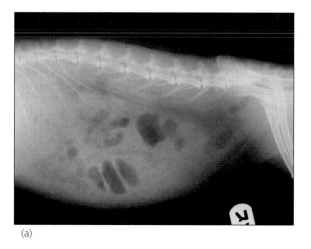

(a)

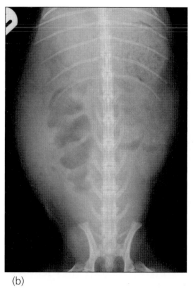

(b)

**Figure 3.3** (a) Lateral and (b) ventro-dorsal radiographs of the abdomen. Note the gas present in the gastrointestinal tract.

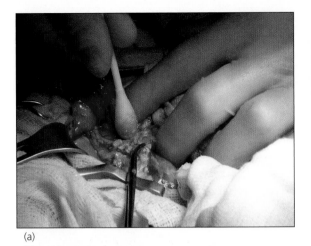

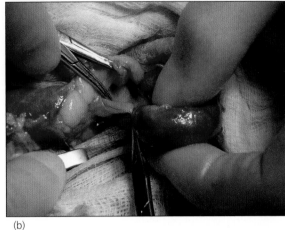

(a)    (b)

**Figure 3.4** Intraoperative images, showing (a) adhesions and (b) dilated ureter.

Based on the ultrasound findings, it was decided to further investigate with an exploratory coeliotomy. Anaesthesia was induced with midazolam (1 mg/kg IV), before the rabbit was intubated and maintained on isoflurane carried in oxygen. Hartmann's solution was administered intravenously at 4 ml/kg per hour. Rectal temperature was monitored throughout the procedure, and supplemental heating provided using a forced warm air blanket and warming of fluids prior to administration.

## Exploratory coeliotomy

Flocculant straw-coloured fluid was present in the peritoneal cavity. Several adhesions were located that had formed at surgical sites of suture placement (Fig. 3.4a). The left ureter entered one of these sites. The suture in the region did not encircle the ureter, but it was not possible to dissect the ureter from the adhesion (Fig. 3.4b). A unilateral nephrectomy was performed (similar to the procedure in other small animals).

## DIAGNOSIS

Adhesions had formed throughout the abdomen, likely in response to the presence of suture material. Obstruction of the left ureter had occurred secondary to physical pressure from one of these adhesions. This resulted in hydroureter and hydronephrosis.

## ANATOMY AND PHYSIOLOGY REFRESHER

In the entire doe (Fig. 3.5), the ovaries lie in the dorsal abdomen with the left ovary just caudal to the left

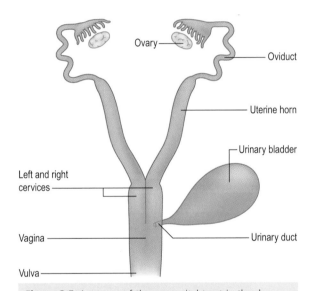

**Figure 3.5** Anatomy of the urogenital tract in the doe.

kidney (the right ovary is at the same level in the body, so not usually in contact with the more cranial right kidney). The fallopian tube transports ova from each ovary to each uterine horn. Often, there is a large amount of fat in the broad and suspensory ligaments. The cervix is bicornuate. The vaginal body is flaccid, and fills with urine during micturition. The cervical body is usually transfixed during ovariohysterectomy, ensuring the ureters and uterine artery (that also supplies the bladder) are not included in the ligature. Damage to the ureters or uterine artery is more likely if a vaginal ligature is placed, but this reduces the risk of future cervical stump neoplasia.

## AETIOPATHOGENESIS OF ADHESIONS AND ILEUS AFTER ABDOMINAL SURGERY IN RABBITS

Catgut is associated with an increased risk of adhesion formation in rabbits, as it requires the immune response of phagocytosis to degrade it. Multifilament suture materials permit 'wicking' of infection through tissues. Multifilament materials and any suture on a threaded needle will also result in more tissue trauma, when compared with monofilament material on a swaged needle. Infection and suture reactions are therefore more likely when multifilament suture is used in the abdomen.

Rabbits are susceptible to gastrointestinal ileus and adhesion formation after surgery. Desiccation of tissues and rough handling (including use of gauze swabs) predispose patients to such problems.

## TREATMENT

During recovery from anaesthesia, the rabbit was monitored for thermoregulation (heat was initially supplemented using a forced warm air blanket) and signs of pain. Analgesia was provided with buprenorphine (which initially also partially reversed the effects of fentanyl used in anaesthesia) at 20 µg/kg q8hr SC for the first 48 hours and then 10 µg/kg q8hr SC for the following 3 days and meloxicam (0.6 mg/kg q24hr PO for 10 days).

Pending culture results of the peritoneal fluid, cephalexin (20 mg/kg q24hr SC) and enrofloxacin

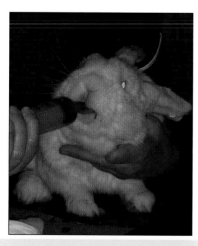

**Figure 3.6** Assist-feeding a rabbit (using a catheter-tip syringe to allow administration of more viscous foods). The syringe tip is placed in the diastema between the incisors and premolar teeth, and food injected slowly into the mouth to permit swallowing.

(10 mg/kg q12hr PO) were administered. No significant growth was cultured from the fluid, and antibiotics were ceased.

Assist-feeding and prokinetics were also continued. Fluids were administered intravenously initially and then subcutaneously when the rabbit became more active and a drip line could no longer be easily maintained.

## CASE MANAGEMENT

### NURSING ASPECTS

- Supportive care is vital in any inappetant rabbit, particularly when faecal production is reduced.
- *Assist-feeding* is easily performed in most rabbits (Fig. 3.6). Products such as Oxbow Critical Care for Herbivores® are excellent replacement foods, and can be syringed slowly into the mouth of conscious rabbits. The syringe tip is placed laterally between the incisors and premolars, and the plunger slowly depressed. If a rabbit is not obviously swallowing, the procedure should be abandoned and consideration given to the use of a nasogastric feeding tube.
- *Prokinetics* should be administered until faecal output (size and number) is normal. For example, metoclopramide (0.5 mg/kg SC/PO q6–12hr), ranitidine (2 mg/kg SC/PO q12hr), or cisapride (0.5 mg/kg PO q8–12hr).
- If dehydration is suspected, *fluids* should be administered (usually subcutaneously or intravenously, depending on the severity of dehydration). This is important if gastrointestinal contents have become dry.
- Monitor body *temperature* (normal range 38.5–40.0°C), and supplement heating or cool the rabbit as appropriate.
- With urogenital disease or after urinary tract surgery, monitor *water intake* (including water drunk and fluids administered) and *urinary output*.

## FOLLOW-UP

The rabbit started eating some vegetables and passing a few small faecal pellets within 48 hours of nephrectomy surgery. Urine was passed the same day as surgery. Fluid administration was stopped when the rabbit began drinking from her sipper bottle.

## CLINICAL TIPS

- Monitor urine output by using incontinence pads in the kennel, weighing before use and after they have been urinated on (1 ml urine weighs 1 g).
- Ensure rabbits have water supplied in a familiar container, e.g. sipper bottle and/or bowl. They may not recognize or use an unfamiliar vessel.
- Intravenous catheters can be placed in several sites, e.g. marginal auricular vein, saphenous vein and cephalic vein. The last two sites are well tolerated by most rabbits. The auricular vein is usually not accessible in breeds with short ears, e.g. the Netherland dwarf. Use of the auricular vein may be associated with disruption of the blood supply to the ear and resultant partial ear necrosis (the author has not personally encountered this problem).

Repetition of haematology showed a mild neutrophilia 5 days after surgery ($5.9 \times 10^9$/l, reference range $1.5–6.6 \times 10^9$/l (30–50% of total white cell count)). Ultrasound at this point demonstrated normal gastrointestinal motility, and a 2 cm diameter mass at the cervical stump (this was palpable before surgery, and had been visualized during surgery as adhesions near the bladder). A thin layer of hypoechoic fluid was present subcutaneously at the incision site.

Urine was red in colour a couple of weeks after surgery, but no dysuria was noted. Urine analysis did not show any erythrocytes present, and it was assumed the colouration was due to dietary pigments. Urine concentrating ability was maintained (specific gravity 1.037, reference range 1.003–1.036, although mineral deposits affect the measurement).

The skin wound healed in 2 weeks. Gastrointestinal function (as assessed by appetite and faecal output) gradually returned to normal over a few weeks, although prokinetics were continued on a reducing dose for 3 weeks after surgery.

Although the rabbit initially lost weight (down to a low of 2.3 kg), this improved with supplemental feeding and tempting with good quality hay and fresh vegetables, reaching the pre-surgery level a couple of months after surgery.

## PREVENTION

- Gentle tissue handling of both the skin and internal organs will reduce postoperative discomfort. Use of analgesics should be routine in rabbit surgery, preferably using a multimodal approach (e.g. using both opioids and non-steroidal anti-inflammatory drugs). Pre-emptive analgesic administration provides superior pain relief.
- Skin wounds in rabbits should be closed using a buried suture pattern, e.g. continuous intradermal sutures, to reduce self-trauma and wound dehiscence. Minimizing excessive activity will reduce stresses on suture lines.
- Use of synthetic monofilament suture of a narrow gauge (with appropriate strength for the site) on a swaged needle will reduce tissue trauma and reaction to ligature and suture placement.
- Synthetic monofilament suture materials should be used in preference to catgut. For example, polyglyconate (Maxon®, Ethicon) is degraded and removed by hydrolysis.
- Flushing the abdomen with copious quantities of warm saline before closure will remove blood clots or potential contamination, reducing the risk of adhesion formation around such material.
- It has been suggested that the calcium channel blocker verapamil (0.2 mg/kg PO/IV q8hr for nine doses) in the immediate postoperative period will reduce the formation of adhesions.
- Gastrointestinal support should routinely include prokinetics and assist-feeding until the patient is self-feeding and passing normal faeces after the procedure. A good quality diet, including meadow hay and leafy green vegetables, should also be offered to encourage self-feeding.

## PROGNOSIS

The prognosis for this rabbit was guarded at the time of renal surgery. Despite the use of narrow gauge monofilament synthetic suture materials, a reaction occurred that resulted in adhesions forming throughout the abdomen. The owner was warned that these may result in either gastrointestinal and/or urinary pathology in the future. As it was not possible to remove the distal portion of the left ureter, the patient is also predisposed to urinary tract infection (although no clinical signs have been noted in 18 months following the procedure).

## ACKNOWLEDGEMENTS

Thanks to the imaging department at the Royal (Dick) School of Veterinary Studies, Edinburgh, for ultrasonography in this case. The nephrectomy was performed by Donald Yool.

# 4 Spinal fracture in a rabbit

## INITIAL PRESENTATION

Acute onset hindlimb paralysis in a rabbit.

## INTRODUCTION

It is common knowledge among veterinary practitioners that rabbits are susceptible to spinal injuries, often associated with handling incidents. Thankfully, training veterinary undergraduates in careful and appropriate handling of rabbits has ensured that this is now relatively uncommon in veterinary practices. This case outlines an unfortunate incident in a teaching hospital where the rabbit sustained a spinal fracture during clinical examination. Good client relations were paramount to a satisfactory outcome from this accident.

### CASE PRESENTING SIGNS

A 7-year-old male entire Netherland dwarf cross-breed rabbit (*Oryctolagus cuniculus*) became acutely paralysed on both hindlimbs after handling for clinical examination and nail clipping.

## HUSBANDRY

The rabbit was housed with another male entire rabbit, and had been in the owner's possession for 6 years. The hutch was in a shed, with access through the day to an exercise pen. The substrate was wood shavings. Several other rabbits were housed in separate hutches in the same air space. The diet offered including *ad libitum* hay, muesli-type commercial rabbit food, and fresh vegetables. Water was offered in a sipper bottle.

## CASE HISTORY

The rabbit presented at the clinic for a routine myxomatosis vaccination. The clinical examination detected overgrown nails, and consent was given for these to be trimmed. A qualified veterinary nurse restrained the rabbit while a veterinary student trimmed the nails. Although the initial examination did not reveal any locomotor deficiencies, it was noted that the rabbit was not placing his hindlimbs appropriately when returned to the carrier after the nail trim.

## CLINICAL EXAMINATION

Examination at this point showed:
- No hindlimb movement
- No deep pain was present in either hindlimb
- A dorsal swelling was palpated in the thoraco-lumbar region of the spine.

A spinal fracture was suspected.

### DIFFERENTIAL DIAGNOSES

The differentials for hindlimb *paralysis* are:
- Trauma: spinal fracture or luxation, intervertebral disc rupture
- Limb deformities, e.g. bilateral fractures, septic arthritis, splay leg
- Spondylosis or spondylitis, osteoarthritis
- Degenerative disc disease
- Spinal neoplasia
- Localized spinal abscess
- Infectious or inflammatory central nervous system disease, e.g. encephalitozoonosis,

toxoplasmosis, neosporosis, meningitis/encephalitis
- 'Floppy bunny syndrome' (flaccid paralysis, of unknown aetiology)
- Congenital neurological dysfunction.

It is necessary to differentiate paralysis from *paresis* or reluctance to move. Aetiologies may vary for general muscular weakness:
- Central nervous system (CNS) infection (see above)
- CNS disease, e.g. brain abscess or tumour, viral haemorrhagic disease (VHD), trauma, encephalitozoonosis
- Metabolic disease (resulting in ataxia or muscular weakness), e.g. hepatic lipidosis or hypokalaemia
- Terminal disease, e.g. septicaemia, renal or hepatic failure, cardiovascular disease, starvation, intestinal obstruction, VHD, predator attack
- Cardiovascular disease
- Congenital or acquired skeletal abnormalities, e.g. splay leg (developmental condition), spondylosis, kyphosis, lordosis
- Nutritional causes, e.g. hypovitaminosis E, hypovitaminosis A
- Severe ulcerative pododermatitis.

Because of the nature of this case and the clinical findings, the main differentials considered were associated with acute trauma.

## CASE WORK-UP

### Neurological examination

This is performed similarly to other small mammals, although the flighty nature of some rabbits and their reluctance to be manipulated in certain ways reduces the comprehensiveness of the examination. For example, tests such as the wheelbarrow test (postural reaction test for strength and coordination of the forelimbs) are resented by rabbits and difficult to perform. It is also important to consider the potential for worsening of pathology if a spinal fracture is manipulated and results in further spinal cord damage.

This patient had bilateral hindlimb paralysis, lacked deep pain in either hindlimb, and had no anal tone. The panniculus reflex was present cranial to the level of the fifth lumbar vertebra, where it abruptly ceased.

## Medical treatment and reassessment

Although the benefits of administering steroids in cases of spinal injury are debatable, it may be useful if given within an 8 hour period in acute cases. Alternatively or in conjunction, strict cage rest may reduce further trauma and damage. If either of these is the sole investigation, treatment response should be reassessed with regular repetition of the neurological assessment to check for any improvement. If none is noted, consideration should be given to imaging modalities to investigate further, or the animal euthanized.

## DIAGNOSIS

Acute injury causing vertebral fracture and spinal cord compression (see below for radiographs).

## ANATOMY AND PHYSIOLOGY REFRESHER

The skeleton in the rabbit is similar to other mammals (Fig. 4.1), with 8 cervical, 12 thoracic, 7 lumbar, 4 sacral and 6 caudal vertebrae. Bone density in rabbits is relatively low, and accounts for only 6% of body mass. There is no cauda equina in rabbits; thus any injury along the vertebral column will affect the spinal cord and result in upper and lower motor neuron damage.

## AETIOPATHOGENESIS OF SPINAL FRACTURES IN RABBITS

Fracture or luxation/subluxation of lumbar vertebrae is common in pet rabbits. It is usually associated with trauma sustained by the spine during incorrect handling. The spine may twist around the lumbosacral junction if the rabbit is held with the heavy hindquarters unsupported, resulting in fractures. Rabbits unused to being handled may struggle during restraint and kick out with the hindlimbs. The fracture is commonly in the lumbosacral region (L6–L7).

Clinical signs of spinal trauma often include loss of the panniculus reflex, and urine and faecal incontinence. Absence of deep pain reflexes carries a poor prognosis.

> **CLINICAL TIP**
>
> Note that the withdrawal reflex is local and its presence does not denote an intact spinal cord.

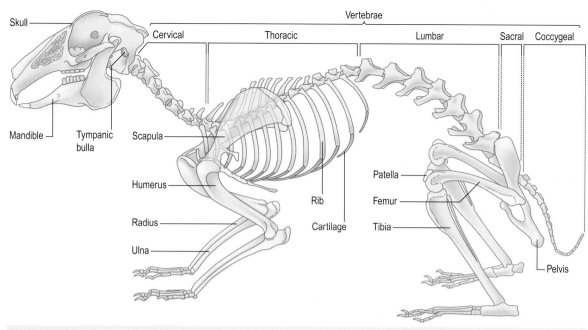

**Figure 4.1** Vertebrae in the rabbit, showing the normal curvature.

## TREATMENT AND OUTCOME

Dexamethasone was administered (30 mg/kg IV) within 1 hour of the incident. The rabbit was hospitalized in a small kennel, and provided with food and water.

Repeating the neurological assessment 1 hour and 4 hours later did not show any improvement. There continued to be no deep pain in either hindlimb, no anal tone, and the rabbit was urinary incontinent. The lack of deep pain sensation 4 hours after the incident carried a poor prognosis, and, after discussion with the owner, the rabbit was euthanized.

Postmortem plain radiographs were taken (Fig. 4.2), confirming the diagnosis of spinal fracture. They showed a fracture of the fifth lumbar vertebra, with obvious deformity of the spinal column that would have resulted in severe spinal cord damage.

## OTHER INVESTIGATION OPTIONS

### Radiography

Plain radiographs may detect an obvious abnormality in bony structures, e.g. vertebral fracture. Contrast medium (i.e. a myelogram) may be required to demonstrate a subtle lesion or one involving soft tissues only, e.g. intervertebral disc herniation, spinal neoplasia or spinal abscesses.

In this case, radiographs were not taken as results would not have affected the outcome – the history and clinical findings were highly suggestive of a vertebral fracture with spinal cord compressions, and the owner did not wish to pursue surgical treatment.

### Cerebrospinal fluid analysis

If a myelogram is to be performed, CSF should be analysed (cytology and protein content) to assess for infection or inflammatory processes. A sample may also be obtained without the need for a contrast study if infection or inflammation is considered more likely than anatomical deformity. The usual sites for access are via puncture of the lumbo-sacral or cisterna magna epidural spaces. It is advisable to analyse the CSF (Box 4.1, Fig. 4.3) before injection of contrast material (Box 4.2) if meningitis is suspected, as the contrast material may exacerbate clinical signs.

### Culture

If bacterial or fungal infection is suspected, it is useful to perform culture and sensitivity testing on samples such as urine, blood and CSF.

### Encephalitozoonosis testing

Detection of the protozoa in urine will confirm infection, but excretion is transient. Serology may demonstrate

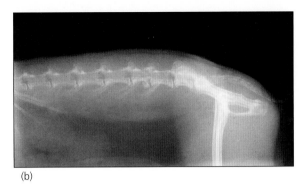

(b)

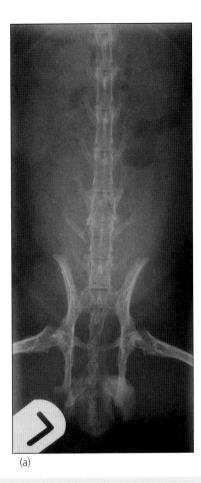

(a)

**Figure 4.2** Plain radiographs of the spine: (a) ventro-dorsal and (b) right lateral views. Note the fracture of the fifth lumbar vertebra and resulting narrowing of the spinal column.

## BOX 4.1 OBTAINING A CSF SAMPLE

- General anaesthesia. Place in lateral recumbency. Clip and aseptically prepare the site
- Atlanto-occipital approach:
  - Flex head (preferably intubated to ensure airway maintained)
  - Site location is half way between the cranial margins of the wings of the atlas (C2 vertebra) and a point 2 mm caudal to the occipital protuberance
  - Insert 38 mm 22 gauge spinal needle, at a 90° angle to the vertebral column
- Lumbar approach:

- Flex the trunk
- Site location is the cranial edge of the dorsal spinous process of the L6 vertebra
- Insert 38 mm 22 gauge spinal needle, directed cranially at a 45° angle
- Advance needle slowly. A 'pop' is felt as the needle penetrates the dura and subarachnoid membranes
- Remove the stylet from the needle and check for CSF in the hub
- Collect the CSF sample from the hub of the needle into a sterile plastic container
- Analyse within 30–60 minutes.

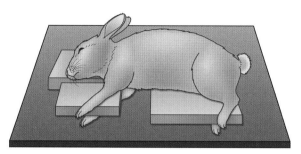

(A) To ensure true lateral recumbency, use foam wedges to separate contralateral limbs and raise the rostral skull

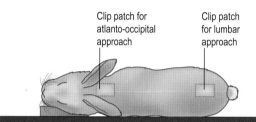

Clip patch for atlanto-occipital approach

Clip patch for lumbar approach

(B) The spine should be flexed in the region for access, i.e. cervical or lumbar area

**Figure 4.3** Sites of puncture for CSF sampling (A) lumbar and (B) atlanto-occipital.

---

> ### BOX 4.2   MYELOGRAPHY
>
> * L6–L7 intervertebral space:
>   * 32–38 mm 23 gauge needle
>   * Use 0.4 ml/kg of iodine-based contrast medium
>   * This will usually extend contrast from L7 to T2
> * Cisternal puncture can be used to assess the cervical/thoracic spinal column.

---

exposure to *Encephalitozoon cuniculi*, but a rising titre (with blood samples taken 4 weeks apart) is required to show active infection.

### Other imaging modalities

Computed tomography (CT) or magnetic resonance imaging (MRI) may be used to assess bone or soft tissue abnormalities. These techniques are currently more expensive than radiography and not readily available to all practitioners, but are useful options to investigate disease affecting the CNS.

## TREATMENT OPTIONS AND MANAGEMENT

> ### NURSING ASPECTS
>
> * Many patients with hindlimb paralysis will continue to eat and drink, providing appropriate food and water is within reach. If the patient is not eating, assist-feeding should be performed as with other ill rabbits (see Chapter 3 for technique).
> * The rabbit will be unable to move away after urination or defaecation (including passage of caecotrophs), and perineal soiling will result. Although handling should be minimized, the patient should be checked twice daily and bathed as necessary to prevent lesions (e.g. urine scalding and faecal matting of fur). After cleaning, the skin and fur should be dried thoroughly using a combination of towel, hairdryer on a cool/warm setting, and a comb or brush. If skin lesions are present or urine scalding severe, a topical antibiotic (e.g. fusidic acid or silver sulfadiazine) or barrier (e.g. petroleum jelly) ointment should be applied.
> * As with other species suffering from paralysis, physiotherapy should be performed for a few minutes several times daily. If complete paralysis is present, this will be passive, ensuring mobility of joints and encouraging stimulation of major muscle groups. As motor function returns, physiotherapy can be more active, for example assisted locomotion. Swimming (providing support using hands and/or an inflatable jacket) can be beneficial, although it should be introduced gradually so as not to stress the patient.
> * Manual expression of the bladder may be required, three or four times daily. Diazepam (0.25–0.5 mg/kg PO) may assist with relaxation of the external urethral sphincter. Over-distension of the bladder wall and urinary tract infection may result in bladder wall damage.
> * The rabbit should be rotated every 4–6 hours to prevent the formation of pressure sores.

## OTHER TREATMENT OPTIONS

### Cage rest

If the spinal lesion is stable, it is advisable to restrict exercise for 6–8 weeks. Nursing should be continued during this time (see above).

### Analgesia

The requirement for analgesics depends on the severity of the condition. Non-steroidal anti-inflammatory drugs (NSAIDs, e.g. meloxicam) are commonly used in rabbits. Opioids such as buprenorphine may be useful in acute cases or as part of a multimodal regime after surgery.

### Surgery

As with other small mammals, surgical repair of vertebral fractures is possible. It should be borne in mind that low bone density will affect the choice of implant, as will the small size of some patients. Patients without deep pain will generally not be considered for surgical treatment owing to the poor prognosis for return of neurological function.

### Support harnesses

Although a selection of hindlimb supports such as carts have been used in various species of pet mammals, the author does not see the use of these as a humane treatment option in the long term for animals with continuing hindlimb paralysis.

### Physiotherapy

Active and passive physiotherapy will be useful for a return to normal function. If available, hydrotherapy can be beneficial in aiding recovery.

### Euthanasia

In cases of severe neurological dysfunction, particularly if owner considerations (including financial ones) preclude any investigation or treatment, euthanasia may be the treatment of choice.

## PREVENTION

It is useful to assess rabbits visually before handling, and to ask the owner if it is accustomed to handling. If the animal is obviously nervous or not regularly handled, it is appropriate to warn the owner that handling may result in injury if the rabbit twists or jumps suddenly.

Practise handling calm rabbits when possible, for example any that are at the veterinary clinic for elective procedures. Experience with these will build confidence in the veterinary clinician for dealing with more difficult patients.

## PROGNOSIS

The prognosis (see Box 4.3) will depend on the severity of spinal cord damage, stability of the vertebral column, demeanour of the patient and capabilities for restricting movement during the fracture healing period (6–8 weeks).

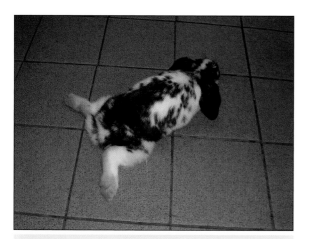

**Figure 4.4** A case of spinal fracture in a dwarf lop rabbit. This individual had some hindlimb movement.

## BOX 4.3   ETHICS

The rabbit's welfare should be considered a priority when dealing with neurological cases. The prognosis as determined by you, the veterinary clinician will have a significant influence on this. It is important to re-evaluate cases regularly, and to consider euthanasia in cases that are deemed to have an extremely poor prognosis early on, or in those that do not improve with treatment and time.

A similar case presented after spinal fracture in the owner's home (Fig. 4.4). This rabbit retained some hindlimb movement, and deep pain was present. Strict cage rest over a period of 8 weeks resulted in recovery.

# 5 Ferret with abdominal mass

**INITIAL PRESENTATION**

Weight loss in a ferret.

## INTRODUCTION

This case embodies a frequent presentation in ferrets of weight loss, along with the common finding of an abdominal mass. The aim is to discuss possible investigations and outline treatment options for common conditions. (See Box 5.1 for a brief guide to ferrets in various parts of the world.)

**CASE PRESENTING SIGNS**

Chronic weight loss in an adult male neutered ferret (*Mustela putorius furo*).

## HUSBANDRY

The current owner had rescued the ferret 2 years prior to presentation. The animal had previously been castrated. He was housed with another ferret in an outdoor hutch on two levels. The animals had intermittent free-range access to a room in the owner's house. The substrate was straw, with fleece material for bedding. During colder weather, the hutch was covered to protect the animals from inclement conditions. Cleaning was performed weekly.

The ferrets were on a commercial dry ferret diet, supplemented with occasional egg and cooked meat. They were offered water in a water bottle, which was changed daily.

Neither ferret had been vaccinated. There was potential for access to wild mink owing to the rural location of the hutch.

## CASE HISTORY

The ferret's appetite had been reduced over the month prior to presentation, particularly with regard to the kibble, although he was still consuming small amounts of commercial cat food and cooked meat. Although the ferret had never been obese, his body condition had deteriorated markedly over the same time period. Historically, the ferret lost some body weight over the winter, but not to the extent seen this time.

The animal's faeces were pale and loose, but no blood was seen. There was no history of vomiting or respiratory signs. Although he drank a considerable amount and urinated frequently, this was considered normal for the individual.

The companion ferret and other pets in the household did not show any signs of illness.

## CLINICAL EXAMINATION

A clinical examination was performed, with the following findings:
- The ferret was bright, alert and responsive
- Body condition was poor (score 3 out of 9), with a weight of 570 g
- Mucous membranes were pink and moist, and capillary refill time was less than 2 seconds
- Teeth were in good condition, although a small chip was present on one canine
- No abnormalities were detected on thoracic auscultation. The heart rate was 360 beats per minute (normal range in an adult ferret is 180–250)
- Superficial lymph nodes were normal on palpation
- The intestines were thickened on palpation, and a mass was detected in the mid-cranial abdomen.

## BOX 5.1   FERRETS AROUND THE WORLD

- In the UK, ferrets are kept for two reasons. Some are purely pet animals, some are used for working ('ferreting' utilizes the animals to hunt wild rabbits), and some are a combination of the two.
- Across the rest of Europe and in Russia, ferrets are variously kept as pets, for fur and for hunting.
- Pet ferrets are popular in Japan.
- Although banned in certain states in the USA, in others, ferrets are extremely popular as pets. They have also been used for medical research and the fur trade for many years.
- New Zealand has banned the keeping of pet ferrets since 2005.
- The black-footed ferret (*Mustela nigripes*) was rated extinct in the wild, but animals bred in captivity have been locally re-introduced in efforts to save the species.

## DIFFERENTIAL DIAGNOSES

The differentials for *anorexia* are wide, with almost any illness resulting in this clinical sign. In many ferrets, only subtle signs of illness will be seen with chronic gastroenteritis.

The differentials for an *abdominal mass* (often with weight loss) in a ferret are:

- Splenomegaly:
  - Idiopathic hypersplenism
  - Neoplasia (see below)
  - Infection (e.g. Aleutian disease (see below), fungal disease)
  - Cardiac disease
  - Endocrine disease (e.g. hyperadrenocorticism)
  - Anaesthesia
- Gastrointestinal foreign body (Fig. 5.1) (common) or gastric trichobezoars
- Neoplasia (often occurs secondary to inflammatory disease):
  - Lymphoma (see Box 5.2)
  - Adrenal gland, e.g. adrenocortical adenoma, adenocarcinoma, teratoma. This case did not show any of the usual signs seen with functional adrenal gland tumours (e.g. alopecia, pruritus or behavioural changes). Adrenal enlargement may be non-neoplastic, e.g. hyperplasia
  - Hepatic, e.g. lymphoma, haemangiosarcoma, adenocarcinoma, hepatocellular adenoma, metastases
  - Splenic, e.g. lymphosarcoma, haemangioma, haemangiosarcoma
  - Pancreatic, adenocarcinoma, insulinoma (although insulinomas are often small and the clinical signs of weakness and seizures do not correlate with this case)
  - Gastrointestinal, e.g. adenocarcinoma
  - Bladder, e.g. transitional cell carcinoma
  - Reproductive tract, ovarian (e.g. leiomyoma, teratoma), uterine (e.g. leiomyoma, adenoma, fibrosarcoma), prostate (e.g. seminoma, carcinoma)
- Abscess (bacterial infection)
- Aleutian disease (viral): mass could be due to splenomegaly, mesenteric lymphadenopathy, hepatomegaly; disease also results in chronic wasting, diarrhoea, lethargy, anorexia and polydipsia
- Thickened intestines may be palpated, e.g. intestinal lymphoma, eosinophilic granulomatous disease (uncommon), proliferative bowel disease (rare, caused by *Lawsonia intracellularis*, mostly animals <1.5 years old)
- Several conditions will result in mesenteric lymphadenopathy that may be palpable, e.g. intestinal lymphoma, inflammatory bowel disease, eosinophilic granulomatous disease (eosinophilic infiltration and granulomas of the abdominal lymphatics and organs), proliferative bowel disease, systemic infection, tuberculosis
- Renomegaly: renal cysts, acute renal failure, hydronephrosis (e.g. associated with urolithiasis obstructing kidney, ureteral or urethral blockage)
- Urolithiasis: uroliths in bladder, or distended bladder associated with uroliths blocking urethra
- Granulomas: tuberculosis (*Mycobacterium bovis*), non-tuberculous mycobacteria (e.g. *M. genavense*)

- Mycotic disease (usually causes lung pathology, but may affect abdominal organs) – blastomycosis (splenomegaly), coccidiomycosis (various organs), histoplasmosis (splenomegaly)
- Gastric bloat (rare): thought to be associated with bacterial overgrowth
- Prostatic disease (hobs), e.g. prostatomegaly with secondary urethral obstruction, prostatic abscess (may be in association with transitional cell tumours of the bladder)
- Pregnant (jills)
- Pyometra (jills).

The differentials for *diarrhoea* include:

- Canine distemper virus (CDV): resulting in diarrhoea and anorexia (other signs include vomiting, respiratory and nervous signs)
- Gastrointestinal infection, e.g. salmonellosis, colibacillosis, bacterial overgrowth, enterotoxaemia, coronavirus (epizootic catarrhal enteritis, ECE), rotavirus (severe disease in kits 2–6 weeks old), *Campylobacter* spp
- Bacterial enteropathies often occur secondary to other disease, e.g. dietary indiscretion or sudden diet change, viral or inflammatory or neoplastic gastrointestinal disease
- Inflammatory bowel disease: may relate to dietary intolerance, hypersensitivity reaction or other immune abnormality
- Toxicoses: many ingested toxins cause gastrointestinal signs (e.g. methylxanthines in chocolate, nicotine in cigarettes)
- Endoparasitism (uncommon):
  - Protozoa, e.g. *Toxoplasma gondii* (signs may include diarrhoea, lethargy and anorexia), *Cryptosporidium parvum* (may be asymptomatic), coccidiosis (*Isospora* and *Eimeria*, usually asymptomatic), *Giardia* spp
  - Helminths (may see diarrhoea with roundworms, threadworms)
  - Cestodes (may result in diarrhoea)
- Human influenza virus: sometimes associated with a transient diarrhoea (along with respiratory disease).

The differentials for *weight loss* include:

- Chronic disease, e.g. pneumonia
- Cardiovascular disease, e.g. dilated cardiomyopathy may result in lethargy and weight loss

- Aleutian disease
- Dental disease
- Neoplasia
- Renal disease, pyelonephritis
- Inflammatory bowel disease
- *Helicobacter mustelae,* with gastritis and ulceration
- Enteritis, bacterial overgrowth
- ECE
- Tuberculosis
- Mycotic disease, e.g. blastomycosis
- Megaoesophagus (poor prognosis)
- Rarely, eosinophilic granulomatous disease, proliferative bowel disease or endoparasites may result in weight loss without loss of appetite.

## CASE WORK-UP

### Supportive care

Owing to the animal's poor condition and the chronicity of the disease, it was deemed appropriate to admit him for nutritional support over 48 hours before further investigation under sedation was performed. A convalescent carnivore diet was administered orally via syringe and offered *ad libitum* in a bowl during this stabilization period.

### Ultrasound

The ferret was sedated with midazolam (1 mg/kg IM), resulting in moderate sedation within 5 minutes.

Physical abdominal examination revealed one large (1 × 2.5 cm) mass caudal to the right kidney, and several smaller (2–9 mm diameter) masses near the main mass and great vessels. Doppler imaging showed the masses to have an excellent vascular supply, precluding the possibility of fine needle aspiration under ultrasound guidance (due to the risks of haemorrhage). The aorta passed close to one of the masses and the architecture of its wall was poorly defined, suggesting that there might be vascular invasion from the mass. It was not clear whether the masses originated from the pancreas or mesenteric lymph nodes.

The gall bladder was almost empty, with hyperechoic contents. A cyst measuring 3 mm diameter was located

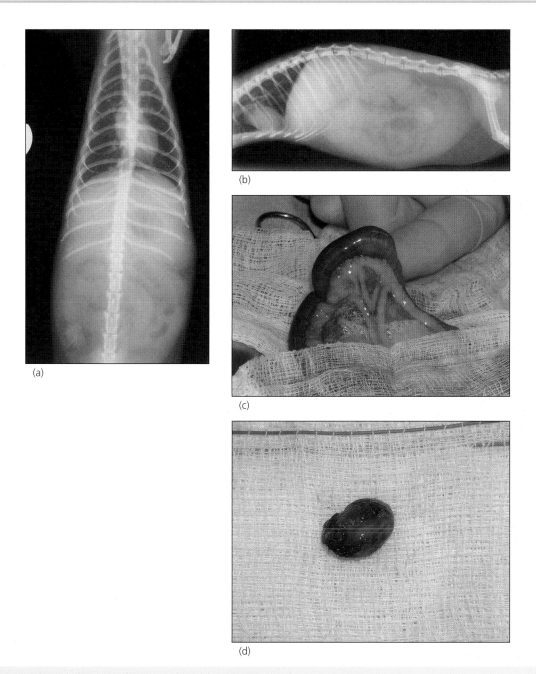

**Figure 5.1** (a–d) Radiographs showing a peanut foreign body in a ferret, and surgical removal.

in a liver lobe. The portal vein was prominent but there was no evidence of shunting. Several mesenteric lymph nodes were enlarged. Both adrenal glands were identified, and both they and the kidneys had a normal ultrasonographic appearance.

**Blood sample**

As insulinomas are common in ferrets, a small sample was taken from the cephalic vein for glucose assessment. The blood glucose was normal at 10.1 mmol/l (reference range in a fasted ferret is 5–6.7 mmol/l,

<11.1 mmol/l if the individual is unfasted; insulinoma is suspected with hypoglycaemia, i.e. <3.9 mmol/l).

After these results and due to the guarded prognosis, the owner elected not to proceed with further investigations.

## FURTHER INVESTIGATIONS POSSIBLE

### Blood sample

Phlebotomy is usually performed from the jugular vein. In habituated or depressed ferrets, this may be achieved conscious. In other individuals, sedation or anaesthesia is used to assist restraint; drugs may affect blood values (e.g. isoflurane will reduce the haematocrit and plasma protein levels as red blood cells are sequestered in the spleen).

Aleutian disease is diagnosed on the finding of hyper-gammaglobulinaemia and by serology.

### Faecal analysis

Wet preparations and flotations can be performed to check for endoparasites. Culture will identify bacterial pathogens that may cause diarrhoea. Assessment for occult blood may be useful.

### Urine analysis

If urinary tract disease is suspected, urine should be analysed for abnormalities by microscopy, refractometry, biochemistry and culture.

### Radiography

Since the ultrasound images suggested that neoplasia was high on the list of differential diagnoses, it would be useful to assess for metastatic spread (i.e. radiograph the thorax).

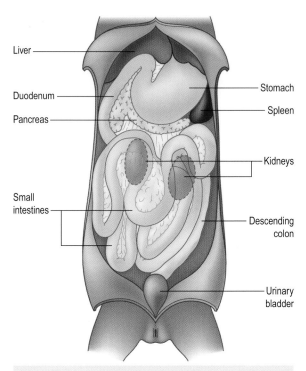

**Figure 5.2** Ventral view of a ferret's gastrointestinal tract.

### Exploratory coeliotomy

This would enable direct visualization of the masses, as well as incisional or excisional biopsy. Exploration of other abdominal organs could also be carried out.

Samples (fine needle aspirate or biopsy) from masses or abnormal organs should be submitted for cytology/histology and culture. Acid-fast stains should be included to rule out mycobacterial disease.

### DIAGNOSIS

Neoplasia of abdominal organ(s) was suspected.

### ANATOMY AND PHYSIOLOGY REFRESHER (FIGS 5.2, 5.3)

Ferrets are carnivorous, and have a short digestive tract. The simple stomach is followed by the small intestine (182–198 cm long), colon and rectum. The ferret liver is relatively large, has six lobes, and normally lies within the curvature of the diaphragm.

The pancreas has two arms with the midpoint near the gastric pylorus. The right arm lies alongside the duodenum. The pancreas shares a common opening into the duodenum with the bile duct. The spleen is crescent shaped, and lies in the left hypogastric area

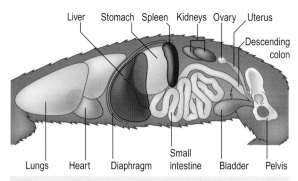

**Figure 5.3** Lateral view of a ferret's gastrointestinal tract.

parallel to the greater curvature of the stomach. The gastrosplenic ligament attaches the spleen to the stomach and liver. The spleen can be large in normal adults.

The kidneys are retroperitoneal, with the right more cranial than the left. The adrenal glands lie at the cranial poles of the kidneys. The left gland is near to the abdominal aorta, while the right gland is adjacent to the caudal vena cava.

## AETIOPATHOGENESIS OF ABDOMINAL NEOPLASIA

Several aetiologies have been proposed for development of neoplasia in ferrets. These include genetics, tumour suppression genes, early neutering, photo-period manipulation (where animals are housed indoors with artificial light cycles, particularly those maintained for breeding), diet (processed foods), viruses, endocrinopathies (e.g. diabetes mellitus, pseudohypoparathyroidism, hyperthyroidism and hypothyroidism). Chemicals and other environmental conditions may also be involved.

Gastrointestinal tract neoplasms include biliary cystadenoma/cholangioma, cholangiocarcinoma, hepatocellular carcinoma and hepatoma. Malignant lymphoma (Box 5.2) is the most common neoplasm of the gastrointestinal tract. Palpation, radiography and ultrasound are used to detect the presence of a mass; biopsy with histology will permit a diagnosis to be made. Primary gastrointestinal neoplasms are usually malignant; for example, adenocarcinomas are usually locally aggressive and metastasize to local lymph nodes.

Adrenocortical neoplasms are usually functional, and associated with a wide range of clinical signs such as alopecia, pruritus, enlarged vulva (in jills), urinary blockage (in males), and splenomegaly. Diagnosis is suspected based on history, clinical signs, ultrasonography and steroid hormonal assays, but is confirmed only by histology of excised adrenal tissue. Surgical removal is currently the preferred treatment option, although research shows depot gonadotrophin-releasing hormone (GnRH) agonists such as deslorelin have promise for medical therapy.

Insulinomas usually present as small nodules, and unlike the disease in dogs and cats are less malignant in ferrets. Blood glucose and insulin levels are used to diagnose the disease, and surgical excision usually results in a prolonged disease-free state.

Endothelial neoplasms may be seen in various abdominal organs (including the liver, spleen and pancreas), lymph nodes or free-floating in the abdomen. Malignancy is reported histologically, but metastases are rare.

Abdominal haemangiosarcomas carry a guarded prognosis. They grow aggressively and may rupture (seeding the abdomen with metastatic tumours or causing a fatal haemorrhage). Early surgical excision may be curative if a single site is affected.

Transitional cell carcinoma (TCC) may arise in the kidney; metastasis is rare and unilateral nephrectomy may be curative. TCC in the bladder carries a poorer prognosis, with local invasion usually occurring before diagnosis; chemotherapy has been used to treat some bladder tumours. Renal carcinomas and adenomas are unilateral and usually incidental findings at postmortem examination.

Most pet animals are neutered, so reproductive tract neoplasms are rare.

## EPIDEMIOLOGY

Most neoplasms (53% reported) in ferrets relate to the endocrine system, with pancreatic tumours the most common (21–38%) and adrenocortical neoplasms the second most common (25%). The most common haematopoietic neoplasm reported is lymphoma, which is also the most common malignancy. Gastrointestinal tract neoplasms are frequent; 50% affect the intestines, with stomach, liver, colon and oral cavity neoplasms less likely. The liver is commonly a site for metastatic spread. Many individuals are affected by multiple tumour types.

## TREATMENT

Owing to the guarded prognosis and risks associated with exploratory surgery, the owner in this case elected to take the ferret home to monitor for further deterioration in his condition. Nutritional support was provided using the convalescent diet.

## TREATMENT OPTIONS AND MANAGEMENT

### Supportive care

Animals suffering from weight loss should be provided with nutritional support (see below). If diarrhoea has also resulted in dehydration, fluid therapy should be commenced (see below).

### Medication

If an infection is suspected, it can be prudent to commence antibiotic therapy before culture results are available. Metronidazole and amoxicillin are common first choices for ferrets with diarrhoea. Protectant drugs may be useful, e.g. ranitidine, cimetidine, famotidine, omeprazole, sucralfate or kaolin/pectin. Motility modifiers such as metoclopramide may be used if an obstruction is not suspected.

## Chemotherapy

The use of chemotherapeutic protocols may be useful for certain cases (e.g. lymphoma).

## Surgery

Surgical excision is possible for some abdominal neoplasms.

---

**NURSING ASPECTS**

- Nutritional support:
  - Offer the ferret a selection of foods, including its normal diet, to encourage self-feeding. As with cats, it may help to moisten the food and/or warm it.
  - Milk ± added cream (to increase milk fat) can be useful to assist with weight gain, although it will cause diarrhoea. Some human baby diets are accepted. There are several carnivore convalescent diets on the market that can be offered and/or syringe-fed to ferrets.
  - The microflora in the ferret gastrointestinal tract is simple, and not involved in digestion. It is therefore uncommon to cause diarrhoea with long-term administration of broad-spectrum antibiotics.
- Fluid therapy:
  - In mild/moderate cases of dehydration, warmed oral and subcutaneous fluids may be sufficient. Oral electrolyte solutions can be given.
  - In ferrets with severe dehydration, the intravenous (or intraosseous) route is necessary. The lateral saphenous or cephalic veins are commonly used for catheter placement.
  - Fluid volumes should include replacement of losses and maintenance requirements, and are calculated as for dogs and cats.
- Hospitalize ill ferrets. Provide supplemental heating, particularly for those with weight loss and low energy reserves (monitoring rectal temperature), as well as a suitable sleeping area (e.g. a soft blanket or towel).

## FOLLOW-UP

The ferret presented at the clinic 2 weeks later. Further weight loss was noted (weight was now 439 g), but the animal had been eating and active until the previous 24 hours. He had become acutely anorexic and lethargic, and was not reacting to stimuli. His mucous membranes were pale, and an acute haemorrhage from one of the masses was suspected. The owner elected for euthanasia of the ferret at this stage (without postmortem examination).

Anaesthesia was induced with isoflurane in a chamber before an overdose of pentobarbitone was injected into the cranial vena cava to complete the euthanasia.

## PREVENTION

Avoidance of the factors listed above for generation of neoplasia is advisable. Early identification and treatment of gastrointestinal disease may also prevent progression to a neoplastic condition.

## PROGNOSIS

The prognosis for abdominal neoplasia depends on the type of tumour (e.g. whether it is susceptable to chemotherapy, whether it has or may metastasize) and the location (including local invasion and vascular supply). Surgical excision may be possible for some tumours. Chemotherapy is an option for other conditions such as lymphoma. Remission periods will vary between chemotherapy protocols and individual response.

# 6 Urolithiasis in a chinchilla

## INITIAL PRESENTATION

Pollakiuria, dysuria and haematuria in a chinchilla.

## INTRODUCTION

Captive chinchillas should be maintained on a high-fibre diet. Commercial mixes for chinchillas may be low in fibre – often resulting in dental disease – and other constituents may vary significantly from the wild diet (Box 6.1). In these diminutive animals, treats should be quantified, as a small amount may be a considerable portion of the diet and result in nutritional imbalance. This case describes a condition that likely developed in response to an aberration of mineral content from the ideal diet.

## CASE PRESENTING SIGNS

A 2-year-old male entire chinchilla (*Chinchilla laniger*) presented with pollakiuria, dysuria and haematuria.

## HUSBANDRY

The owner had another chinchilla, but they were housed separately and allowed to mix daily only under direct supervision. The chinchilla's enclosure was constructed of wire mesh and measured approximately 1 m wide × 1 m deep × 1.5 m high. Two wooden shelves were provided along with a small wooden nest box. He had access to a dust bath daily for 15 minutes.

The diet mainly comprised Timothy grass hay and proprietary grass-based chinchilla pellets. A small amount of treats including apples, rosehips and green vegetables was given twice weekly. Water provided was human-grade mineral water. The owner weighed the chinchilla weekly.

## CASE HISTORY

The chinchilla had previously been seen at the clinic after trauma resulted in a superficial leg wound. This healed uneventfully. The companion chinchilla had no previous medical history. Both animals had been in the owner's possession for more than 1 year.

The owner reported that the chinchilla (Fig. 6.1) had clinical signs for 3 days prior to presentation:
- Difficulty passing urine
- Small amounts of urine were passed, containing some blood
- Otherwise no problems were noted. The chinchilla was active, eating, drinking and passing faeces as normal.

## CLINICAL EXAMINATION

The chinchilla was well habituated to restraint and a full clinical examination was possible. Findings included:
- Bright, alert and reactive
- Good body condition, with a weight of 670 g
- No skin lesions detected
- Normal locomotion
- Thoracic auscultation normal
- Resented abdominal palpation slightly; the owner suggested this was normal for this animal. The bladder appeared comfortable
- No preputial damage or haemorrhage detected.

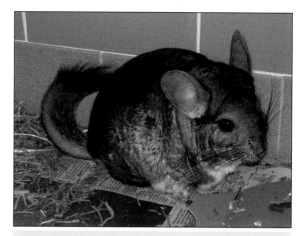

**Figure 6.1** The chinchilla was behaving relatively normally on presentation.

## DIFFERENTIAL DIAGNOSES

The clinical signs were suggestive of urinary tract disease. The differentials for *haematuria* were:
- Cystitis
- Urolithiasis
- Bladder neoplasia
- Renal infarcts
- Trauma to the distal urinary tract, for example attack on the prepuce from the con-specific animal
- Disseminated intravascular coagulation
- In a female, reproductive tract disease – pyometra, uterine hyperplasia or neoplasia.

## CASE WORK-UP

### Urinalysis

A free-flow urine sample was collected and analysed. Using a refractometer, the urine specific gravity was 1.046. On dipstick, significant amounts of protein and blood were identified, and the pH was 8.5. On microscopic examination, red blood cells were evident. Bacteria were suspected to be contaminants owing to the method of urine collection, as no white blood cells were seen. No crystals or renal casts were detected.

### Ultrasound

Abdominal ultrasound was performed with the chinchilla conscious. A mineralized urolith measuring approximately 5 mm in diameter was detected in the bladder. Cystitis was also present. Both kidneys had a normal shape, internal structure, opacity and size (approximately 1.9 cm in length).

### Other possible investigations

These could include evaluation of blood chemistry, such as blood urea nitrogen (BUN), creatinine, calcium, phosphorus, albumin and total protein. It is useful in cases of urinary tract disease to determine whether azotaemia is present. Haematology may be useful, for example to determine whether renal disease or the urinary blood loss was causing anaemia.

Another imaging modality that could be of use to investigate the urinary tract would be radiography. Plain radiographs would detect a radiodense urolith. Contrast studies can be performed as in other species, for example a retrograde cystogram or an intravenous urogram (IVU).

If a urinary tract infection were suspected, it would be useful to perform culture on a urine sample. The sample would ideally be collected aseptically, for example using ultrasound-guided cystocentesis (a difficult technique with the small size of a chinchilla's bladder).

## DIAGNOSIS

A urolith was detected using ultrasound. The resultant cystitis explained the clinical signs noted. In similar cases in other individuals, such discomfort may result in other signs such as reduced appetite and lethargy.

Mineralized stones are relatively easy to detect on radiography or ultrasound. Ultrasound is a more sensitive tool for assessment of kidney structure, although radiography is more likely to detect mineralized calculi within ureters or the urethra.

Urine analysis is rarely reported in chinchillas, but comparison with published results for other small herbivores suggests that the parameters assessed were within the normal ranges except for the presence of protein and blood. (Murinae such as mice and rats naturally have proteinuria.)

## ANATOMY AND PHYSIOLOGY REFRESHER

The penis is obvious just cranial to the anus, and can be everted 1–2 cm manually. An os penis is present in chinchillas. Males do not have a true scrotum and the testes are found within the inguinal canal or abdomen, with the caudal epididymis dropping into two small sacs next to the anus. The female's prominent urinary papilla can be confused with the penis, but the ano-genital distance is greater in the male.

As in other mammals, the kidneys lie retroperitoneally to the left and right of the midline. The urinary bladder can be relatively small in chinchillas, and usually contains alkaline urine. In females, the external urethra is separate to the vagina. The slit-like vulva lies between the urinary papilla and anus, and is closed by a membrane except during oestrus and parturition.

Free-ranging chinchillas are reported to rarely drink. They obtain most of their water from plants, and from licking dewdrops.

## AETIOPATHOGENESIS OF UROLITHIASIS

In another hystricognathi – the guinea pig – calculi are regularly associated with ascending infections and bacterial cystitis. In this species, crystals are principally formed from calcium carbonate, and diets high in calcium and oxalate are a risk factor. Calculi may form in the kidneys, ureters, bladder or urethra.

Clinical signs associated with urinary tract disease may be quite specific for this body system, including polydipsia, polyuria or anuria, isosthenuria, stranguria, dysuria and haematuria. The animal may vocalize during attempts to urinate. In other cases there may be quite vague signs of illness, such as reduced appetite or complete anorexia, cachexia and dehydration. Signs associated with discomfort may include a hunched posture, or sensitivity to palpation or movement of the dorsum or spine.

## EPIDEMIOLOGY

Although relatively common in lagomorphs and guinea pigs, urolithiasis is infrequently reported in chinchillas.

## TREATMENT

### Anaesthesia

Acepromazine (0.75 mg/kg) and ketamine (40 mg/kg) were administered IM to induce anaesthesia. After 5 minutes, this resulted in a surgical depth of anaesthesia for approximately 45 minutes. During this period, oxygen was administered via a close-fitting facemask. At the end of this period, anaesthesia was maintained with isoflurane (1–3%) until the end of surgery. Glycopyrrolate (0.02 mg/kg SC) was administered to reduce respiratory secretions after induction.

Anaesthesia was monitored using ECG pads on the patient's feet. The heart rate varied between 120 and 250/min and the respiratory rate between 36 and 44/min during the procedure. The surgical depth of anaesthesia was primarily assessed by using the toe pinch reflex.

### Surgery

Owing to the small size of the patient, an operating microscope was used for magnification during the surgical procedure. A midline coeliotomy was performed to remove the urolith. The bladder was gently elevated using stay sutures during the procedure. The bladder wall appeared thickened and inflamed. Unfortunately, the bladder was too small to safely take a sample of the wall for culture prior to closure. The bladder incision was closed with a simple continuous pattern of poliglecaprone 25 (5/0 USP, 1 metric). The same suture material and pattern were used to close the muscle and subcuticular layers. An intradermal pattern was placed in the skin, with a small amount of tissue glue to oppose the wound edges (Fig. 6.2).

### Perioperative supportive care

The chinchilla's rectal temperature dropped to 34.3°C, and a forced warm air blanket was utilized to try to increase this (normal range 38–39°C). The chinchilla was recovered in an incubator – with an environmental temperature of approximately 35°C – with supplemental oxygen. The patient was moving around well after 20 minutes.

A period of apnoea during the recovery period was treated by administration of doxapram intravenously (1 mg/kg, into the lateral auricular vein) and intermittent positive pressure ventilation (IPPV) via the facemask.

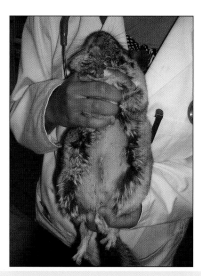

**Figure 6.2** Abdominal wound postoperatively, with intradermal sutures.

Fluids were administered at the end of surgery (20 ml of warmed Hartmann's solution SC). Prokinetics – metoclopramide (0.5 mg/kg PO or SC q12hr) and cisapride (0.5 mg/kg PO q12hr, no longer available in the UK) – were administered postoperatively for 24 hours until the patient was passing normal droppings. Analgesia was provided postoperatively using buprenorphine (0.05 mg/kg SC q8hr for 24 hours) and meloxicam (0.3 mg/kg PO q24hr). Antibiosis was commenced with trimethoprim potentiated sulphonamide (30 mg/kg PO q12hr).

## TREATMENT OPTIONS AND MANAGEMENT

### Diet

Dietary modifications were made to reduce the formation of further calculi, aiming to reduce high urinary calcium and oxalate levels. The owner was advised to avoid alfalfa-based pellets and hay that are high in calcium. Kale, spinach, celery, parsley and strawberries are high in oxalates, so should be given in small quantities only. A Timothy hay-based diet is relatively low in calcium and high in fibre, and should reduce urolith formation.

### Supportive care

This was similar to that given for other illnesses in small rodents. Gastrointestinal support may include assist-feeding, prokinetics such as metoclopramide and ranitidine, and appetite stimulants such as diazepam (0.2–0.3 mg/kg PO or SC q12hr) or vitamin B complex

(5–10 mg/kg SC or IM). Some authors may use steroids (prednisolone at 0.5–1.0 mg/kg PO q12–24hr) as an appetite stimulant and anti-inflammatory, but caution should be exercised over such drugs that may cause immunosuppression.

## OTHER TREATMENT OPTIONS

If uroliths are present elsewhere in the urinary tract – such as the ureters or urethra – they are often milked into the bladder before surgical removal. It can be helpful to pass a small urinary catheter to prevent small stones migrating into the urethra during the cystotomy.

In animals with acidic urine, dissolution therapy may inhibit calcium stone crystallization in the urine. Potassium citrate (150 mg/kg divided q12hr) binds calcium and thus reduces the urinary saturation of calcium salts, reducing ion activity and alkalinizing the urine. Although most herbivores have alkaline urine, the citrate may help inhibit calculi formation following surgical removal of a stone.

Where renal dysfunction is present, it is beneficial to provide diuresis. A reduced protein diet, phosphate binders, and vitamin and iron supplementation (to support red blood cell regeneration in the bone marrow) may also be appropriate.

Potentially nephrotoxic medications should be avoided. These include NSAIDs and aminoglycosides. (A low-dose NSAID was administered in this case as hydration appeared to be good and renal dysfunction – based on urine analysis – was not suspected. Ideally, blood chemistry would have been performed to assess for azotaemia prior to NSAID use.) Antibiotics may be indicated.

## FOLLOW-UP

Antibiosis and NSAID administration were continued for 2 weeks postoperatively. Although initially haematuria was still present, this was to be expected with the degree of cystitis noted at surgery. The haematuria gradually reduced and resolved over 2 weeks. The dysuria and pollakiuria stopped within 2 days of surgery.

Laboratory analysis of the urolith (Fig. 6.3) was as follows:

- Size = 3.4 × 3.3 × 3.2 mm
- Weight = 0.05 g
- Composition = 100% calcium carbonate.

## PREVENTION

The previous diet of the chinchilla was assessed, and modified slightly to reduce the mineral content. Timothy hay is a good quality grass-based hay that is relatively low in calcium, and should form the majority of the animal's diet. Significantly, the owner was advised to

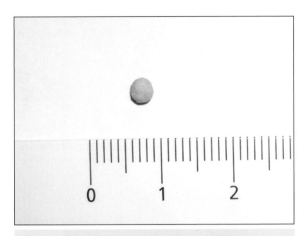

**Figure 6.3** Urolith removed via cystotomy (cm scale).

provide the chinchilla with non-mineral water, as this was thought to be a potential predisposing factor in the formation of the urolith.

## PROGNOSIS

The chinchilla fared well after surgery. However, it is not possible to completely remove minerals from the animal's diet and there is a risk of recurrence of the urolithiasis.

## ACKNOWLEDGEMENTS

I would like to thank the imaging and surgical departments at the Royal (Dick) School of Veterinary Studies for their assistance with this case, in particular Regine Hagen for ultrasonography and Donald Yool for surgical expertise.

# 7 Cheilitis in a guinea pig

## INITIAL PRESENTATION

Crusting on the lips in a guinea pig.

## INTRODUCTION

Guinea pigs generally fare well in captivity (Box 7.1), but are susceptible to many stressors. Careful attention should be paid to husbandry conditions both to reduce various diseases and also to optimize the environment during recovery.

### CASE PRESENTING SIGNS

A 15-month-old female entire guinea pig (*Cavia porcellus*) presented with crusting around the lips (cheilitis) and reduced appetite.

## HUSBANDRY

The guinea pig was housed with a sibling companion – another female – mainly in an outdoor hutch with an attached run over grass. During the winter months, the animals were moved to an indoor enclosure to protect them from inclement weather. They had sawdust as the substrate in the main enclosure, with some straw in the bedding area.

They were fed on hay and proprietary guinea pig concentrate pellets, along with fresh vegetables (cabbage, carrot and cucumber) daily and occasional fruit. Water was offered in a water bottle. No specific vitamin C supplement was given.

## CASE HISTORY

The guinea pig presented in the autumn (late September). Both guinea pigs had been seen 4 months previously with ectoparasites (lice), which had been treated with topical application of fipronil, off licence. For the week prior to the current presentation, the owner had noticed crusts around the lips of this guinea pig. The lesions appeared to wax and wane. Her appetite was slightly reduced.

## CLINICAL EXAMINATION

The guinea pig (Fig. 7.1) was examined with the following findings:

- Good body condition, weighing 724 g
- Auscultation of chest and abdominal palpation revealed no abnormalities
- Skeleto-muscular assessment – no sign of lameness or limb discomfort
- General coat condition good, with no evidence of the previous ectoparasites
- Crusting around lips, particularly at commissures.

The companion animal had some lesions, but these were much less severe.

### DIFFERENTIAL DIAGNOSES

The differential causes for these *crusting lesions* were:

- Secondary to a diet of abrasive and acidic food
- Bacterial infection, which may be primary or secondary
- Fungal infection: dermatophytosis mostly affects the nose, face and ears, and results in alopecia and scaling. Other fungal infections,

such as *Cryptococcus neoformans, Candida albicans* and *Malassezia ovale,* may result in ulcerative dermatitis

- Poxvirus
- Nutritional deficiency, for example hypovitaminosis C
- Ectoparasite lesions are common: sarcoptic mange (*Trixacarus caviae*) lesions are usually over the dorsal neck and thorax, but may become disseminated. *Demodex caviae* typically results in lesions on the head, forelegs and trunk. The fur mite *Chirodiscoides caviae* usually affects the dorsum
- Stress, such as old age, concurrent disease or hypovitaminosis C, may affect skin and coat condition
- Neoplasia (not common at this site in guinea pigs)
- Trauma, such as from the animal's enclosure, resulting in cuts that scabbed over during healing.

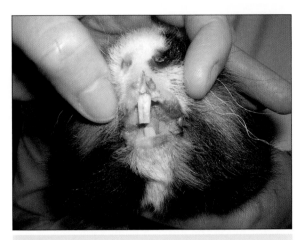

**Figure 7.1** Guinea pig on presentation with crusting around lips.

## BOX 7.1 ECOLOGY OF GUINEA PIGS

- Originally from the Andes, guinea pigs are domesticated descendants of wild cavies. Therefore they do not exist naturally in the wild
- Normal habitat of cavies: grassy plains. Seek shelter in burrows, crevices or tunnels in vegetation. Crepuscular activity
- Social groups, usually consisting of several sows, one boar and offspring. Communicate primarily using vocalization
- Susceptible to heat stress
- Average weight: 0.7–1.2 kg
- Length: 20–25 cm
- Free-ranging diet: predominantly grasses. Perform caecotrophy
- Reproduction: gestation 59–72 days (average 63–68 days). Litter of 1–6 pups (average 3). Precocial young. Pelvic symphysis usually fuses at 9–12 months of age in the female, and dystocia is likely if the initial pregnancy occurs after this
- Longevity: up to 8 years (longest recorded lifespan in captivity 14 years).

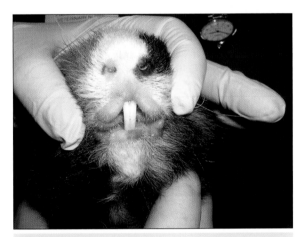

**Figure 7.2** Guinea pig after cleaning crusts with dilute chlorhexidine.

## CASE WORK-UP

The initial diagnosis was based on clinical signs, although this did not identify the aetiology of the lesions. The lesions were cleaned with dilute chlorhexidine (Fig. 7.2). This revealed inflammation around the lips. Ulceration was present at the commissures of the mouth.

## DIAGNOSIS

The guinea pig was suffering from cheilitis.

## ANATOMY AND PHYSIOLOGY REFRESHER

The oral cavity is small in guinea pigs, with a small rostral opening. The labio-nasal sulcus (or philtrum) allows the upper lip to be mobile between left and right, aiding food prehension. The lower lip is not divided.

Guinea pigs have an absolute requirement – as do primates – for daily vitamin C as they lack the enzyme L-gluconolactone oxidase, which is involved in vitamin C synthesis from glucose (see Box 7.2). Adult guinea pigs require 10 mg vitamin C/kg per day, although this increases to 30 mg/kg per day during pregnancy.

## BOX 7.2   HYPOVITAMINOSIS C (SCURVY) IN GUINEA PIGS

- Although most proprietary foods for guinea pigs are manufactured to contain vitamin C, it is rapidly degraded (particularly if improperly stored, e.g. >22°C) and the diet fed may be deficient. Fresh vegetables, particularly leafy greens, peppers, broccoli and tomatoes, are a good source of vitamin C. It is advisable to supplement vitamin C in guinea pigs, usually by adding it to the drinking water (at 1 g vitamin C per litre of water). The vitamin is degraded (oxidized) by contact with metal, so should not be offered in a metal water bowl. Oxidization will also occur rapidly in direct sunlight or if organic material is present (such as dirt in the water). The supplemented water should therefore be changed daily.
- Vitamin C is required throughout the body for the formation of collagen, and a deficiency rapidly (within 4 days) results in pathology. The epiphyseal region of long bones and the costochondral junctions may appear enlarged on radiographs. A reduction in blood vessel integrity may result in haemorrhage, e.g. into joints – particularly the stifles – skeletal muscle, gingivae, intestine and subcutaneous tissues.
- Clinical signs of hypovitaminosis C in guinea pigs include anorexia, hypersalivation, lameness or a stiff gait or paresis, unkempt coat, and lethargy. Because of joint pain, animals may vocalize when handled. Swellings at costochondral junctions and joints may be palpated. Pathological fractures may occur. Immunosuppression may result in diarrhoea, oculo-nasal discharge, and bacterial infections.

## AETIOPATHOGENESIS OF CHEILITIS

The differentials for causing this condition are listed above. Damage to the integument locally results in ulceration and exudates, and thence crust formation. Inflammation will be present.

## EPIDEMIOLOGY

Owing to common aetiologies of this condition involving either husbandry and/or infectious agents, in general, animals housed together in the same conditions will all develop cheilitis. However, it may be that one animal is more susceptible than others – as noted in this instance – and shows more severe lesions.

## TREATMENT

### Conservative

Initially, conservative treatment was instigated. The owner was advised to supplement dietary vitamin C by adding it to drinking water daily, at an increased dose of 50–100 mg/kg/d. The lesions were cleaned with dilute antiseptic (chlorhexidine) daily.

### Medication

At the revisit 1 week later, the cheilitis had improved a little. The nasal planum was clear – although a mild inflammation was still present – but the lips were still affected with crusting. Systemic antibiosis (trimethoprim potentiated sulphonamide at 30 mg/kg PO BID) and an anti-inflammatory (meloxicam at 0.3 mg/kg PO SID) were given at this point.

## TREATMENT OPTIONS

For some cases, it can be useful to apply water-resistant muco-protectant ointments (such as petroleum jelly). If lesions are severe and appetite is reduced due to discomfort, analgesia may be required until the condition has healed.

### NURSING ASPECTS

- If the guinea pig does not eat readily soon after recovering from anaesthesia, assist-feeding is advisable to reduce the occurrence of ileus. This should be continued until the appetite is more normal. Offering a variety of foods may also tempt the patient to eat.
- If faecal output is reduced, prokinetics such as metoclopramide should also be administered (0.5 mg/kg PO or SC q12hr).

## FOLLOW-UP

The lesions improved significantly. However, they remained present – with intermittent increases in severity – and major crusts recurred 2 months later. At this point, it was decided to investigate further in an attempt to identify the aetiology of the lesions.

### Biopsies

After a pre-medicant injection of buprenorphine (0.05 mg/kg SC), the guinea pig was anaesthetized with sevoflurane – using a chamber for induction and a small facemask for maintenance of anaesthesia. Incisional biopsies were taken from the lesions on the lips and philtrum. Samples of the crusts were also taken for bacterial and fungal culture.

The lesions resolved with topical cleaning, systemic antibiotic therapy and improved husbandry.

## DIAGNOSTIC RESULTS

The histological diagnosis was of dermatitis with both bacterial and fungal elements identified. Colonies of bacteria were seen, and suspected to be the most likely aetiological agent. There was no evidence of an immune-based reaction or viral aetiology.

A DNase negative *Staphylococcus* species was cultured. It was sensitive to several antibiotics, including sulphonamide co-trimoxazole.

## PREVENTION

Husbandry conditions should be optimized, including provision of sufficient vitamin C in the diet. Good hygiene in the enclosure – including food and water containers – will reduce the risk of infection. New animals should be quarantined for a period, enabling monitoring for disease before mixing with others.

## PROGNOSIS

This condition is usually not life-threatening, although it may be extremely uncomfortable for the individual animal. In many cases, lesions are self-limiting and no treatment is required. If stressors are involved, these may predispose to other conditions or make the animal susceptible to more serious infections.

# 8 Skin neoplasia in a hamster

## INITIAL PRESENTATION

Skin lesion in a Syrian hamster.

## INTRODUCTION

Historically, owners of small rodents have been reluctant to consult veterinary clinicians for treatment of illnesses in their pets. However, there is often a close bond between owner and pet, particularly if a child is the predominant carer, and the veterinary clinician will now regularly be called upon to treat these animals. It is important to provide an attentive and professional service, as this is an opportunity to imprint the importance of animal welfare and veterinary care of pets in the child's formative years.

## CASE PRESENTING SIGNS

An 18-month-old male Syrian hamster (*Mesocricetus auratus*) (see Box 8.1) presented as a second opinion case with a non-healing lesion on the lateral body wall.

## HUSBANDRY

The hamster was housed in a commercial hamster cage approximately 80 × 40 × 30 cm, comprising coated metal bars with a plastic base and tubing. A running wheel was provided. Newspaper covered the floor of the cage, with shredded paper as a burrowing substrate. The plastic hide contained cloth-based nesting material. The hamster used a glass jar on its side – containing soiled bedding – as a latrine. The hamster was handled daily, with extra exercise in a plastic hamster exercise ball twice a week. There were no other pets in the household.

A commercial rodent mix was provided as the main proportion of the diet. Small amounts of fresh fruit and vegetables – including apple and broccoli – were offered from time to time. Water was provided in a sipper bottle.

## NURSING ASPECT

- Do not use cotton wool or synthetic fibres as nesting material for hamsters. The fibres may wrap around limbs, causing constrictions, or become impacted in cheek pouches.

Fresh food and water were provided daily, and the cage was cleaned out once a week.

## CASE HISTORY

The hamster was purchased from a local petshop and had been in the owner's possession for 15 months. The owner noticed a mass on the hamster's flank 1 month before presentation. The hamster had been seen by another veterinary clinician for treatment, but no improvement was seen after a course of enrofloxacin.
- No previous history of medical problems
- Hamster bright, active and eating well. Normal urine and faeces passed
- Mass on left flank: initially a smooth surface and approximately 0.5 cm diameter, but it had increased in size since noted and the surface had become irregular and moist. No pruritus noted.

## BOX 8.1  ECOLOGY OF SYRIAN HAMSTERS

- Hamsters are members of the Muridae family, with 12 species of hamster in the sub-family Cricetinae
- Syrian hamsters are also known as golden hamsters
- Range in the wild: small area of north-western Syria. Classified as Endangered (at risk of extinction) by the IUCN
- Normal habitat: arid or semi-arid areas, from rocky mountain slopes and steppe to cultivated fields. Nocturnal/crepuscular (more nocturnal in captivity). Excavate a burrow <2 m long
- Solitary animal. Aggressive towards other hamsters (fight if kept in a group)
- Average weight: 100–125 g
- Length: 13–13.5 cm, tail 1.5 cm
- Free-ranging diet: herbivorous – mainly seeds and nuts. Sometimes take insects such as ants, flies, cockroaches and wasps. Perform caecotrophy
- Reproduction: hamsters become sexually mature soon after weaning, between 56 and 70 days old. Male and female meet briefly to copulate. Usually breed only once annually in the wild (although can breed year round in captivity). Gestation 15–18 days. Litter of 8–10 pups on average (can be up to 20) Altricial young, being born hairless and blind, are cared for by the female. Weaned around 3 weeks of age
- Longevity: 2–3 years
- Hibernate if environmental temperature <5°C
- Use incisors and fore-feet for self-grooming
- Use scent glands to mark territory
- Can hoard up to half the animal's body weight in food within the cheek pouches
- Extensively used in research, particularly using the cheek pouches that are immunologically privileged sites.

## CLINICAL EXAMINATION

As the hamster was habituated to handling, a reasonably complete examination was possible. Findings included:

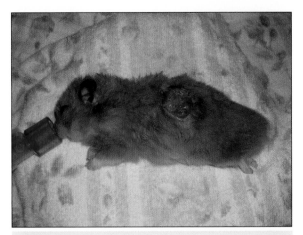

**Figure 8.1** Large ulcerated mass on the Syrian hamster's flank.

- Good body condition, weighing 110 g
- Incisors normal length and shape
- No sign of respiratory disease – no oculo-nasal discharges, and thoracic auscultation (using an infant-size stethoscope) was unremarkable
- No abnormalities detected on abdominal palpation
- Locomotion normal
- Single large (approximately 2 cm diameter) flattened ulcerated skin mass on left body wall (Fig. 8.1). Not palpably extending into tissues underlying the skin.

## DIFFERENTIAL DIAGNOSES

The differentials for the *skin lesion* were:
- Infection: bacterial, fungal (typically dermatophytosis will produce dry lesions), viral
- Neoplasia: benign or malignant. Hamster polyomavirus infection may result in skin tumours
- Trauma: resulting in wounds, often become secondarily infected resulting in pyoderma and abscessation
- Sebaceous scent glands: which may become inflamed after rubbing on abrasive cage equipment or if housed on wood shavings
- Ectoparasites: pruritus is rare but may result in self-trauma and open lesions that are susceptible to secondary bacterial infection
- Contact dermatitis: from cedar or pine wood shavings. A granulomatous inflammatory response may occur (usually on the face or feet).

## CASE WORK-UP

The non-healing nature of the lesion – despite broad-spectrum antibiosis – was suspicious for neoplasia. However, infection unresponsive to the antibiotic used (enrofloxacin) was also possible.

### General anaesthesia

Anaesthesia was induced using isoflurane in an induction chamber (Fig. 8.2) and maintained via a small facemask. Surgical depth was monitored using the toe pinch reflex. Respiratory rate and depth, and heart rate and rhythm were also monitored using a stethoscope during anaesthesia.

### Radiography

Lateral (Fig. 8.3a) and ventro-dorsal (Fig. 8.3b) body radiographs were taken to assess for the presence of systemic disease. No abnormalities were detected.

### Other investigative procedures that may have been performed

Abdominal ultrasound may have been used to detect visceral metastases or other pathology. This would require a high-frequency probe owing to the small size of the patient; a stand-off may also be useful in this instance.

An impression smear from the mass could have been examined cytologically. Equally, culture could have been performed from a superficial swab of the moist area.

## DIAGNOSIS

Skin neoplasia (see details below in Laboratory investigations).

## ANATOMY AND PHYSIOLOGY REFRESHER

Hamster fur is soft and smooth. Hair is sparse on the feet and tail, and almost totally lacking from the pinnae. The skin is loosely attached around the neck.

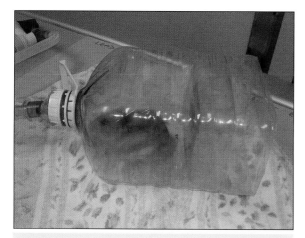

**Figure 8.2** Induction of general anaesthesia in a chamber.

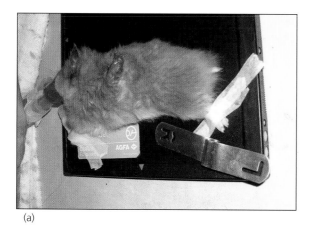

(a)

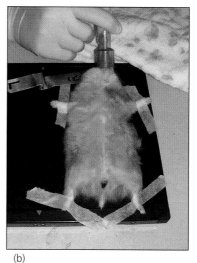

(b)

**Figure 8.3** Positioning for (a) lateral and (b) ventro-dorsal radiographs of the hamster.

The flank glands are situated in the costo-vertebral region. They comprise sebaceous glands, short sparse hairs and pigment cells. The gland size and pigmentation increases with age, particularly in males.

## AETIOPATHOGENESIS OF SKIN NEOPLASIA

Neoplasms of the skin can be associated with viral agents or may occur spontaneously.

Hamster polyomavirus (HaPV) may result in a subclinical infection in some animals. In other cases, cutaneous neoplasms – epithelioma or trichoepithelioma – or multicentric lymphoma may result. In colonies with endemic infection, cutaneous tumours are more common, usually affecting the periocular, oral or anal regions. T-lymphocytes are the neoplastic cells involved. The lesions are wart-like, but may progress to ulcerate and form crusts. High numbers of trichoepitheliomas can be debilitating.

Melanomas (melanotic or amelanotic) and melanocytomas are often found on the head, back and flank gland. Malignant neoplasia such as melanomas can metastasize widely. Epitheliotropic lymphoma results in pruritus and exfoliative erythroderma. Systemic illness results in lethargy, anorexia and weight loss.

## EPIDEMIOLOGY

Melanomas and melanocytomas are the most common skin neoplasms in hamsters. Males appear to have a higher incidence of these neoplasms. Epitheliotropic lymphoma is the second most common skin neoplasm. Less common neoplasias include carcinoma and pilomatrixoma.

The hamster polyomavirus is spread in urine, is highly resistant to disinfection, and epizootics cause high mortality.

## TREATMENT

### Anaesthesia

This was performed as for the investigation above.

### Surgery

A large area of skin was clipped around the lesion and prepared for surgery. It is important not to over-wet small patients as hypothermia secondary to heat loss from evaporation is a risk. The mass was excised using an elliptical incision. The mass did not grossly extend into the underlying muscle layer, and the skin and

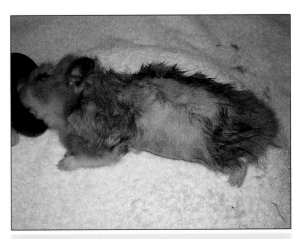

**Figure 8.4** Postoperative photograph showing intradermal suture closure of the skin.

subcutaneous layers only were removed. The wound was closed in two layers using polyglecaprone 25, with a continuous pattern (3/0 USP, 3 metric) in the subcutaneous layer and an intradermal pattern (4/0 USP, 2 metric) in the skin (Fig. 8.4).

### Perioperative supportive care

Analgesia was provided using buprenorphine (at 0.05 mg/kg SC q8hr for the initial 24 hours perioperatively) and meloxicam (at 0.6 mg/kg SC at the time of surgery). The hamster was closely monitored during recovery from anaesthesia, particularly to check that he was eating. During this period (lasting a couple of hours) the patient was housed in an incubator until he was moving around well.

### Laboratory investigations

The mass was submitted for culture and histology. A poorly differentiated carcinoma was diagnosed. *Staphylococcus intermedius* was cultured, thought to be a secondary infection in the ulcerated tumour.

---

**CLINICAL TIPS**

- It is important to closely monitor rodents after surgery.
- They will often chew sutures and open wounds. Appropriate choice of suture pattern (usually intradermal) in the skin and analgesia will reduce this problem. In some cases, mild sedation can be given for a short period.

- To avoid hypoglycaemia, it is vital that small animals begin eating soon after recovery from anaesthesia. Assist-feeding should be provided if necessary.
- To avoid hypothermia, recovery is best performed in an incubator. A heat mat or other supplemental heating should also be provided during surgery.

## TREATMENT OPTIONS AND MANAGEMENT

### Medication

Analgesia was continued using meloxicam (0.3 mg/kg PO q24hr for 5 days after surgery).

### Husbandry

The hamster was bedded on newspaper with a small amount of soft shredded paper (kitchen towel) for 1 week after surgery, to prevent irritation of the wound. In order to minimize the risk of wound dehiscence during this period, handling was restricted and exercise reduced (by removing the exercise wheel and avoiding use of the exercise ball).

## OTHER TREATMENT OPTIONS

### Surgery

If local infiltration of neoplasia occurs, more extensive surgery may be required. With small animals such as rodents, the clinician should carefully gauge any stresses, possible side-effects (such as wound dehiscence after self-trauma), and the animal's quality of life before performing more radical surgery. Magnification can be useful when performing intricate surgery on small patients.

### Supportive care

If the hamster had not started to self-feed shortly after surgery, assist-feeding would have been performed (using baby food). In some cases, analgesia may be required for a longer period. Antibiosis may be required if infection is present.

## FOLLOW-UP

The hamster recovered well from surgery, and was self-feeding within 2 hours. No self-trauma was observed following surgery or after ceasing opioid analgesia. The patient was discharged the following day.

Reassessment 10 days after surgery showed the skin wound to be healing well. Although slightly subdued for 2 days after surgery, the hamster had been behaving normally during the previous week.

## PREVENTION

In cases of neoplasia due to viral infection, biosecurity and isolation from other hamsters will prevent disease.

## PROGNOSIS

Histology showed clear margins around the tumour. However, a guarded prognosis was given with this malignant tumour and the owner advised to monitor closely for recurrence.

# SECTION 2

# BIRDS

# 9 Birds – an introduction

## INTRODUCTION

Birds such as parrots and canaries have been kept as pets for many centuries, for their beauty, song and mimicry. Raptors are more usually kept for hunting. It is impossible to provide details of all species (there are around 10 000), but the rudimentary principles of captive avian husbandry will be covered. This chapter will also outline clinical assessment and elementary investigations.

## TAXONOMY

Taxonomic classification of birds in the superorder Neognathae is given in Table 9.1.

## BIOLOGY

Basic internal anatomy for birds-including gastrointestinal, respiratory and cardiovascular – is given in Figs 9.1–9.3.

### Psittaciformes
#### African grey parrot (Psittacus erithacus)

These parrots originate from sub-Saharan Africa, and are commonly seen as pet birds. They often respond to attention and stimulation by forming a close bond with owners. Cages marketed for parrots are often too small for anything more than temporary accommodation at night. Ideally, an outdoor aviary should be provided to permit free flight. A sheltered area is necessary for sleeping and to protect the bird from adverse weather conditions. If an outdoor enclosure is not a viable option, exercise may be provided in a secure room indoors. The enclosure should be made of non-toxic materials, avoiding heavy metals such as zinc and lead, and sited away from sources of toxic fumes such as polytetrafluoroethylene (PTFE, from heated non-stick cooking materials).

Various perches should be provided in the enclosure, and toys added (and changed regularly to retain interest). Parrots are sociable, and should be paired with a conspecific if possible. If parrots are left alone, a radio can be switched on to provide some stimulation. Full spectrum UV lighting should be provided for African greys housed indoors, to help prevent behavioural problems and hypocalcaemia.

Although free-ranging birds eat a large amount of nuts and seeds, over-feeding of these foodstuffs in captivity results in malnutrition due to differing energy requirements (lower in captive animals). It is advisable to feed a proprietary pelleted diet, supplemented with fresh fruits and vegetables (10% of the diet), and some sprouted pulses (Box 9.1). Grit may help with digestion. Vitamin and mineral supplements may be additionally required, particularly for breeding birds (Box 9.2). Fresh water should be provided in a bowl for drinking; many birds also appreciate a shallow water container for bathing.

#### Budgerigar (Melopsittacus undulatus) and cockatiel (Nymphicus hollandicus)

These two species both originate from Australia. Budgies congregate in large flocks over semi-arid plains. Cockatiels are small members of the cockatoo family, and are also a social species.

In captivity, both are ideally housed in an outdoor aviary enabling flight. It should be made of strong wire mesh, with a sheltered sleeping area. As with all outdoor enclosures, construction should be solid to prevent predator access, and a double entry door is advisable to prevent escapes. If housed indoors, accommodation should permit exercise through daily flight. Perches and toys are provided as for other parrots.

Adult male budgerigars of most colour varieties have a blue cere while adult females have a pink/brown cere. Adult male cockatiels have bright red/orange cheek

**Table 9.1** Taxonomic classification of birds in the superorder Neognathae*

| Order | Types of bird | Family | Subfamily | Species examples |
|---|---|---|---|---|
| Columbiformes | Pigeons | Columbidae | – | Rock dove, feral pigeon or racing pigeon (*Columba livia*) |
| Falconiformes | Vultures, hawks, eagles, and falcons | Cathartidae Sagittariidae Pandionidae Falconidae Accipitridae | – | New World vultures, e.g. black vulture (*Cathartes atratus*) Secretary bird (*Sagittarius serpentarius*) Osprey (*Pandion haliaetus*) Falcons, e.g. common kestrel (*Falco tinnunculus*), peregrine falcon (*F. peregrinus*) Hawks and eagles, e.g. bald eagle (*Haliaeetus leucocephalus*), golden eagle (*Aquila chrysaetos*), red kite (*Milvus milvus*) |
| Passeriformes | Passerines | 82 families | – | e.g. hill mynah (*Gracula religiosa*), canary (*Serinus canaria*), zebra finch (*Poephila guttata*) |
| Psittaciformes | Parrots | Psittacidae | Psittacinae | True parrots, e.g. blue-and-yellow macaw (*Ara ararauna*), budgerigar (*Melopsittacus undulatus*), African grey parrot (*Psittacus erithacus*), rosy-faced lovebird (*Agapornis roseicollis*) |
| | | | Loriinae | Lories and lorikeets, e.g. rainbow lorikeet (*Trichoglossus haematodus*) |
| | | | Nestorinae | Keas |
| | | | Strigopinae | Owl parrot |
| | | | Cacatuinae | Cockatoos, e.g. sulphur-crested cockatoo (*Cacatua galerita*), galah or rose-breasted cockatoo (*Eolophus roseicapillus*) |
| | | | Nymphicinae | Cockatiel (*Nymphicus hollandicus*) |
| | | | Micropsittinae | Fig and pygmy parrots |
| Strigiformes | Owls | Strigidae Tytonidae | – | Eagle owl (*Bubo bubo*), snowy owl (*Nyctea scandiaca*) Barn and bay owls, e.g. barn owl (*Tyto alba*) |

*The other taxonomic superorder of birds is the Palaeognathae, which includes ratites such as ostriches and emus.

## BOX 9.1 TOXIC FOODS FOR PARROTS

These include avocado, caffeine (in tea or coffee), alcohol, chocolate and salty foods.

## BOX 9.2 HYPOCALCAEMIA

This is extremely common in African grey parrots. It is often associated with malnutrition and a lack of access to UV light. Clinical signs typically include ataxia and seizures.

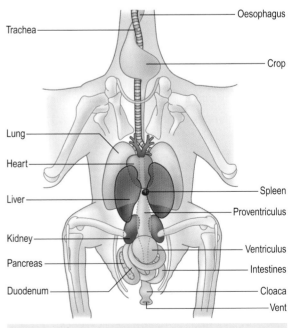

**Figure 9.1** Ventro-dorsal view of internal organs.

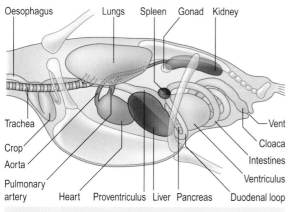

Oesophagus    Lungs    Spleen    Gonad    Kidney

Trachea

Crop

Aorta

Pulmonary
artery    Heart    Proventriculus    Liver    Pancreas

Vent

Cloaca

Intestines

Ventriculus

Duodenal loop

**Figure 9.2** Lateral view of internal organs.

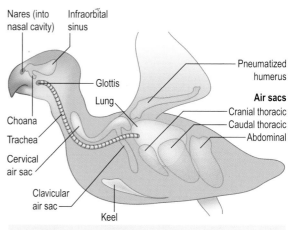

Nares (into    Infraorbital
nasal cavity)    sinus

Glottis

Lung

Choana

Trachea

Cervical
air sac

Clavicular
air sac

Keel

Pneumatized
humerus

**Air sacs**
Cranial thoracic
Caudal thoracic
Abdominal

**Figure 9.3** Air sacs in birds.

---

### BOX 9.3    IODINE DEFICIENCY

This is common in budgerigars fed on all seed diets, resulting in thyroid pathology. Providing an iodine supplement, e.g. an iodine block, prevents the condition.

---

patches, and females retain horizontal bars on their tails; some features of sexual dimorphism will not be visible in certain varieties (such as cheek patches in the lutino).

Captive diets may include small seed mixes, although commercial formulated pellets are better balanced. Fresh green food (e.g. chickweed, dandelion or lettuce leaves), small amounts of fruit, and cuttlefish bone should be provided. Vitamin and mineral supplementation is advised if the bird is on a seed diet (Box 9.3).

### Blue-and-yellow macaw (Ara ararauna)

This bird originates from South and Central America. Its large size (up to 1.3 kg in weight) means accommodation should also be spacious. Providing there is sufficient interaction, macaws will bond closely to their owners. Dietary requirements are similar to the African grey parrot.

## Passeriformes

### Canary (Serinus canaria)

These small birds (10–40 g) originated from the Canary Islands. Housing is similar to budgerigars.

Free-ranging individuals eat various seeds. Captive diets should avoid larger fatty seeds such as sunflowers, but mixes commonly contain millet seed. Vitamin and mineral supplementation is necessary with seed diets.

Balanced proprietary pelleted diets are available. Fresh green food, small amounts of fruit, cuttlefish, and grit (to aid digestion and provide minerals) should also be offered.

### Zebra finch (Poephila guttata)

This small (10–20 g) bird originates in Australia. The species breeds readily in captivity and many colour forms exist. Free-ranging birds eat grass seeds, and individuals in captivity often receive a mainly seed-based diet, although extruded pellets provide a more balanced diet.

### Greater hill mynah (Gracula religiosa)

This bird is a member of the starling family, and originates from the hill regions of South Asia. It is medium-sized, with a body weight of 180–250 g. This species is a good mimic and therefore a popular pet.

Hill mynahs are a typical 'softbill', feeding on fruit and insects in the wild. Captive insectivore diets are available, and fruit can be added to this. The species is susceptible to iron overload disorders (haemochromatosis). Citrus fruits should be fed at a different time to foods high in iron (e.g. meat-based products), as vitamin C increases iron uptake.

## Falconiformes

This order includes hawks, falcons, eagles and vultures. These species are chiefly diurnal. Most are solitary except during the breeding season, although Harris' hawks (Parabuteo unicinctus) are gregarious. Raptors may be kept for hunting, demonstration flying, clearing airfields and rubbish dumps of other birds, pest control and breeding for conservation or commercial reasons.

Birds are either kept tethered or housed in an aviary (Box 9.4). Tethered birds are attached to a perch by a leash (Box 9.5) during the flying season (typically winter for hunting and summer for birds used in public demonstrations), and normally moved to an aviary during the close season for moulting. Some birds may be 'free-lofted' (being housed in and flown from aviaries), in particular vultures that may find tethering stressful. Substrates in enclosures vary from bare earth to gravel to bark chip; all should be hygienically maintained to reduce the risk of disease.

---

### BOX 9.4   PERCHES FOR RAPTORS

- Bow perches are used for hawks, buzzards and eagles.
- Falcons are maintained on block perches.

---

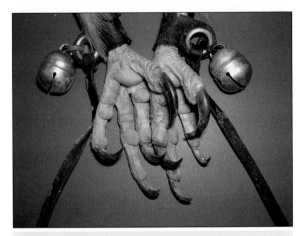

**Figure 9.4** Falconry equipment on the legs of a peregrine-saker hybrid. Aylmeri wrap around the tibiotarsus, to which jesses are attached.

Although all are carnivorous, the food eaten depends on the species (and may include vertebrates, invertebrates and carrion). Falconiformes have a crop, and cast (regurgitate) indigestible material including fur and feathers. Water should be provided, usually in a large shallow bowl that permits drinking and bathing. Sexual dimorphism may be obvious, with differences seen in size (e.g. peregrine males are smaller), colour and markings (e.g. common kestrels).

---

### BOX 9.5   FALCONRY EQUIPMENT

- Jesses: leather thongs around tibiotarsi for restraint (Fig. 9.4)
- Aylmeri: popular type of jess, bracelet joined by riveted brass ring
- Swivel: rotating metal joint between jesses and leash
- Leash: attaches between swivel and perch or gauntlet
- Gauntlet: leather glove worn on falconer's left hand (or right hand if left-handed)
- Hood: a close-fitting leather cap, blindfolds and calms birds
- Lure: imitation bird on a line, used to exercise and train falcons.

---

### Harris' hawk (Parabuteo unicinctus)

This species comes from the southern USA, and Central and South America. Harris' hawks are commonly kept for hunting owing to their social hunting behaviour. Males may reach 880 g and females 1.2 kg.

## Strigiformes

This order includes owl species, which are, for the most part, nocturnal. Owls are solitary or form loose pairs, except during the breeding season. Flying is limited with owls, and most captive birds are maintained for personal pleasure or 'line' breeding of colour variants. Owls are usually 'free-lofted', as in general they find tethering stressful.

These carnivorous birds are usually fed once daily (as are falconiformes). They do not possess a crop, and, as bones are not digested, cast material includes fur, feathers and bones from prey. Sexual dimorphism is slight in the main, although obvious in some species such as the snowy owl (Fig. 9.5).

### Barn owl (Tyto alba)

This species is distributed worldwide (aside from polar and desert regions), with several subspecies identified. Females of the European subspecies (Tyto alba alba) usually have more spotting over ventral feathers than the male, whose underparts are white. They feed predominantly on small vertebrates, particularly rodents.

### Eagle owl (Bubo bubo)

This large bird may reach 3 kg (males) to 4.2 kg (females). They originate from Eurasia. Prey items in the wild include animals up to 10 kg, including foxes and young deer.

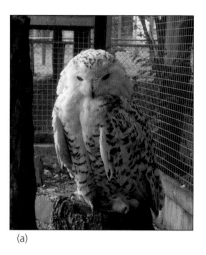
(a)

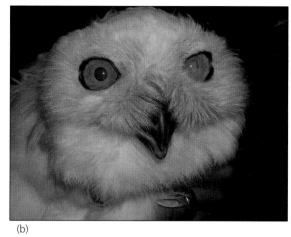
(b)

**Figure 9.5** Snowy owl. (a) The female has brown flecks on her ventral feathers whereas (b) the male is white.

## Columbiformes

### Racing pigeon (Columba livia)

Domesticated European pigeons have descended from the wild rock pigeon (*Columbia livia*) from Asia and the Mediterranean. Pigeons may be kept for several reasons – exhibition, racing, performance flying, or for meat. The racing season in central Europe generally runs from April until September.

Most commonly, pigeons are group-housed in lofts, usually with facilities to separate birds in compartments such as for breeding. Environmental conditions (including temperature, humidity and ventilation) in lofts are paramount to good health of the birds. As with other bird accommodation, good hygiene should be maintained by regular cleaning and disinfection.

Dietary requirements vary depending on the use of the pigeon and season, for example differing between rearing, racing, moulting and resting periods. Proprietary mixes are available, as are nutritional supplements.

## HISTORY

Although a full clinical examination is possible on most medium- to large-sized birds, it is still important to take a full history (see Box 9.6). Husbandry changes or inadequacies commonly contribute to disease. In addition, companion birds are often prey species and will hide signs of illness, so any clinical changes seen may be subtle.

> ### BOX 9.6 SUGGESTED TOPICS TO COVER DURING HISTORY TAKING FOR BIRDS
>
> - Species
> - Age
> - Gender
> - Source, e.g. petshop or breeder, imported, captive-bred or wild-caught, relevant paperwork (e.g. CITES)
> - Period in owner's possession (if this is relatively short, husbandry details from the previous carer may be important)
> - Reproductive history
> - Housing (cage/room/flight/aviary): size, construction materials, location, substrate, cleaning regime, indoors/outdoors, free flight
> - Exposure to potential toxins, e.g. cigarette smoke, household chemicals
> - UV-B access: either exposure to sunlight or the use of UV bulbs, including when the bulbs were last changed. (UV meters may be used to assess UV output in older bulbs or tubes, as visible light is still produced even when UV production has waned.)
> - Day to night cycle, use of 'black-out' cover at night
> - Presence of nest boxes/nest material
> - Perches: number, material and size

- Toys: description, rotation or continuous presence in enclosure
- Diet: what food is offered (including supplements) and what is eaten, frequency of feeding
- Water provision: for drinking (any supplements), bathing/spraying (to encourage preening, any 'tonics' in the water), and swimming (in waterbirds)
- Moulting: frequency, date of last moult, any problems noted
- Wing clip (current or previous)
- Handling frequency and any training given
- Previous medical history (including any treatments)
- Current problem: time period, outline of clinical signs and progression noted by owner
- Current physiology: appetite and thirst; faecal, urine and urates output (including number/ size, frequency/volume and description)
- Question owner further about the pet's current health: any other clinical signs of disease or changes in behaviour (these may be subtle until disease is severe)
- Companion animals in the same enclosure/ airspace/indirect contact: any health problems (current or previous).

For raptors, it is important to ask relevant questions pertinent to the bird's working or training history. Some birds will be 'free-lofted' in an open aviary, or tethered. If tethered, the bird will wear 'equipment' (usually leather) on its legs to attach to the bow or block perch. The substrate of perches is very important for raptors as many succumb to bumblefoot due to inappropriate or unhygienic substrate. Raptors will produce a pellet ('cast') after feeding, containing indigestible material (feathers and fur in Falconiformes, also bone in owls).

## CLINICAL EXAMINATION

It is important to initially observe the bird without restraint if possible. While taking the history, the patient's demeanour can be assessed. Look for any dyspnoea, or obvious neurological or motor deficits (Box 9.7). Birds typically hide illness, particularly prey species such as passerines and psittacines, and do not show clinical signs until disease is quite far advanced. This is especially true in a strange environment such as the veterinary clinic on first presentation. The patient may relax after some time in the clinic, and begin to display clinical signs.

*Small passerines and psittacines* such as budgerigars may be grasped without any equipment, or a thin paper towel may be used. The bird is grasped from behind with its head between the clinician's first and second fingers, and the palm and thumb surrounding the body to restrain the wings (Fig. 9.6a). Care should be taken not to put excessive pressure around the thoracic region; restricting keel movement will also restrict breathing (potentially fatally).

It is useful to employ a towel to restrain *larger psittacines* such as Amazon parrots or macaws (Fig. 9.6b). Towels are preferred to thick gauntlets as they allow the handler to feel the bird and apply adequate (and not excessive) pressure, and, once restrained, the bird may be distracted by allowing it to chew on a loose corner of towel. Towels also hide the hand and reduce the risk of a 'hand phobia' developing in the pet parrot. The handler should beware of attack from the beak, since most parrots are capable of inflicting deep and painful bites. The bird is approached from behind, and the head restrained just below the mandible using an incomplete circle formed between thumb and first finger. The bird will be calmer if the towel covers the head. The towel is gently wrapped around the body to restrain the wings. During the examination, the handler grasps around the tarsometatarsal region to restrain the feet. Although injury is possible from the claws, it is not usually serious from most species. The towel can be partially unwrapped to permit full clinical examination, for example to assess each wing.

### BOX 9.7 PSITTACOSIS

- This zoonotic disease is common in pet parrots, and is caused by *Chlamydophila psittaci*.
- Clinical signs in birds can be vague, but often involve the respiratory system.
- Infection in humans (chlamydophilosis or ornithosis) usually causes flu-like symptoms, but may be chronic and severe in immunocompromised individuals (including the young and elderly).
- New birds should be tested for infection. Usually a polymerase chain reaction (PCR) is performed on a pooled faecal sample to check for *Chlamydophila* antigen, although

shedding is intermittent and a negative result does not guarantee that the bird is free of infection. Positive birds may be re-infected or the organism may re-activate after treatment.

- PPE (personal protective equipment) such as examination gloves, a facemask and goggles should be worn in suspicious cases. Owners should be informed of the potential for human infection. Good personal hygiene is important when dealing with any animal that may be carrying a zoonotic infection.
- If therapy against psittacosis is to be administered, all birds in the collection should be treated. The positive bird should be quarantined and treated separately. Doxycycline (e.g. 75 mg/kg IM q5d for six doses, then q4d for three doses is suggested for many parrots) or enrofloxacin (e.g. 15 mg/kg IM or PO q12hr for 45 days) are the antibiotics of choice. Medication is ideally administered on an individual bird basis, although chlortetracycline in food (2500–5000 mg/kg in feed for 45 days) may be useful in large collections.

Most captive *raptors* wear leg equipment and are trained to the fist. A partial examination may be performed while the bird is on the gauntlet. However, the bird must be 'cast' using a towel to complete a full clinical examination (Fig. 9.6c). Raptors will be quieter if they are hooded during casting, but the hood should be removed to permit examination of the head. As with parrots, the bird is approached from behind. The main difference with raptors is that, in general, the clinician should be aware of the potential for injury from the talons (although the beak in larger birds such as eagles may cause injury to handlers). The towel is used to cover the wings to restrain them, before the tarsometatarsal or tibiotarsal regions are grasped through the towel to restrain the feet. After grasping, it is usually possible to restrain both feet with one hand, while using the other hand to support the body against the handler's chest and hold the towel edges loosely wrapped around the bird.

Birds may become warm during restraint, particularly if a towel is used. The procedure should therefore be as brief as possible to prevent hyperthermia. Collect all examination and sampling equipment prior to handling to minimize the time of the procedure. In birds with obvious existing respiratory problems, it may be prefer-

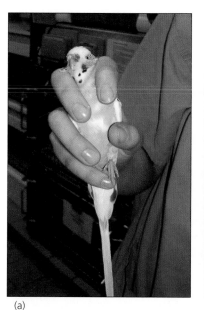
(a)

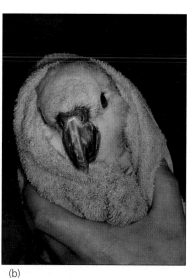
(b)

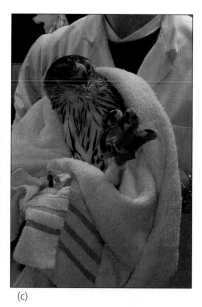
(c)

**Figure 9.6** Handling birds. (a) Passerines and small psittacines may be restrained either with the naked hand or using a thin paper towel. Avoid putting excess pressure around the thoracic region that may restrict breathing movements. (b) Medium or large psittacines should be restrained using a towel. Ensure the beak is controlled. (c) Raptors should be cast using a towel. Ensure the feet are controlled.

able to postpone clinical examination until after stabilization (e.g. a period in an oxygen chamber).

## INVESTIGATION

### Phlebotomy

Although venous access is usually possible in conscious birds, restraint for the procedure may be stressful. It is often preferable to anaesthetize using gaseous agents or sedate the bird to reduce the stresses of physical restraint. Avian blood vessels are fragile and susceptible to laceration and subsequent haemorrhage; a small needle (usually 25 gauge) is used and pressure is applied for a few minutes after the procedure to ensure haemostasis.

In most species, the right jugular vein is accessed for phlebotomy (Fig. 9.7). The bird is placed in lateral recumbency and pressure applied at the base of the neck to raise the vein. Alternative sites include the superficial ulnar or superficial plantar metatarsal veins (the latter are particularly useful in long-legged birds such as waterfowl); both of these are ideal sites for placement of intravenous catheters (Fig. 9.8).

Blood volume in a healthy bird is approximately 10% of body weight (i.e. 100 ml/kg). Up to 10% of the blood volume (i.e. 10 ml/kg, or 1 ml/100 g) may be sampled at one time. In ill birds, the volume should be smaller, and it can be helpful to maintain circulatory volume with replacement fluids after phlebotomy. For a haematology and biochemistry panel, blood is usually collected into ethylenediamine tetraacetic acid (EDTA) and heparin tubes, and a fresh smear prepared. Haematological

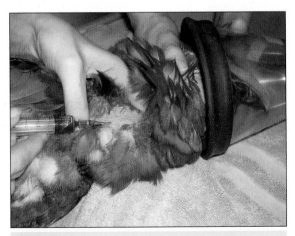

**Figure 9.7** Jugular phlebotomy in a green-winged macaw.

analysis may be performed on the heparin sample, which is useful if only a very small volume is taken. Blood smears are used to assess for haemoparasites as well as the morpholog of leucocytes. An estimated and differential white cell count can also be performed on the smear.

### Radiography

General anaesthesia is routinely used for restraint of birds during radiography. However, in certain circumstances (e.g. if a bird is in severe respiratory distress or if a gastrointestinal contrast study is being performed), conscious radiographs may be taken. In these instances, the bird is placed on a perch in a radiolucent box and a horizontal beam used to obtain a lateral radiograph. Obviously image quality will be reduced owing to suboptimal positioning, with the wings overlying the body.

The most common radiographic views taken of birds are lateral and ventro-dorsal images of the body. For the lateral view, the legs are pulled caudally so they do not overlie the middle of the coelomic cavity. If the caudal coelomic cavity is the focus of interest, the legs can be restrained more cranially in the lateral position. For the ventro-dorsal view, the bird is placed in dorsal recumbency with the wings extended and restrained (using adhesive tape or sandbags) laterally and the legs restrained caudally. The wings may be folded around each other (at the elbows and carpi) to retain them in a dorsal position in many deeply anaesthetized birds, although this position puts some pressure on the joints, and may result in self-injury if the anaesthetic becomes light and the bird struggles.

Care should be taken during any positioning that undue pressure is not placed on any body parts that may result in injury (the wings are particularly susceptible to damage). The preferred position of the anaesthetized bird for ease of breathing is lateral recumbency, enabling ease of keel movement (that may be restricted in ventral recumbency) and without excessive pressure from internal organs on the air sacs (that occurs during dorsal recumbency). Periods in other positions should be minimized.

For examination of more peripheral body parts, adhesive paper tape is used to position the site and enable two orthogonal views to be obtained. Foam wedges or sandbags may be useful to support the body for positioning.

### Sampling

Faecal analysis is frequently performed in birds. In all species, but particularly those housed outdoors that may be exposed to faeces from wild birds, faecal examination should be performed regularly to assess for endoparasites. Culture may be of interest in cases of suspected gastrointestinal bacterial or fungal (yeast) infection. Some clinicians routinely perform in-house microscopy of Gram-stained samples to assess gastrointestinal microflora; although results are very dependent on the bird's current diet, this test can be a screening tool to investigate dysbiosis or yeast infections.

Other samples may be analysed microscopically. As with other species, impression smears from lesions or fine needle aspirates (using ultrasound to guide the needle into deeper lesions) may be assessed. Crop washes are regularly performed (using sterile saline) to investigate upper gastrointestinal tract disease. Tracheal washes and bone marrow aspirates may also be executed to obtain samples. Tissue samples are frequently obtained via endoscopy or surgery, and submitted for culture or histology.

### BOX 9.8   ENDOSCOPY

- Endoscopy is an extremely useful tool in avian medicine.
- Many systems may be assessed, including:
  - Both upper and lower gastrointestinal tracts
  - Upper airways: often as far as the tracheal bifurcation and syrinx
  - Lower airways: air sacs and the caudal lung regions can be assessed from the coelomic cavity
  - Coelomic organs, such as the liver, serosal surfaces of the gastrointestinal tracts, pancreas, kidneys and ureters, gonads and reproductive tract
  - The cloaca, involving terminations from the gastrointestinal, reproductive and urinary tracts.
- General anaesthesia is usually required, in part to protect the equipment from trauma!

## TREATMENT

### Basic procedures

#### Drug administration

*Topical* ointments and creams are rarely used in birds, as they may damage the plumage or be toxic if ingested.

The *oral* route is by far the easiest route to administer fluids or medication to birds (Box 9.9). Some supplements or drugs may be taken in food or water, but many birds will refuse such items owing to the difference in taste. For some pet birds, particularly those that were reared on egg food, food (with or without drugs as appropriate) offered on a spoon may be voluntarily taken. Small volumes may be syringed directly into the oral cavity, taking care not to allow the bird to chew and ingest the tip of the syringe.

For larger volumes, such as those required for nutritional support, crop tubing (more correctly called gavage in species such as owls that do not possess a crop) is advised. If a plastic tube is used, a gag should be used to hold the mouth open. An assistant restrains the conscious bird while the clinician passes the tube caudolaterally in the oral cavity, avoiding the central glottis at the base of the tongue. The tip of the tube is palpated in the crop or oesophagus at the base of the neck before the medication is administered.

### BOX 9.9   FLUIDS

- Large volumes should be warmed prior to administration.
- Typical volumes administered by gavage are <20 ml/kg.

*Intramuscular* injections are typically administered in the pectoral muscles. The needle is inserted in the caudal third of the muscle, directed cranially. The plunger should be withdrawn to ensure a blood vessel has not been inadvertently entered before the medication is injected. In larger birds, the iliotibialis lateralis (not advised for nephrotoxic agents due to the renal portal system Box 9.10) or biceps femoris muscles may be used.

### BOX 9.10   RENAL PORTAL SYSTEM

- A dual afferent blood supply exists to the kidneys.
- As with mammals, the renal arteries (cranial, middle and caudal) supply the kidneys. Birds and reptiles also possess a renal portal vein.
- The renal portal system may drain the drug directly to the kidneys when medication is injected into the caudal part of the body. For this reason, potentially nephrotoxic agents or those that undergo significant renal metabolism are not injected in this region.

Although commonly employed in other species, the *subcutaneous* route is difficult to use in birds. Avian skin is thin and there is a relatively small potential subcutaneous space. Sites for injection (in order of preference) include the precrural fold or inguinal region, the dorsal neck or interscapular areas, the lateral flank, over the pectoral muscles, the axillary region, or in the propatagial skin fold of the wing. The intracoelomic route is not used for fluid administration in birds (Box 9.11).

In small birds venous access may be technically difficult, and the jugular vein is utilized for *intravenous* injections. However, it is easier to maintain an intravenous catheter in vessels such as the ulnar, brachial or superficial plantar metatarsal veins. For the former, the catheter may be secured using adhesive tape to the feathers or suture material to the skin; for the latter site, adhesive tape around the leg will secure the catheter.

Injection of medications or fluid *intraosseously* is equivalent to entry to the circulation via intravenous administration (Fig. 9.9). General anaesthesia is usually required for this painful procedure, and surgical preparation is necessary to reduce the risk of infection. Pneumatized bones such as the humerus should be avoided.

Commonly, the distal ulna or proximal tibiotarsal bones are used. The joint is flexed before a needle is inserted into the bone. A bung or administration set is attached before securing the needle to the limb. Fluids or medication may be administered in boluses or via CRI (continuous rate infusion).

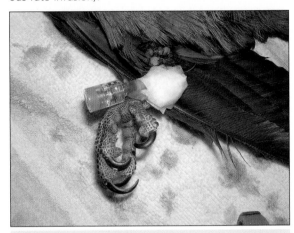

**Figure 9.8** Intravenous catheter placed in the superficial plantar metatarsal vein of a male eclectus parrot (*Eclectus roratus*).

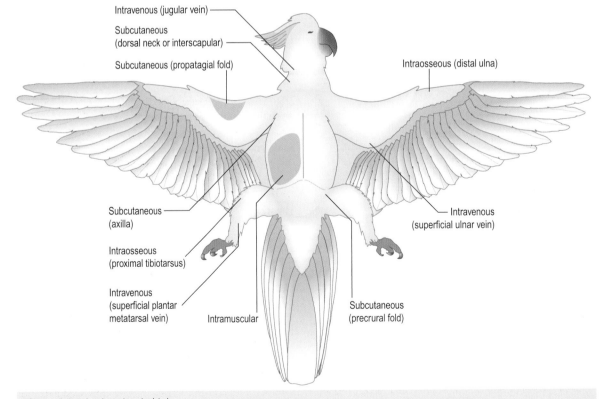

Intravenous (jugular vein)

Subcutaneous (dorsal neck or interscapular)

Subcutaneous (propatagial fold)

Intraosseous (distal ulna)

Subcutaneous (axilla)

Intravenous (superficial ulnar vein)

Intraosseous (proximal tibiotarsus)

Intravenous (superficial plantar metatarsal vein)

Intramuscular

Subcutaneous (precrural fold)

**Figure 9.9** Injection sites in birds.

### BOX 9.11  WARNING

- Do not administer fluids by intracoelomic injection in birds. The air sacs fill most of the cavity between organs, and injection of fluids will effectively drown the bird as the respiratory tract is flooded.
- Small volumes of medication (such as antimicrobials for treating air sacculitis) may be deliberately injected into the air sacs to provide local treatment.

The respiratory tract may be entered by intratracheal administration (e.g. saline used for sampling from a tracheal wash) or *nebulization*. The latter is frequently utilized to administer medications deep into the airways.

### Assist-feeding

As described in the section above, some birds will take food offered in a spoon. For others, gavage-feeding is the easiest route for providing nutritional support (Fig. 9.10). Avian convalescent diets are available, providing easily digestible sources of nutrition. In general, adult crop capacity is approximately 3% of the bird's body weight (e.g. 9 ml in a 300 g bird). Most will require 30–60 ml/kg per day, although this should be altered depending on body condition, and weight loss or gain. The total daily dose should be divided into three or four doses.

A duodenostomy feeding tube may be placed in cases requiring more intensive nutritional support, or an oesophagostomy tube used where chronic support is envisaged. Care should be taken to prevent the patient from traumatizing the wound or tube.

## Anaesthesia

### Pre-anaesthesia

It is imperative to make a judgement on whether the avian patient is sufficiently healthy to undergo general anaesthesia. This judgement will be based on the animal's history, clinical findings, and the clinician's experience. If in any doubt, ill birds not requiring a life-saving procedure under anaesthesia should be stabilized before anaesthesia is induced. Alternatively, consider whether the procedure could more safely be completed under sedation and/or analgesia.

Severely dyspnoeic birds should be placed into an oxygenated chamber. Dehydrated or collapsed birds may

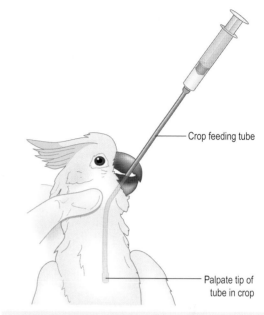

**Figure 9.10** Gavage in birds.

Crop feeding tube

Palpate tip of tube in crop

benefit from fluids (preferably intravenous or intraosseous, but the oral or subcutaneous routes may be accessed with less stress). Those in poor body condition may be hypoglycaemic or have other metabolic derangements that require nutritional support.

Birds may regurgitate if they have food material or liquid in their crops. Fasting periods vary between species and between individuals (as animals with a slowed gastrointestinal transit time or crop impaction will not empty their crop so rapidly). In general, gastrointestinal transit time is rapid. If the crop is full of liquid and anaesthesia is urgent, it may be emptied by suction before induction. Small birds (<100 g) should not be fasted due to the risks of hypoglycaemia; conversely raptors are usually fasted for at least 12 hours (permitting egestion of casting material before anaesthesia is induced).

### Pre-medication

Typically, no pre-medication is administered before a short non-painful procedure requiring anaesthesia in a bird (such as phlebotomy or radiography). However, there are several reasons for pre-medicating certain cases. These include provision of analgesia, sedation reducing the stresses of handling and induction, and lowering the requirement of general anaesthetic agents (and thus their side-effects). Some of these benefits will also result in a smoother recovery period.

**Table 9.2** Commonly used pre-medicants in birds

| Drug | Dose (mg/kg) | Route | Comment |
|------|--------------|-------|---------|
| Butorphanol | 1.0–4.0 | IM, IV | Sedative, analgesic; 2–3 hours duration |
| Diazepam | 0.2–0.5 | IM, IV | Aqueous solution can be administered IM or IV; propylene glycol solution is IV only. Tranquillization |
| Midazolam | 0.25–0.5 | IM, IV | Sedative, anti-anxiety |
| Ketamine | 2.5–20 | IM | Low doses used for sedation |

IM, intramuscular; IV, intravenous.

**Table 9.3** Gaseous anaesthetic agents used in birds

| Drug | Concentration (%) | | Comment |
| | Induction | Maintenance | |
|------|-----------|-------------|---------|
| Isoflurane | 4–5 | 2.5–3.0 | Induction in 2–3 minutes |
| Sevoflurane | 7–8 | 4 | Smoother induction due to lack of respiratory tract irritation |

Note: Lower concentrations will be required if pre-medication has been administered.

It is usual to combine agents to produce a smooth sedation and provide analgesia. A frequently used combination is butorphanol with midazolam (Table 9.2).

### Inhalation agents

Most birds are restrained in a towel for mask induction of anaesthesia using one of the agents listed below (Table 9.3, Box 9.12). The mask should be close fitting to reduce environmental contamination; where the mask is of an inappropriate size, an examination glove may be placed over the end and a small hole incised to contain the bird's head. It is customary to pre-oxygenate (providing 100% oxygen for a few breaths) prior to introducing the anaesthetic agent. After induction, most avian patients are easily intubated for maintenance on gaseous agents (Box 9.13).

---

### BOX 9.12 HALOTHANE

- The use of halothane is contraindicated in birds due to the ease of overdosage.
- Side-effects include myocardial depression and sensitization to catecholamine-induced cardiac arrhythmias.
- Cardiac and respiratory arrest are simultaneous with this agent.

---

### BOX 9.13 INTUBATION IN BIRDS

- Intubation protects the bird's airway (e.g. from aspiration if regurgitation occurs), allows continuous provision of gases (oxygen and anaesthetic agents) and permits ease of IPPV (intermittent positive pressure ventilation). This is especially important if positioning of the patient compromises keel movement or the air sacs are compressed.
- The glottis lies midline in the oral cavity at the base of the tongue. Tongue anatomy varies between avian species, being large and fleshy in psittacines but long and thin in raptors.
- The tracheal lumen is relatively large in birds, e.g. a 3 mm endotracheal tube (ETT) may be used in a 300 g parrot. Avian tracheal cartilage rings are complete, and so an uncuffed ETT should be used. Once placed, the ETT is secured to the lower beak using adhesive tape (Fig. 9.11).
- Since the diameter of the tracheal lumen narrows towards the syrinx, ETTs should not be advanced too deeply. Damage to the trachea may result in stricture formation.

---

### Injectable agents

Injectable anaesthetic agents are rarely used to anaesthetize birds in veterinary clinics, although they still have some use for field anaesthesia. Some diving species (such as ducks) may breath-hold during induction with

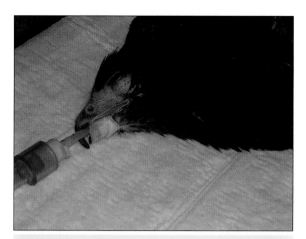

**Figure 9.11** Anaesthetized Harris' hawk, intubated. Note the adhesive tape around the lower beak to secure the endotracheal tube.

**Table 9.4** Commonly used injectable anaesthetic protocols in birds

| Drug | Dose (mg/kg) | Route | Species |
|---|---|---|---|
| Etomidate | 1.0–2.0 | IV | Use with a benzodiazepine |
| Ketamine | 50–100 | IM | Safe, but rough induction and recovery if sole agent |
| Ketamine + midazolam | 10–40 + 0.2–2.0 | SC, IM | Anaesthesia |
| Propofol | <14 | IV | Induction, dose to effect; can administer incremental boluses to prolong anaesthesia. Intubate and IPVV |

IM, intramuscular; IV, intravenous; SC, subcutaneous.

gaseous agents, and injectable anaesthetics (or pre-medication with sedative agents) may smooth anaesthetic induction in these birds (Table 9.4).

Ketamine at high doses will safely produce anaesthesia, although induction and recovery are rough and effects are variable in different species. Propofol may be used to induce anaesthesia, although the resulting respiratory depression necessitates intubation and IPPV. Incremental boluses may be administered to prolong anaesthesia. Some clinicians have used etomidate to anaesthetize critical patients. Administration is intravenous and effects are short-lived. It must be combined with a benzodiazepine to reduce tremors.

### Monitoring anaesthesia

Unsurprisingly, the best pieces of monitoring equipment are the anaesthetist's eyes, ears and fingers. Respiratory rate and depth can be directly visualized, heart rate and rhythm monitored using a stethoscope (oesophageal in larger patients), mucous membrane colour visualized (easiest on a section of everted vent), and capillary refill time assessed by digital compression of mucous membranes.

Respiratory monitors modified for small patients may be used to assess respiratory rate. Doppler probes or electrocardiograms permit hands-free monitoring of heart rate. Digital temperature probes may be placed in the crop or cloaca. Systolic blood pressure can be monitored indirectly using an inflatable paediatric cuff around the wing, a sphygmomanometer and Doppler probe on the ulnar artery. Capnography may be used to measure exhaled carbon dioxide, using side-stream sampling, although correlation with arterial carbon dioxide levels may be poor particularly in small (<100 g) patients. Despite the routine use of pulse oximetry in mammals, output from this technology shows poor correlation with arterial oxygen saturation of haemoglobin in birds.

### Peri-anaesthetic care

Heat loss from anaesthetized birds is significant, and care should be taken to preserve body temperature. Insulating materials such as bubble-wrap are useful, and supplemental heating (e.g. using heat pads or warm-air blankets) should be provided particularly for more prolonged procedures. If recovery from anaesthesia is likely to be prolonged, for example if injectable sedatives were used or the anaesthetic period has been long, place the bird in an incubator after the procedure. Oxygen supplementation may be required after the procedure for dyspnoeic patients.

Fluids are administered to most patients undergoing anaesthesia for longer than 20 minutes. A bolus of 10–20 ml/kg is usually sufficient, but a CRI will be more appropriate for longer procedures. If possible, blood pressure should be monitored during anaesthesia and fluids administered to maintain circulatory pressure.

The time period without food should be minimized, particularly in small birds that may succumb to hypoglycaemia after relatively short periods of fasting. If small birds are not self-feeding within 1–2 hours, they should be assist-fed (e.g. by crop-gavage).

Analgesics should be given to patients undergoing a painful procedure or those with any condition likely to cause discomfort. Agents used may include any or a combination of opioids, local anaesthetics, and non-steroidal anti-inflammatory agents (NSAIDs). Butorphanol has been demonstrated in several species to be an effective analgesic, while buprenorphine may have limited effectiveness. Lidocaine and bupivacaine may be administered concomitantly (at 1 mg/kg of each administered locally) to provide local anaesthesia. Meloxicam (at 0.2 mg/kg q24hr) is a commonly utilized NSAID.

## Surgery

Taper-point needles are preferred for most avian skin and soft tissues, while cutting needles may be used in thicker skin (such as over the legs and feet) and tendons. Do not use catgut, as a granulomatous reaction results. Polyglactin 910 also results in an inflammatory response. Monofilament sutures are preferred, and polydioxanone causes minimal tissue reaction, although absorption may take longer than 120 days. Birds rarely remove sutures, although the risk is increased if the wound is uncomfortable (so provide analgesia as outlined above).

Magnification is recommended for avian surgery, as are microsurgical instruments. Bipolar electrosurgery is extremely useful, for both incisions and haemostasis. The use of retractors will improve visualization of the surgical field. Transparent drapes will permit better visualization of the patient by the anaesthetist during surgery.

Routine approaches to the coelomic cavity in birds include left lateral, central midline, flaps (extending the ventral midline incision with parasternal and/or parapubic incisions), and the transverse abdominal approach. The surgeon should be aware that respiratory changes will occur once the air sacs have been penetrated, usually requiring an increase in anaesthetic gases to maintain a surgical plane of anaesthesia.

## Euthanasia

For most birds, anaesthesia is induced with volatile agents before injecting an overdose of barbiturates. If possible, pentobarbitone is injected intravenously. If this is not achievable, the drug may be injected into the liver or intra-coelomically (although both these routes will result in carcase changes that may affect postmortem analysis).

# Regurgitation in a cockatoo

## INITIAL PRESENTATION

Regurgitation and haematochezia in a bare-eyed cockatoo (or little corella).

## INTRODUCTION

As avian species hide signs of illness, the onset of clinical signs is often acute, regardless of whether the disease process is acute or chronic. Supportive care is vital in patients that are unwell. This case demonstrates the need for a complete investigation to diagnose the underlying condition.

### CASE PRESENTING SIGNS

A 15-year-old male little corella (*Cacatua sanguinea*) (Box 10.1) presented with acute onset regurgitation, haematochezia/melena, lethargy and inappetence.

## HUSBANDRY

The cockatoo had been rescued by the current owner while still a juvenile. Historically it had chronic feather damage associated with parental mutilation when a chick. The diet was mainly seed-based but with fresh fruits added. The cockatoo was caged on its own, but shared airspace with other parrots (there had been no new additions in the previous 6 months).

## CASE HISTORY

On the day prior to presentation, the cockatoo regurgitated once. Frank blood had been present in the faeces. On the day of examination, the faeces was almost black (Box 10.2). The owner reported him to be lethargic and inappetent (Box 10.3).

## CLINICAL EXAMINATION

Some weight loss was noted since the previous examination (weighing 586 g, compared with 612 g 3 months earlier). The rhinotheca (sheath of the upper beak) was slightly overgrown, although not sufficiently so as to result in difficulty prehending food. Some 'clicks' were auscultated over the ventral abdominal region but as there was no evidence of dyspnoea it was suspected these related to organomegaly rather than respiratory disease. As with many avian patients, it was difficult to assess demeanour during the consultation – during this time the cockatoo appeared bright, alert and responsive. After admittance and settling into the hospital, he did become more quiet and lethargic.

### CLINICAL TIPS

**Assessment of bird demeanour**

- If a client advises that their pet bird is quiet or subdued at home, believe them!
- It is in a bird's best interests to hide signs of illness, and many will rally to create a false impression of health in a novel environment (your consulting room).
- If possible, it is useful to visit the bird in its home environment to observe natural and relaxed behaviour – this will give a truer impression of the bird's demeanour.

## BOX 10.1   ECOLOGY OF COCKATOOS

- The bare-eyed cockatoo (also known as the little corella) belongs to the sub-family Cacatuinae, the white cockatoos.
- They are native to Australia. In the wild, they congregate in flocks of up to several thousand birds. They are diurnal, roosting overnight in trees and foraging in daylight. They chew bark off the trees in which they perch.
- The free-ranging diet comprises mostly seeds including cereal crops, and the birds feed mostly on the ground.
- Although experienced breeders may be able to differentiate sexes by size of head/body, they are generally considered sexually monomorphic. As such, sex determination requires either DNA sampling (from blood or feather pulp) or surgical sexing by endoscopy.
- In the wild, they may bathe in the rain (hanging upside down or flying around) or flutter in wet leaves of trees.
- One individual was reported to have lived 46.9 years in captivity.
- Housing in captivity usually comprises either an aviary or a large cage with regular exercise in a larger space such as a room.
- Diets offered to captive parrots are often seed-based, but this may lead to malnutrition. It is usually more appropriate to base the diet on a formulated pellet feed with additional fresh fruit and vegetables.

## BOX 10.2   COMPONENTS OF NORMAL BIRD DROPPINGS

- Urine: clear liquid
- Urates: white/off-white insoluble, uric acid is the major nitrogenous waste in birds
- Faeces: colour and consistency will vary depending on species and diet fed, usually dark green or brown.

## DIFFERENTIAL DIAGNOSES

*Lethargy* is a vague clinical sign and can be attributed to general ill health in a bird.

The differentials for vomiting or *regurgitation* are:

- Ingestion of irritants (e.g. certain houseplants) or rancid food
- Gastrointestinal infection (more likely upper tract): bacteria, fungal/yeast (e.g. candidiasis [*Candida albicans*], megabacteriosis [*Macrorhabdus ornithogaster*]), protozoa (trichomoniasis)
- Diseases affecting gastrointestinal motility: toxicity (e.g. lead, zinc), proventricular dilatation disease (PDD, caused by avian bornavirus)
- Foreign body in gastrointestinal tract (GIT), particularly upper GIT (crop or in oesophagus at thoracic inlet)
- Other causes of gastrointestinal obstruction, e.g. neoplasia
- Acute metabolic disease, including causes of dehydration or polydipsia
- Renal failure
- Hepatopathy
- Pancreatitis
- Septicaemia
- Motion sickness
- Goitre (in budgerigars with iodine deficiency).

*Blood in droppings* may originate from urine, faeces, the reproductive tract or the cloaca. Haematuria is produced in renal disease, commonly with toxicity or neoplasia; if seen transiently after restraint, haematuria may relate to fragile blood vessels associated with hepatic or gastrointestinal disease. If blood is present in the droppings separate from the faeces or urine, it originates from either the reproductive tract or cloaca.

The differentials for *blood in faeces* (fresh or changed) mainly pertain to hepatic or gastrointestinal disease, and include:

- Severe bacterial or viral gastroenteritis
- Severe parasite infection: protozoa (e.g. *Giardia*), nematodes (unusual, more commonly seen in birds in outside aviaries with contamination from wild birds)
- Heavy metal toxicity (lead, zinc) may result in frank blood or haemoglobinuria
- Coagulopathy, e.g. associated with hepatopathy
- Haemorrhage from gastrointestinal neoplasia, including papillomas (in South American psittacines – diagnosed by cloacal examination)
- Intestinal haemorrhage associated with a foreign body, e.g. with necrosis or rupture

- Reproductive disease or cloacitis may cause haematochezia
- Blood in faeces may originate from meat products in the diet of some birds
- *Melena* is commonly seen in cases of advanced hepatic disease, gastrointestinal ulceration or starvation. Less common causes include gastric and hepatic adenocarcinoma or pancreatitis.

## CASE WORK-UP

It is important to identify and correct the underlying cause of the clinical signs to enable long-term treatment.

### Supportive care

In an acute episode where finances are of concern, it can be beneficial to offer nursing care in the first instance. This will involve hospitalization in a warm environment, to reduce the energy requirements of the ill bird. The use of incubators or brooders (Fig. 10.1) is recommended in this case, although the use of an airing cupboard in the owner's home will suffice if hospitalization is not possible.

Fluids should be administered to replace fluids lost in regurgitation and also maintenance requirements. Ideally, these should be administered parenterally (SC/IV/IO [intraosseous]) to rehydrate the bird before the gavage route is utilized (as oral fluids may be regurgitated). It can be useful to flush the crop, particularly if necrotic debris or infection is present. Oral nutritional support should be administered in a form that is high in energy and easily digestible, gavage-feeding small amounts of non-viscous easily digestible formula. Birds should be tempted to eat with a variety of good quality foods, including those they are accustomed to receiving and recognize.

### Medical treatment

If regurgitation persists, a gastrointestinal motility modifier may be trialled if an obstruction is not suspected, for example metoclopramide (0.5 mg/kg PO/IM q8–12hr). Again, the metoclopramide should initially be administered parenterally. Bacterial or yeast infections commonly occur in birds secondarily to other disease, including individuals with immune suppression. Crop swabs or dropping samples can be analysed using in-house stains to assess for excessive quantities of bacteria or yeast, and culture and sensitivity utilized if deemed appropriate. It can be useful to treat these and assess the response before more expensive investigations are performed.

> **CLINICAL TIP**
>
> Metoclopramide may cause seizures in macaws.

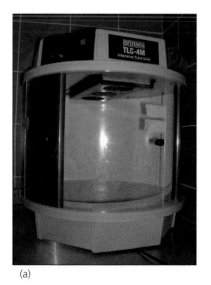
(a)

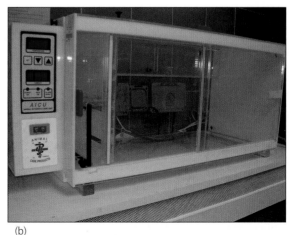
(b)

**Figure 10.1** Various (a) brooders and (b) incubators are available, providing a convenient way of ensuring ill birds are maintained in a warm environment.

## BOX 10.3   WHEN SHOULD YOU INVESTIGATE AN ILL BIRD?

Many factors will assist with this decision.

- Client financial considerations are often important, although many pet birds are now insured.
- As prey species, parrots often conceal signs of illness until they are severely compromised. For this reason, it is usually advisable to investigate any ill health and obtain a diagnosis to enable appropriate treatment to commence as soon as possible.
- In some instances, the bird will be severely compromised (e.g. in collapsed individuals) and supportive care should be given to stabilize the patient before further investigation. Excessive handling (even for a thorough examination) in these birds may well result in more rapid demise than if the pathology was permitted to run its course. Owners should be warned of the risks associated with handling such individuals.

## Lateral and ventro-dorsal radiographs (performed under anaesthesia with isoflurane)

Material present within the body cavity reduced the air sac space (Fig. 10.2). Differential diagnoses included free fluid, organ enlargement or gut distension. Contrast studies with barium may be useful to outline the gastrointestinal tract (barium sulphate may also provide some medical benefit as a protectant and anti-inflammatory).

## Blood sample

A general health profile was performed, with haematology and biochemistry (Table 10.1). This showed signs of:

- Dehydration (elevated haematocrit and uric acid)
- Tissue damage (elevated lactate dehydrogenase)
- Mild anaemia (with some hypochromic red blood cells)
- Changes in white cells suggestive of infection (leucocytosis with a marked heterophilia, monocytosis (with some atypical monocytes) and moderate lymphopenia).

Lead and zinc levels were both within normal limits.

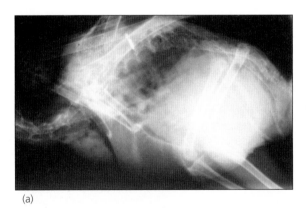
(a)

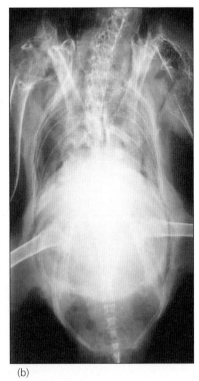
(b)

**Figure 10.2** (a) Lateral and (b) ventro-dorsal radiographs showing soft tissue/fluid density in abdominal region of coelomic cavity.

**Table 10.1** Blood results (with reference ranges for comparison)

|  | Result | Reference range |
|---|---|---|
| Haemoglobin* | 12.4 g/dl | 14.4–19.2 |
| Haematocrit* | 0.33 l/l | 0.45–0.62 |
| Red blood cells* | $2.26 \times 10^{12}$/l | 2.44–3.23 |
| MCV | 146.0 fl | 166.5–209.0 |
| MCHC | 37.6 g/dl | 27.9–35.3 |
| MCH | 54.9 pg | 50.1–68.5 |
| White blood cells* | $22.9 \times 10^9$/l | 1.5–10.3 |
| Heterophils* | 95%; $21.76 \times 10^9$/l | 1.47–10.33 |
| Lymphocytes* | 2%; $0.46 \times 10^9$/l | 0.00–3.40 |
| Eosinophils | $0 \times 10^9$/l | 0.00–0.69 |
| Monocytes* | 3%; $0.69 \times 10^9$/l | 0.00–0.52 |
| Basophils | $0 \times 10^9$/l | 0.00–2.02 |
| Thrombocytes | $18 \times 10^9$/l | 0–24 |
| Fibrinogen | 1.00 g/dl | – |
| Total protein* | 26.3 g/l | 28–43 |
| Albumin | 11.8 g/l | 9–15 |
| Globulin | 14.5 g/l | 12–36 |
| Calcium | 2.20 mmol/l | 1.90–2.20 |
| AST | 104 U/l | 32–180 |
| CK | 192 U/l | 27–253 |
| Uric acid* | 456 µmol/l | 190–327 |
| LDH* | 977 U/l | 130–353 |
| Zinc | 29 µg/l | 0–200 |
| Lead | 0.29 µmol/l | 0–1.21 |

* Abnormal values outside reference range.
AST = aspartate aminotransferase; CK = creatinine kinase; LDH = lactate dehydrogenase; MCV = mean corpuscular volume; MCHC = mean corpuscular haemoglobin concentration; MCH = mean corpuscular haemoglobin

## Crop swab

Cytology showed clumps of bacteria of various types, and no evidence of parasites. Culture was performed on a swab and a crop wash. *Esherichia coli* was cultured; this was sensitive to amoxicillin/clavulanate, co-trimoxazole, cephalexin, gentamicin and ciprofloxacin, but resistant to tetracycline. An unidentified Gram-negative bacillus was also cultured; this was sensitive to tetracycline, amoxicillin/clavulanate, cephalexin and gentamicin, but resistant to co-trimoxazole and ciprofloxacin.

If regurgitated material had been produced, it would have been useful to analyse this by cytology and culture also.

## Faecal analysis

A wet preparation and Gram-stain were performed. No parasites were present, but as with the crop sample some clumps of mixed bacteria were present. The test for occult blood was strongly positive. No pathogens were cultured from a cloacal swab.

## Reshaping of the beak

This was performed using a slow-speed burr, taking care to dampen the beak to prevent overheating and discomfort.

## TREATMENT AND PROGRESS

### Medication and supportive care

Metoclopramide was administered, initially subcutaneously and then orally. Antibiotics (amoxicillin clavulanate at 125 mg/kg q12hr PO) were instigated. An easily assimilated avian recovery diet was gavage-fed (10 ml TID). Vitamin K1 injection may be useful in cases of melena where a coagulopathy is suspected.

The cockatoo regurgitated once during hospitalization for 3 days and faeces were more normal in colouration. He was then discharged. A gastrointestinal infection was suspected and treatment continued with gastrointestinal motility modifier (metoclopramide) and antibiotic (amoxicillin clavulanate at 125 mg/kg PO q12hr).

Some improvement was seen on this treatment protocol. No further regurgitation or haematochezia was noted in the patient, he began to eat some food, and his demeanour improved a little. However, he was still lethargic and began passing undigested seeds in his faeces so further investigation was warranted.

## FURTHER INVESTIGATION

### Ultrasound

The abdominal region was examined by ultrasound in the conscious bird. (This will stress some individuals, either resulting in the need for anaesthesia or a reduction in the period of restraint and thus the range of examination possible.) Assessment of the coelomic cavity was impeded by the air in the air sacs. The liver, spleen and kidneys were partially visualized. The ventriculus was briefly visualized and was of normal size. No significant amount of free fluid was identified. The intestines contained mainly gas and some motility was present. No significant abnormalities were detected, but coelomic structures were incompletely visualized using ultrasound (as is often the case when intestinal gas is present).

### Endoscopy

It was elected to perform endoscopy to permit direct visualization of the intra-coelomic organs. The cockatoo was anaesthetized and placed in right lateral recumbency to allow coelomic endoscopy. This showed the gastrointestinal tract to be enlarged and distended, precluding complete assessment of the cavity. The gonads, kidneys, lungs, air sacs and heart had a normal appearance.

---

### CLINICAL TIPS

**Anaesthesia**

- Induction: isoflurane via a closely fitting facemask
- Intubation: 3 mm diameter endotracheal tube
- Maintenance: isoflurane (3%).

**Peri-anaesthetic monitoring and supportive care**

- Oesophageal stethoscope
- ECG leads attached: one either side of the heart on the ventral wing and one on the left lateral thigh
- Intravenous catheter placed in superficial plantar metatarsal vein, and warmed Hartmann's solution administered through out procedure (4 ml/kg per hour)
- Supplemental heating: heat pad under bird.

---

### CLINICAL TIPS

**Endoscopy of the coelomic cavity**

- Place anaesthetized bird in right lateral recumbency (Fig. 10.3a). (This allows visualization of the left-hand side of the coelomic cavity – if the right side needs to be examined, the bird can be moved to left lateral recumbency and the procedure repeated.)
- Secure both wings dorsal to the body and extend the uppermost leg caudally.
- Identify the area (incision site is between the last two ribs, ventral to the uncinate process) and surgically prepare the site (Fig. 10.3b). Often this does not require much/any plucking of feathers. Minimize the use of antiseptic liquids, particularly alcohol-based ones, which will contribute to cooling and potential hypothermia. It can be helpful to use paper adhesive tape to secure adjacent feathers down to reduce their chance of contaminating the site.
- A small incision is made in the skin using a scalpel blade. Small scissors or forceps are used for blunt dissection through the muscle layers. The rigid endoscope (usually a 2.7 mm scope with a sheath) is then inserted into the coelomic cavity (entering with a 'pop' as the peritoneal membrane is breached).
- After internal assessment is complete, the skin wound is usually closed with a single suture.
- Coelioscopy is contraindicated in cases of coelomitis, ascites or organomegaly.

---

## DIAGNOSIS

Based on the endoscopic and other findings, the main differential diagnoses were proventricular dilatation disease, other neurogenic causes of gastrointestinal hypomotility or dilation, or neoplasia of the gastrointestinal tract.

## ANATOMY AND PHYSIOLOGY REFRESHER

The oral cavity leads to the oesophagus, which lies on the right-hand side of the neck. The crop is a dilation of the oesophagus at the base of the neck (the crop is not present in all avian species), which functions to store

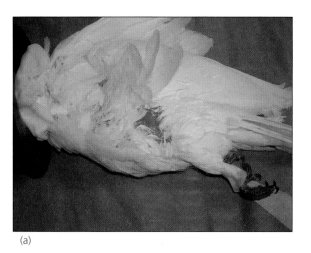

(a)

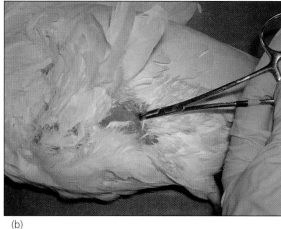

(b)

**Figure 10.3** (a) Positioning and (b) site for coelioscopy on left-hand side. With both legs extended, the incision site will enter the caudal thoracic air sac.

food when the stomach is full. The stomach is divided into two portions, the glandular proventriculus and the muscular ventriculus (gizzard). Ingesta moves forward and back between the two parts of the stomach during digestion, with food that does not require grinding bypassing the ventriculus. The rest of the avian gastro-intestinal tract includes the small intestine and large intestine (including the caeca). The pancreas and liver assist with digestion.

## AETIOPATHOGENESIS OF GASTROINTESTINAL NEOPLASIA

As in human medicine, lifestyle and environment are thought to play a role in the risks of developing neoplasia, for example exposure to various chemicals and toxins. Where viruses are associated (e.g. papillomas in South American psittacines are thought to be caused by herpesvirus), contact with affected individuals is a source of infection.

## TREATMENT OF THIS CASE

After discussion of the results with the owner, it was elected to euthanize the cockatoo.

As the owner wished to bury the bird, a cosmetic necropsy only was performed, removing the gastrointestinal tract for histology. A fibrosarcoma was evident in the ventriculus (Fig. 10.4), with mucosal ulceration (the

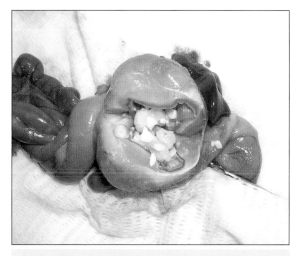

**Figure 10.4** Fibrosarcoma of ventriculus at postmortem.

likely origin of blood in the faeces). The distal intestine also showed mucosal atrophy and dilation. The postmortem examination did not show any myenteric ganglioneuritis or leiomyositis, both of which are characteristic for PDD.

## OTHER TREATMENT OPTIONS

Although unlikely to affect the ultimate prognosis in cases of neoplasia, improving husbandry conditions and diet may assist with quality of life. Controlling secondary infections will also help. Immunomodulatory medications or herbal remedies have been suggested to be useful therapies in some cases. Some tumours may be surgically resectable (although thought should be given to the gastrointestinal function after removal of large portions).

## NURSING ASPECTS

### Crop-feeding

- Restrain the bird in a soft towel, extending the head and neck to straighten the oesophagus.
- Use a gag to keep the beak open, or use a metal crop-feeding tube (soft tubes may be bitten).
- Insert the tube into the mouth and pass down the oesophagus on the right-hand side of the neck.
- Check positioning by palpating the tip of the tube in the crop and the trachea separately.
- Instil fluid/food slowly, checking for regurgitation. If any reflux is seen, aspirate any material in the mouth and allow the bird to swallow or spit out excess material.

## PREVENTION

Avoidance of carcinogenic agents and introduction of new birds with potentially contagious disease (e.g. papillomas) will reduce neoplastic disease. However, for most neoplasms we do not know the aetiology and prevention is not possible.

## PROGNOSIS

The prognosis for birds with regurgitation depends very much on the aetiology. Many of the infectious agents are treatable. Heavy metal toxicities respond well to removal of ingested metal along with chelation therapy. Proventricular dilatation disease carries a poor long-term prognosis, although some patients respond well in the short-term to control of gastrointestinal infection with antibiotics, nutritional support, and the NSAID celecoxib.

In general, the prognosis with gastrointestinal neoplasia in avian species is guarded. Some 3–4% of submissions from psittacines for histopathology are neoplastic, with most from budgerigars. In the gastrointestinal tract, reports include papillomas, squamous cell carcinomas, fibrosarcomas, infiltrative adenocarcinomas, leiomyomas and leiomyosarcomas, melanomas and lymphoma. Approximately half of alimentary tract neoplasms in psittacines are malignant.

# 11 Harris' hawk with bumblefoot

## INITIAL PRESENTATION

Bilateral foot lesions in a Harris' hawk.

## INTRODUCTION

This case outlines the combination of husbandry factors and veterinary treatment of skin lesions in raptors. Unless hygiene issues are addressed, lesions may become chronic. Regular assessment is necessary to monitor for progression to more severe pathology.

## CASE PRESENTING SIGNS

A 7-year-old male Harris' hawk (*Parabuteo unicinctus*) presented with skin lesions on both feet.

## HUSBANDRY

The Harris' hawk (Box 11.1) was bred in captivity in the UK, and had been in the current owner's possession for 1 month. He was housed in a covered aviary with three perches, of artificial turf-covered wood. The pea gravel substrate was cleaned as necessary. The bird was not tethered, but did wear leather leg equipment (aylmeri and jesses, Fig. 9.4). The diet comprised various whole carcases, including day-old chicks, rabbit and quail. Water was provided in a wide shallow bath (changed regularly). The owner was an experienced falconer who owned and worked other raptors besides this Harris' hawk.

## CASE HISTORY

During catch-up for a training session, the owner noticed some lesions on the hawk's feet. No change in appetite, demeanour, or perching or flying abilities had been noted. The owner thought there might have been some trauma from the enclosure, as the bird had been noted grasping the nylon netting of the aviary roof.

## CLINICAL EXAMINATION

Harris' hawks are relatively relaxed birds, particularly those accustomed to human contact. A full clinical examination was performed conscious:

- Good body condition for flying (pectoral muscles present but keel easily palpable), weighing 700 g
- No abnormalities on auscultation or palpation
- Skin lesions: smoothing of dermal papillae on plantar surface of feet, some superficial cracks and inflammation in skin
- Right foot: same as left foot, also minor lesions on 3rd digit (Fig. 11.1a).
- Left foot: 1st and 2nd digits affected, distal phalanges (Fig. 11.1b)

## CLINICAL TIPS

### Physical examination of raptors

- Trained birds can usually have a general physical examination performed while the bird is standing on the owner's fist (using a falconer's glove and leg equipment) (Fig. 11.2a). It is helpful if the bird is hooded for this procedure, although this should be removed for examination of the head and oral cavity (Fig. 11.2a).
- Further examination, including detailed assessment of the feet, is best performed with the bird 'cast'. The bird is approached from behind and a towel is wrapped around the body to restrain the wings. The legs should be grasped to avoid injury to the handler from talons (Fig. 11.2b). Larger birds may require general anaesthesia to relax the foot muscles and permit a full examination of the feet (Fig. 11.2b).

## BOX 11.1   ECOLOGY OF HARRIS' HAWKS

- Range in the wild covers south-west USA and as far south as Chile and Argentina in South America
- Normal habitat: sparse woodland, semi-desert, some marshes
- Average weight: male, 700 g; female, 1 kg (i.e. sexual dimorphism)
- One female may mate with more than one male
- Birds are flown at a slightly light weight to encourage them to return to the owner for feeding. Birds coming into moult are allowed to put on weight to cope with metabolic demands
- Popular birds for falconers as hunt in packs of 2–6 (most raptors are solitary hunters). Larger prey taken if group-hunting (e.g. jackrabbits)
- Free-ranging diet: birds, lizards, mammals, and large insects
- Relatively easy to train.

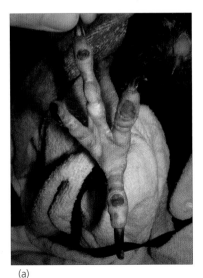
(a)

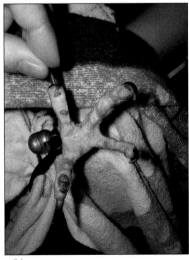
(b)

**Figure 11.1** Grade 2 bumblefoot lesions in the Harris' hawk (*Parabuteo unicinctus*). (a) Right foot, (b) left foot.

## DIFFERENTIAL DIAGNOSES

The differentials for *foot lesions* in raptors are:
- Bumblefoot, including corns
- Talon disorders: injuries, abnormal growth
- Toe injuries
- Wounds
- Dislocations
- Fractures
- Soft tissue injuries, e.g. tendon
- Abscesses: often on the dorsal aspect of the foot
- Dry gangrene: due to compromised blood supply after surgery or electrical injury
- Avipox virus (dry form): papules/vesicles/crusts, often with secondary bacterial, fungal or *Chlamydophila* infections
- Constriction injuries, e.g. from thin jesses or pox scabs
- Haematomas: after fighting with quarry
- Self-mutilation
- Tendon sheath infections
- Septic arthritis
- Frostbite: in tropical species housed in very cold conditions
- *Erysipelothrix rhusiopathiae* infection
- Cutaneous mycobacteriosis.

## CASE WORK-UP

In this case, clinical examination provided the diagnosis.

## OTHER POSSIBLE INVESTIGATIONS

### Radiography

It is advisable to radiograph the raptor's feet to assess for bone involvement in the condition.

### Culture

Where possible, swabs should be taken from exudates for microbiology (bacteriology and mycology) and cytology. If organisms are cultured, sensitivity testing should be performed.

### Blood sampling

In some cases, haematology and biochemistry may be performed to assess for systemic signs of infection or concomitant disease processes.

### Ultrasound

In some cases it may be useful to use ultrasound to assess soft tissues underlying the skin or lesion. A stand-off will be required to optimize image quality. Doppler ultrasound probes can also be utilized to monitor blood supply to the digits if vascular compromise is suspected (Fig. 11.3).

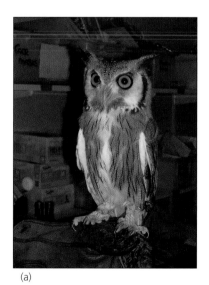
(a)

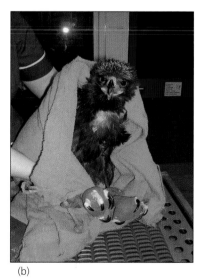
(b)

**Figure 11.2** Restraint and examination of raptors (a) on the fist (scops owl, *Otus* spp) and (b) cast with a towel (steppe eagle hybrid, *Aquila nipalensis* hybrid).

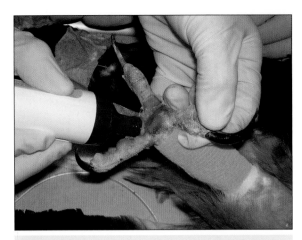

**Figure 11.3** Assessment of the blood supply to the foot of a hawk eagle (*Hieraaetus* spp) using a Doppler probe after tibiotarsal fracture.

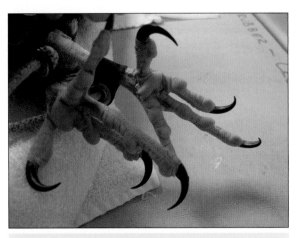

**Figure 11.4** Normal healthy skin on the foot of a gyr–peregrine falcon hybrid (*Falco rusticolus/F. peregrinus*). Note the rough surface with papillae that help cushion the foot.

## DIAGNOSIS

The clinical findings were consistent with grade 2 bilateral bumblefoot lesions.

## ANATOMY AND PHYSIOLOGY REFRESHER

Birds of prey have an anisodactyl arrangement of digits. The first digit (or hallux) faces backwards and the other three forwards. This enables them to perch and hold prey.

Scales on the distal leg are dermo-epidermal modifications. These are larger on the dorsal foot, and smaller on the lateral and palmar surfaces. Skin on the plantar surface of the foot has a rough surface, with dermal papillae that protect the foot (Fig. 11.4). The toe pads are local skin modifications, with a cushioning layer of connective tissue; these are closely adhered to underlying bone.

## AETIOPATHOGENESIS OF BUMBLEFOOT

Bumblefoot is a multifactorial disease. Several factors interact to affect the integrity of the skin and deeper tissues of the foot.

- Husbandry issues most commonly contribute to the condition:
  - Hard abrasive or inappropriately shaped perches result in damage to the foot

- Inactivity both increases time spent perching and results in reduced circulation to the feet. Overweight birds will also put more pressure on the feet
- Dietary deficiencies (e.g. hypovitaminosis A) may weaken the epithelium and result in easily damaged skin
- Overgrown talons will affect weight bearing, with more pressure on the metatarsal pad making it susceptible to damage. The talons may also puncture the plantar surface of the foot, as may foreign bodies present within the environment.
- Anything affecting balance and perching capabilities of the contralateral foot may predispose pathology in the other foot as weight distribution becomes asymmetrical. For example, an injury affecting one foot or leg will force the bird to use the other in preference. For this reason, it is usual to bandage both feet even if pathology is unilateral.

Characteristics of the condition include superficial abrasions and ulceration, progressing to cellulitis or abscessation of the plantar epithelium of the foot (Box 11.2). Without treatment, the pathology further develops to involve other tissues locally, including tendons, joints and bones. In some cases, systemic disease may be seen, for example amyloidosis, valvular endocarditis, and infection in distant joints.

## BOX 11.2 GRADING BUMBLEFOOT LESIONS (REMPLE 1993)

Prognosis deteriorates with each grade.
Grade 1 – Flattening of dermal papillae, or proliferation with corn formation. Possible hyperaemia.
Grade 2 – Infection without gross swelling.
Grade 3 – Infection without apparent involvement of deep structures. Hot, painful, swollen.
Grade 4 – Infection of deep structures, e.g. tenosynovitis, arthritis, osteomyelitis.
Grade 5 – End-stage, loss of function of foot.

## BOX 11.3 AIMS OF THERAPY

- Reduce inflammation and swelling
- Remove necrotic tissue, usually by surgical debridement
- Provide drainage where infection is present
- Remove pathogens
- Protect the lesion from further infection
- Use of dressings to encourage granulation and healing
- Use of bandages to protect the foot (and the contralateral foot) from further insult.

## BOX 11.4 SUMMARY OF TREATMENT OPTIONS

- Husbandry/management changes, correcting any predisposing factors:
  - Optimize diet
  - Provide suitable perches
  - Maintain hygiene of perches
  - Keep at flying weight
  - Increase exercise
- Topical ointments massaged into foot
- Systemic antibiotics
- Bandages
- Surgical debridement
- Euthanasia.

## EPIDEMIOLOGY

The most common sites for lesions are the pads, particularly the large metatarsal pad, the pads under the middle phalangeal joint of 2nd/3rd/4th digits, and the distal digital pads of 1st/2nd digits.

Species differences exist with the disease, such that broadwings (accipiters, red-tailed hawks and Harris' hawks) usually respond better to treatment that falcons.

## TREATMENT

There were two main approaches necessary for treatment of this case.

### Husbandry changes

The owner was advised to improve perch hygiene. This involved spraying the perches daily with dilute disinfectant (e.g. quaternary ammonium compounds).

### CLINICAL TIP

It can be useful in some cases to tether a bird to retain it on the perch for longer periods if the surrounding environment is less clean. However, this will reduce exercise capabilities and may affect blood flow to the lesions, predisposing progression of pathology. It is usual to continue flying birds, but to a lure rather than hunting (as the latter will involve trauma to the feet during catching).

### Medical therapy

The feet were cleaned daily using dilute antiseptic solution (e.g. chlorhexidine or povidone–iodine), the owner wearing gloves to prevent contamination with human skin commensal bacteria (Boxes 11.3 and 11.4). Topical antibiotic ointment was used to soften the skin and prevent further cracks forming as well as providing local antibiosis.

As the surface of the skin was breached, systemic antibiotic was also administered (marbofloxacin at 10 mg/kg PO q24hr). Inflammation was treated with a systemic NSAID (meloxicam at 0.1 mg/kg PO q24hr).

## TREATMENT OPTIONS AND MANAGEMENT

There was some difficulty in keeping the bird's feet clean without dressings. This may have been a combination of dirty perches and prey/food items being caught in the skin and talons. A new lesion developed at the base of one talon (3rd digit of left foot on medial surface).

In this case, initial therapy did not resolve the lesions. It was considered that further trauma was occurring from the perches, and a decision was taken to bandage the feet. This has its drawbacks, reducing the frequency of topical cleaning and medication, as well as precluding daily inspection of the lesions.

The systemic antibiotic was changed to amoxicillin clavulanate (125 mg/kg PO q12hr). If possible, antibiosis should be based on culture and sensitivity results.

The perch was changed to a rubber bow perch, as it was difficult to maintain good hygiene on the artificial turf perch. Food items were presented in smaller pieces to reduce the necessity of the bird grasping to tear it apart.

## NURSING ASPECTS

### Bandaging

- Raptors will usually leave bandages alone.
- As there is very little soft tissue overlying vital structures such as blood vessels and bone in the distal limb, care should be taken to ensure dressings are not applied too tightly.
- In cases with severe bumblefoot lesions, including those where surgery has been necessary, ball bandages are often used to enclose the foot and provide protection from further pressure.
- If a corn or similar lesion is present, a doughnut-shaped ring of foam or other support material may be used to support surrounding tissues while releasing pressure on the lesion.
- In lower grade cases such as this, the aim is for a light dressing that will provide some cushioning, and protect the foot from dirt and further minor trauma.
- For this case, the bandage consisted of: a non-adhesive dressing, synthetic padding material, and non-adhesive elastic wrap. This thin dressing permitted normal perching.
- If a single foot is affected, the contralateral should also have a light bandage to protect it from pressure due to the extra load bearing as weight is shifted from the affected foot.

## CLINICAL TIPS

- It is vital to correct husbandry, particularly hygiene, to prevent recurrence or progression of bumblefoot lesions.
- Wear gloves when examining raptors' feet. Many infections are associated with *Staphylococcus* spp that may originate from the owner's hands.

## OTHER TREATMENT OPTIONS

### Diet

The diet should be assessed. Multivitamin and mineral supplementation is advisable during treatment of lesions.

### Perches

Artificial turf should be used to cover all perching surfaces. The turf can be wrapped in soft leather, towels, or non-adhesive elastic wrap bandaging material if the bird's feet are painful. These coverings can be easily removed for cleaning.

### Body condition and exercise

If the bird is not already at its flying weight, it should be reduced to this level to minimize pressure on the feet. To this end and to increase blood circulation through exercise, trained birds should still be flown.

### Topical ointments

Massaging ointments into the feet helps improve the local circulation. Preparations such as those containing aloe vera are useful. Topical antibiotics may be beneficial, particularly where the skin integrity has been breached. Povidone–iodine will harden skin during the healing process. Some practitioners advocate the topical use of antibiotics (e.g. piperacillin or fusidic acid) in combination with DMSO (dimethylsulphoxide) to increase their uptake.

### Antibiotics

Systemic antibiotics should be given to cases with swollen or obviously infected feet. Suggested options include marbofloxacin, amoxicillin clavulanate, or lincomycin. These should be continued for at least 1 week (often a longer course is required).

### Analgesia

NSAIDs or opioids are useful in cases of obvious lameness, or in conjunction with surgery.

### Bandaging

Bandages may be used in more minor cases to protect against further insult. In severe cases, they are employed to protect a wound from contamination and relieve pressure from the plantar surface by providing support around the foot. In the latter cases, soft materials such as foam or neoprene are used. Hydrogels and collagen ointments are often used underneath bandage materials to promote healing. In infected lesions, daily wet-to-dry dressings should be used. As with other species, sufficient padding should be used to prevent pressure necrosis from bandages that are too tight.

## Debridement

If the skin has been breached, debridement should be performed. In most cases, this will necessitate surgery under anaesthesia. A small Volkmann's curette is used. The wound should be irrigated. If closure is possible without tension, a simple interrupted suture pattern is used, but tension-relieving sutures may be required. In many cases, it is advisable to allow closure of the resulting wound by secondary intention, or to delay closure until the infection has been cleared and surrounding tissues are well vascularized and viable. Initially after surgery, the bird is housed on a soft padded surface (e.g. thick foam pads covered with artificial turf). The foot is always dressed after surgery (as is the contralateral foot), and systemic antibiotics administered for at least 2 weeks (or until first intention healing has occurred). Sutures are removed after 21 days, over a period of a few days to allow for gradual return to full skin strength at the wound site. Dressings are changed every 2–3 days, and removed after a month.

Antibiotic-impregnated polymethylmethacrylate beads may be surgically inserted to provide long-term local antibiosis. These are principally used for cases where tendons and joints are affected. Antibiotics commonly used include piperacillin, ceftazidime, and amikacin. The beads are usually removed after 7–10 days.

## Euthanasia

In cases where foot function has been lost (e.g. such that the bird is unable to perch, or cannot grasp food), euthanasia is recommended. This is often the best option if systemic infection and pain cannot be controlled in cases with osteomyelitis.

## FOLLOW-UP

As the inflammation reduced and the bird was perching without apparent difficulty, the NSAID was discontinued after a few weeks. Antibiotics were continued for a total of 12 weeks.

At one point during treatment, purulent material was present in one of the lesions. It would have been useful to culture this, but the other treatments resolved this in a few days.

Bandages were changed every 3–5 days, depending on how the lesions appeared at each check. After a few weeks, the owner was able to perform this at home and veterinary visits were less frequent. Dressings were removed after 10 weeks. The topical treatments were continued until all cracks had closed over.

Re-epithelialization was rapid once the dressings had been removed, although it was several weeks before a normal papillated appearance to the skin was present. While healing was continuing, perch hygiene was important.

## PREVENTION

Good husbandry conditions, especially perch choice and hygiene, are important in prevention of development of bumblefoot lesions. Regular assessment of raptor feet should be performed by the owner, preferably wearing gloves to prevent transfer of bacteria from the person's skin to the bird's skin.

## PROGNOSIS

Healing is often prolonged even in low-grade bumblefoot lesions. This is due to pressure necrosis, reduced vascular perfusion, and poor systemic antibiotic delivery to the site. Recovery commonly takes 2–6 months.

> ### CLINICAL TIP
>
> Environmental conditions play a massive role in the condition and must be addressed to ensure a good outcome and prevention of recurrence.

Systemic conditions may adversely affect the healing process, for example aspergillosis, hepatic lipidosis and chronic renal disease. Conversely, bumblefoot is a chronic inflammatory condition treatment of which requires prolonged management, and the disease may predispose pathology such as amyloidosis, aspergillosis and clostridial enterotoxaemia.

### Reference

Remple JD (1993): Raptor bumblefoot: a new treatment technique. In: Redig PT, Cooper JE (eds) Raptor Biomedicine II. University of Minnesota Press, Minneapolis, pp. 154–160.

# 12 Tibiotarsal fracture in a dove

## INITIAL PRESENTATION

Acute onset unilateral lameness in a Socorro dove.

## INTRODUCTION

The avian skeleton is light but strong. Fractures frequently result if a bird sustains trauma. However, bone healing is rapid and most cases heal well if appropriately supported.

## CASE PRESENTING SIGNS

A 6-month-old Socorro dove (*Zenaida graysoni*) presented with suspected tibiotarsal fracture.

## HUSBANDRY

The dove was part of a breeding colony held in a zoological collection as part of an international *ex situ* conservation project (Box 12.1). It was housed individually in an indoor aviary at the time of the incident. The aviary was approximately 2 × 2 × 3 m, and comprised solid walls with a wire mesh front. Several natural branches were present for enrichment and perching. The diet provided was a proprietary pigeon seed mix supplemented with chopped fruit and greens.

## CASE HISTORY

The bird was noted to be 10/10ths lame on its left leg late one evening. A brief conscious examination revealed a palpable fracture in the tibiotarsus. Analgesia was provided using meloxicam (0.1 mg/kg PO). No other signs of illness were noted.

## CLINICAL EXAMINATION

Reassessment of the bird the following day was performed:
- Body weight 98 g, good body condition (keel palpable but good pectoral muscle coverage)
- Plumage in good condition
- Oral examination, palpation of abdominal region, auscultation of air sacs – no abnormalities detected
- Orthopaedic examination:
  - Nails appropriate length, no foot lesions
  - Left leg: non-weight bearing, bruising evident mid-tibiotarsus, skin intact, tibiotarsus unstable (suspected fracture site), deep pain present
  - No abnormalities on right leg or either wing.

## DIFFERENTIAL DIAGNOSES

Although it may not be possible to easily differentiate lameness from ataxia in a small bird, the differential diagnoses lists (for avian species) are slightly different.

The differentials for *lameness* are:
- Trauma resulting in fracture, dislocation, or soft tissue injury
  - Note that systemic illness (e.g. hypocalcaemia, central nervous system lesions) may result in weakness, ataxia or seizures and predispose to injuries after falling

- Metabolic bone disease (MBD) or neoplasia will also result in bone weakness and predispose to pathological fractures
- Overgrown claws
- Infection, e.g. bumblefoot, septic arthritis
- Arthritis, e.g. older bird, after traumatic injury
- Neoplasia (particularly budgerigars): renal (e.g. adenocarcinomas, embryonal nephromas), gonadal (e.g. ovarian or testicular tumours) or adrenal. Neoplasms act as a space-occupying lesion, pressing on the sciatic or pudendal nerves that run between these organs and the bony synsacrum
- Other causes of organomegaly (commonly renomegaly) pressing on sciatic nerve intra-coelomically
- Intra-articular gout
- Bruising in the pelvic regions after or during egg laying (females)
- Spinal pathology.

The differentials for *ataxia* are:

- Infectious diseases:
  - Viruses, e.g. paramyxoviruses (there are at least nine known serotypes), polyomavirus, central lesions with proventricular dilatation disease (PDD, mostly affecting psittacines), togaviruses (e.g. West Nile virus), influenza A, reovirus
  - Bacteria, e.g. *Chlamydophila psittaci* (especially chronic infections), granulomas or abscesses (with *Listeria monocytogenes* and *Mycobacterium* spp), septic arthritis (e.g. at joints between notarium and synsacrum, with abscess compressing spinal cord), encephalitis (with *Staphylococcus aureus, Enterococcus* spp, *Pasteurella* spp, *Klebsiella* spp)
  - Fungi, e.g. aspergillosis (due to secondary cerebral infarction or toxin-induced peripheral neuropathies), mycotoxins in food
  - Parasites, e.g. CNS infection with *Filaroides* spp and *Sarcocystis* spp, cerebrospinal *Baylisascaris procyonis* (in North America)
- Toxicity: heavy metal toxicity
- Metabolic disease: hypocalcaemia, hepatic encephalopathy, renal disease, hypoglycaemia
- Malnutrition, e.g. hypovitaminosis E/selenium, hypovitaminosis B2 (riboflavin deficiency), hypovitaminosis B1 (uncommon)

- Trauma (as above)
- Neoplasia, e.g. peripheral neuropathy (including aetiologies outlined above, and also schwannomas and malignant schwannomas), central nervous system pathology (e.g. astrocytomas, oligodendrogliomas, teratomas, lymphosarcomas and meningiomas)
- Congenital defects (uncommon).

### BOX 12.1   ECOLOGY OF SOCORRO DOVES

- Socorro doves originate from the island of Socorro in the Revillagigedo Islands, Mexico. Previously they were common in forest areas higher than 500 m above sea level.
- Socorro doves are frugivores, with free-ranging birds depending on ferns and euphorbias.
- The bird is highly terrestrial, and they have been extirpated by feral cats. Other factors such as human predation and grazing of the bird's food sources by sheep may have also contributed to their decline. The IUCN now describes Socorro doves as Extinct in the Wild.
- The species are predominantly solitary, with pairs forming for breeding. Young are chased away as soon as they can fend for themselves, and the male and female separate outside the breeding season.
- *Ex situ* breeding programmes are expected to provide stock for reintroduction after cats and sheep have been eradicated from the island.

## CASE WORK-UP

The dove was anaesthetized with isoflurane (see box on page 91).

### Radiographs

Lateral and ventro-dorsal views of the body (Fig. 12.1) were taken to assess for any concomitant illness – no evidence was seen. Further views with the X-ray beam collimated on the left leg confirmed the presence of a mid-shaft transverse fracture of the left tibiotarsus (Fig. 12.2).

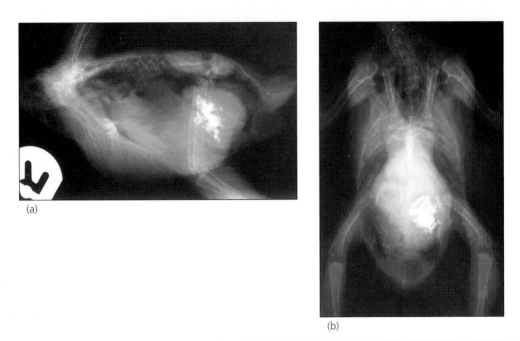

(a)

(b)

**Figure 12.1** (a) Lateral and (b) ventro-dorsal radiographs of the Socorro dove's body, with no obvious systemic disease. Note the (normal) presence of radio-dense grit in the ventriculus.

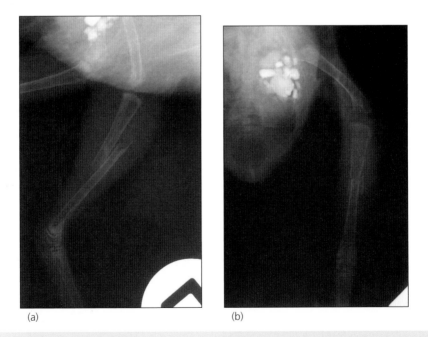

(a)                              (b)

**Figure 12.2** (a) Lateral and (b) cranio-caudal views of the left leg, showing a transverse fracture in the mid-shaft of the tibiotarsus. Soft tissue swelling is also present at the site.

## CLINICAL TIPS

### Anaesthesia

- Birds are usually restrained in a small towel and anaesthesia induced with isoflurane (3–4%) using a close-fitting facemask.
- If possible, an endotracheal tube is then inserted to maintain anaesthesia. This permits intermittent positive pressure ventilation (IPPV) to ensure pulmonary perfusion is maintained. Care should be taken during IPPV not to over-inflate and rupture the delicate avian air sacs.
- During recovery, oxygen is administered until the bird is breathing normally. Extubation is performed once the bird is voluntarily moving, such as lifting its head.

## CLINICAL TIPS

### Monitoring anaesthesia

The depth of anaesthesia is assessed by testing the bird's reflexes:

- Withdrawal: toe pinch or muscle tone (e.g. in wing); lost at surgical depth of anaesthesia
- Corneal reflex: should remain present during anaesthesia, but movement of the nictitans membrane over the cornea will be slowed at deeper levels of anaesthesia
- Response to stimulation of cere and peri-cloacal skin: responses lost at a light-to-medium plane of anaesthesia.

Respiratory system:

- Respiratory rate and character are monitored
- Capnography: an indirect measure of arterial carbon dioxide
- Blood gas analysis: gold standard for assessment of respiratory function, small patient size and financial considerations preclude common use.

Cardiovascular system:

- Blood pressure: indirect measurement using an inflatable cuff
- Capillary refill time (should be <1 second) can be assessed on non-pigmented skin on the feet, or on the basilic or ulnar veins at the medial elbow

- Mucous membrane colour is not a reliable assessment of peripheral oxygenation
- Heart rate can be assessed by a variety of methods:
  - Palpation of a pulse, e.g. the brachial artery in the axillary region; this also gives an assessment of peripheral circulation. (Peripheral circulation is better assessed by checking capillary refill time on featherless areas such as non-pigmented skin on the feet.)
  - Bell stethoscope – positioned over the heart (over the pectoral muscles)
  - Oesophageal stethoscope (in larger birds).
  - ECG – pads are placed across the heart, e.g. one on either wing and one on the left lateral thigh; self-adhesive pads are preferred to clips as they will damage delicate avian skin less.

Monitor body temperature with a cloacal or oesophageal probe.

## OTHER INVESTIGATIONS POSSIBLE

### Blood sample

It would be useful to perform haematology and biochemistry to assess for systemic illness, including metabolic derangements that may have resulted in ataxia and predisposed the injury.

## DIAGNOSIS

Simple closed mid-shaft fracture of left tibiotarsus.

## ANATOMY AND PHYSIOLOGY REFRESHER

Although most medullary cavities in growing birds contain active bone marrow, some adult avian bones contain air (i.e. are pneumatized) to further reduce weight and increase flight capabilities. The femur is pneumatized in many species. The tibia and proximal row of tarsal bones are fused to form the tibiotarsus. The proximolateral fibula is short, associated with a reduction in rotational ability. The distal row of tarsal bones is combined with the second, third and fourth metatarsal bones to form the tarsometatarsus. The first metatarsal bone remains separate. The main muscles of the leg are close to the body, with long tendons of insertion distally.

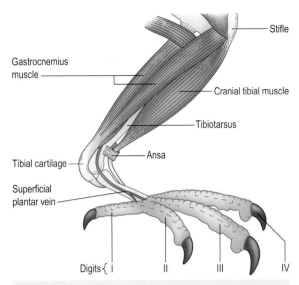

**Figure 12.3** Avian leg anatomy, including craniomedial surgical approach.

The hindlimbs of birds are modified for bipedal locomotion, perching, leaping for takeoff and absorbing shock during landing. The tibiotarsus is the major weight-bearing long bone.

The cranial tibial muscle (which flexes the hock joint) originates from the lateral femoral condyle and the lateral cnemial crest on the tibiotarsus (Fig. 12.3). Fibularis longus and cranial tibial muscles are cranial on the bone, gastrocnemius caudally – leaving the medial and distal bone surfaces exposed. The cranial tibial artery lies over the distal tibiotarsus on the flexor surface at the hock joint, and the medial metatarsal vein emerges cranial to the plantar tendons at the hock.

Avian bones heal rapidly. In most cases with appropriate stabilization, healing will be present within 3–4 weeks. Healing occurs by callus formation.

## AETIOPATHOGENESIS OF TIBIOTARSAL FRACTURES

As the tibiotarsus is an important load-bearing bone, it is commonly involved in fractures, usually after external trauma. The weakest point is just distal to the fibular crest, approximately one-third of the bone's length below the stifle joint, and this is a common site for fractures. Fractures frequently occur after bating accidents in raptors (where a bird on a short leash jumps forcefully from a perch). A spiral comminuted fracture in the distal third of the tibiotarsus may result if identity rings are caught on protruding enclosure materials.

Relatively large muscle masses protect the tibiotarsus to a degree, and fractures are usually closed. Tibiotarsal fractures are prone to rotational stresses from soft tissues. Repair should usually involve internal fixation as well as anti-rotational stabilization.

Problems that may be associated with tibiotarsal fractures (particularly wild birds) include nerve damage, accompanying spinal injury, and bumblefoot development on the contralateral foot due to uneven weight bearing during the healing process.

Bruises are common after trauma that results in avian bone fractures. If the cutaneous vasculature has been disrupted by trauma, dry gangrene may ensue.

## EPIDEMIOLOGY

Tibiotarsal fractures in the proximal one-third are frequently seen following bating. These fractures are generally low energy, and typically result in transverse fractures. Wild birds usually suffer high-energy fractures that are often comminuted. In psittacines, middiaphyseal or distal tibiotarsal fractures are usually seen. Trauma will be more likely if enclosures have protruding wires or other materials.

## TREATMENT

### Surgery

Under the same anaesthetic as for radiography, the Socorro dove was transported to theatre and prepared for surgery. A craniomedial approach to the left leg permitted access to the fracture. An intramedullary pin was placed in the left tibiotarsus using a retrograde technique. (The pin may be placed in a normograde manner, but with more difficulty.) Polydioxanone, 1.5 metric (4/0 USP), was used to suture muscles in a continuous pattern. The skin was closed with poliglecaprone 25 suture, 1.5 metric (4/0 USP), using a continuous pattern.

> **CLINICAL TIPS**
>
> **Avian surgery**
> - Pluck feathers rather than cutting them.
> - Do not over-wet patients during skin preparation, as small patients will be susceptible to hypothermia.

Labels on Figure 12.3: Stifle, Gastrocnemius muscle, Cranial tibial muscle, Tibiotarsus, Ansa, Tibial cartilage, Superficial plantar vein, Digits { I, II, III, IV

- Use transparent (e.g. sterile plastic) drapes to allow the anaesthetist to monitor respiratory movements.
- Provide adequate analgesia, e.g. use local anaesthetic such as lidocaine (at 1–3 mg/kg topically/IM/SC, calculate dose accurately to avoid toxicity), as well as an NSAID such as carprofen (at 2–4 mg/kg PO/IM/SC/IV q8–12hr) and an opioid such as buprenorphine (at 0.01–0.05 mg/kg IM q8hr).

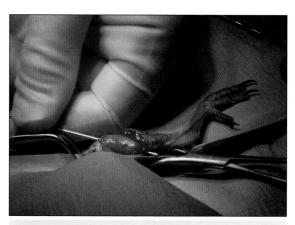

**Figure 12.4** Placement of intramedullary pin.

## CLINICAL TIPS

### Tibiotarsal fracture repair

- Rigid stabilization is necessary for rapid bone healing, with rotational alignment important.
- Use an IM pin with a diameter 50–65% of the marrow cavity (Figs 12.4, 12.5).
- In preference, use positive profile threaded pins for the external fixator.
- The end of the IM pin protruding from the stifle can be attached to the external fixator (i.e. it becomes a 'tie-in fixator').
- Stabilize the limb postoperatively for 1–3 days to improve patient comfort.
- Perform passive physiotherapy 3–5 days after surgery, twice weekly during the healing period.

## BOX 12.2   POTENTIAL POSTOPERATIVE COMPLICATIONS

- Transitory paralysis for 3–5 days, due to injury or surgery. 'Knuckling over' is common
- Abrasion of the foot in the injured limb: prevent by protecting with a dressing
- Bumblefoot in the contralateral limb: prevent by protecting with a dressing.

## Supportive care and medication

An intravenous catheter was placed in the right superficial plantar metatarsal vein, and Hartmann's solution administered (at 10 ml/kg per hour) throughout the procedure.

Antibiosis was administered preoperatively with amoxicillin clavulanate (125 mg/kg IM), and continued orally (same dose q12hr) for 1 week after surgery. Meloxicam (0.1 mg/kg) and butorphanol (0.5 mg/kg) were administered intramuscularly to provide analgesia. Meloxicam was continued orally (same dose q24hr) for 1 week.

The bird was assist-fed a convalescent formula once it had fully recovered from anaesthesia.

A light dressing was placed on the leg to cover the wound for 24 hours postoperatively to limit postoperative swelling. The leg remained bruised for several days; this is normal for birds, and the green colouration is quite apparent due to their thin skin.

Exercise was restricted for 3 weeks after surgery. The dove was assessed daily by keepers, and weekly by the veterinary practitioner (Box 12.2).

## OTHER TREATMENT OPTIONS

### Alternative surgical options

The use of external fixation will prevent rotation. If an external fixator is used solely for the repair, three pins should be used above and below the fracture site for maximum stability; each pin should penetrate both cortices. In some cases, it may be appropriate to use external fixation in combination with an intramedullary pin (i.e. a 'tie-in' fixator).

The most proximal and distal pins with external fixators should be sufficiently far from the ends of the bone to avoid iatrogenic damage. For example, the distal pin should be 2–3 mm proximal to the condyles to avoid

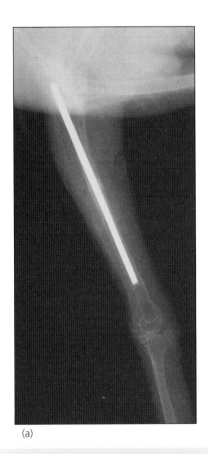

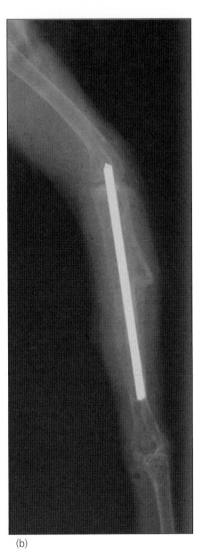

(a)                                                          (b)

**Figure 12.5**   Postoperative radiographs. (a) Lateral and (b) cranio-caudal.

entering the intercondylar sulcus or causing trauma to the tendon of the long digital extensor in the supratendinal ridge. The proximal pin is inserted from craniolaterally, just distal to the tibial plateau and cranial to the fibula, and directed caudomedially to avoid neurovascular bundles (which lie medially and laterally on the proximal tibiotarsus).

Some surgeons prefer type II external fixators. This is certainly the treatment of choice for severely comminuted fractures. Whenever external fixation is used, pins should be removed in a staged fashion to permit gradual increases in stressors on the healing bone.

Other surgical techniques described for fracture repair in birds include intramedullary polydioxanone rods, shuttle pins, plates and screws.

### Non-surgical support

In small birds such as budgerigars or cockatiels, an external splint may be fashioned for fractures distal to the hock, using adhesive tape such as zinc oxide tape. This is less likely to be effective for the tibiotarsus due to movement possible within overlying soft tissues, particularly rotation associated with tension from digital flexor muscles.

## Nutritional supplementation

If there is any doubt over the diet of the bird, supplemental minerals (particularly calcium and phosphorus) should be administered during the healing process.

## FOLLOW-UP

Although the dove was not using the leg normally on the day after surgery, the digits were moving. A common complication of limb fractures in birds is devitalization or denervation.

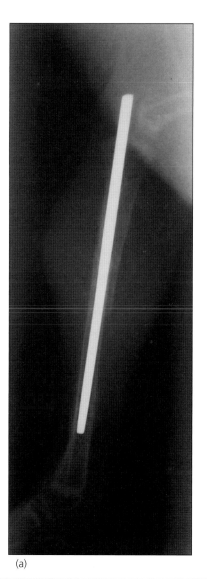
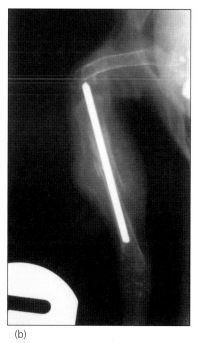

(a)    (b)

**Figure 12.6** Follow-up radiographs showing callus formation at the fracture site. (a) Lateral and (b) cranio-caudal.

Four days after surgery, a degree of rotation of the foot was present. This is a potential complication when a single intramedullary pin is used to repair a fracture. The limb was temporarily splinted, with a bandage including joints proximal (stifle) and distal (tibiotarsal–tarsometatarsal) to the fracture. Restriction of joint movement for prolonged periods of time will result in loss of function. This bandage was removed a few days later, by which time there was more rotational stability at the fracture site.

Three weeks after surgery, the leg was re-radiographed under general anaesthesia (Fig. 12.6). Callus formation was present around the fracture site and new bone growth was evident. The intramedullary pin was removed. Meloxicam was administered at the time of the procedure. Mobility in the limb was reasonable, although the restriction of joint movement even for a few days had resulted in some reduction in movement of the tibiotarsal–tarsometatarsal joint. There was a mild valgus present due to rotation at the fracture point during healing. This was not deemed to be clinically significant in this individual, but could well be in a working raptor that requires fully functioning limbs to capture prey. Heavier birds will be more prone to bumble-foot lesions if uneven weight bearing is present.

## PREVENTION

Provision of an appropriate diet and aviary conditions permitting regular exercise should prevent formation of weak bones. The enclosure should also be checked for any potential sources of traumatic injuries. In the case of raptors, perching should be provided in a safe manner, without inappropriately long tethers.

## PROGNOSIS

As avian bone healing is rapid, the prognosis is excellent, providing accurate apposition of the fracture ends can be achieved. The necessity for surgery is dependent on the species, the fracture, and the proposed use of the individual bird.

If the fracture site had been open, the risk of infection and osteomyelitis is high. These cases carry a more guarded prognosis.

# 13 Feather plucking in a parrot

## INITIAL PRESENTATION

Acute onset feather plucking in an Amazon parrot.

## INTRODUCTION

Many companion species (e.g. dogs, cats and rabbits) present regularly at the veterinary clinic for routine vaccinations, thus giving the veterinary practitioner an opportunity to perform a full health assessment (including history and clinical examination). On the other hand, avian pets are often not seen at the clinic until significant signs of illness are noted. It is wise to nurture avian clients and encourage 'well-bird checks'. If clients present a new bird, take the opportunity to obtain a detailed history and perform a full physical examination.

### CASE PRESENTING SIGNS

A 1-year-old orange-winged Amazon parrot (*Amazona amazonica*) (Fig. 13.1, Box 13.1) was presented for nail clipping. It became evident during the consultation that the bird had been plucking feathers for the previous 2 weeks.

## HUSBANDRY

The parrot had been in the owner's possession for 8 months. It was housed indoors in a large (1 m × 1.5 m × 2 m) metal cage, with free flight permitted in the living room for a total of 2 hours daily. A number of perches were present in the cage; all were round wooden dowel rods. Commercial parrot toys were provided on a rotational basis, of both plastic and wooden construction. The floor of the cage was lined with newspaper, which was changed daily.

The diet mainly comprised a dried seed and nut mix, sold for parrots. The bird also ate a small selection of fruit from time to time, including oranges and grapes. Fresh water was provided daily in a metal bowl.

A friend of the owner had been caring for the parrot 3 weeks previously, for a period of 1 week, while the owner was on holiday. The bird had remained in the owner's home for the duration, but there had been some change in daily routine associated with the visiting carer.

The owner did not possess nor had come into contact with other birds. The carer did not have contact with other birds.

## CASE HISTORY

The owner noticed the Amazon's claws becoming overgrown, and presented it for a nail trim. During the consultation, a history was taken and the bird examined. It transpired that the bird had started to pluck feathers from its sternal region 2 weeks previously (after the owner returned from holiday). The owner was persuaded to permit further investigation of the feather plucking problem.

## CLINICAL EXAMINATION

Examination showed:
- Bird bright and alert
- Weight 480 g, overweight (keel not palpable due to fat layer overlying, usual weight range for the species is 440–470 g)
- Auscultation of air sacs was unremarkable

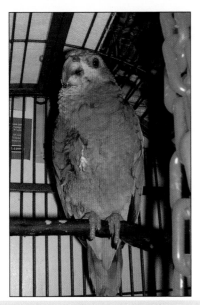

**Figure 13.1** Orange-winged Amazon parrot.

## BOX 13.1   ECOLOGY OF AMAZON PARROTS

- Amazon parrots (*Amazona* spp) originate from central South America. Orange-winged Amazons are located in Columbia, Trinidad and Tobago, with their range extending south to Peru and central Brazil. They reside in forest and semi-open country.
- Amazons are sexually monomorphic. Gender identification is by DNA analysis of blood or feather pulp, or visualization of the gonads via coelioscopy.
- There are about 30 subspecies of Amazon parrot.
- They are generally quiet, feeding in treetops.
- The diet in the wild consists of various seeds and fruits, including fruit from palm trees and sometimes cocoa.
- Flocks accumulate for night roosting. Mated pairs usually pair for life, and stay close together.
- Although the species are not endangered in the wild, it is persecuted as an agricultural pest and captured for the pet trade. Some are hunted by locals as a food source. Orange-winged Amazons are listed on CITES Appendix II, restricting trade.

- Feather loss over the ventral sternum and axillary regions, with wings and legs unaffected
- Feathers present on sternum showed some dystrophy
- No locomotory problems detected.

## DIFFERENTIAL DIAGNOSES

There are two main groups of aetiologies for feather plucking in birds – medical diseases and behavioural problems. It may be possible to suspect one or the other during the initial consultation, history taking and physical examination. However, in many cases, behavioural disease is diagnosed after ruling out medical problems. As this can be expensive for the owner, the list of differential diagnoses and investigations required should be discussed in full at the outset.

The *medical* differentials for feather plucking were:

- Malnutrition ('stress' marks (horizontal bars or weaknesses) are usually present on the feathers, associated with interrupted feather growth): general malnutrition or specific (e.g. omega-3 fatty acid deficiency, excess salt)
- Systemic disease, e.g. hepatic disease
- Chlamydophilosis
- Air sacculitis
- Toxins, e.g. nicotine exposure (other signs may include excitability, vomiting, diarrhoea, and seizures), heavy metal toxicosis
- Environmental factors, e.g. low humidity, inappropriate photoperiod, noxious aerosols
- Metabolic disease, e.g. hypocalcaemia (principally grey parrots)
- Allergy, e.g. inhaled, contact, food (e.g. peanuts, sunflower seeds), insect hypersensitivity
- Endoparasites, e.g. giardiasis (common in cockatiels)
- Pain, e.g. over an arthritic joint
- Infectious causes of feather dystrophy (may present similarly to self-feather plucking, but the head may also be involved): psittacine beak and feather disease (PBFD, circovirus), polyomavirus (in older budgerigars that survive infection), 'French moult' (budgerigars, caused by PBFD or polyomavirus)

- Reproductive disease, e.g. ectopic egg, egg-related peritonitis
- Dermatitis, e.g. skin irritation, skin desiccation, folliculitis (bacterial or fungal), polyfolliculosis in lovebirds (usually ventral neck or dorsum, may be infectious aetiology (e.g. polyomavirus) or secondary to self-trauma)
- Uropygial gland infection
- Pancreatitis
- 'Colic'
- Genetic, e.g. feather deformities (e.g. 'feather duster disease' in budgerigars)
- Neoplasia
- Hypothyroidism (few documented cases; 'normal' avian total thyroxine levels vary with species and season, so diagnosis is difficult)
- Ectoparasites (rare): mites and lice (highly host-specific).

The *behavioural* differentials for feather plucking were:

- Inadequate socialization (especially hand-reared birds)
- Failure to learn normal preening behaviours (again, especially hand-reared birds)
- Inappropriate daily routine, resulting in bird being 'overtired' (e.g. prolonged daylight period)
- Boredom
- Iatrogenic, e.g. after poor wing trim
- Reproduction-related, e.g. nesting frustration
- Fear/panic after a traumatic episode, cage-mate aggression.

## CASE WORK-UP

### History

Similar to other dermatological investigations, a detailed history should be obtained to gain as much information about the feather plucking bird's current and previous environment. Suggestions for pertinent topics to cover include:

- Signalment: age, species, reproductive history, source
- Gender: some species are sexually dimorphic, in monomorphic species sexing is performed on DNA analysis of blood/feather samples or by endoscopy; reproductive history (particularly egg laying in females)
- Rearing history: parent- or hand-reared, alone or in a creche

- Environment, e.g. cage, perches, toys, other pets (particularly other birds), exposure to potential toxins (e.g. smokers, air fresheners or other sprays, cooking fumes or open fires), heating, access to UV light (e.g. outside or artificial light indoors), hygiene routine
- Diet: it is important to determine what is eaten (rather than just what food is offered)
- Daily routine: including time in cage, free movement indoors or outside, interactions with owners and other birds, photoperiod (is a black-out sheet used at night?)
- Spraying/bathing (in water or with added products)
- Moulting history
- Wing clipping (current or historical)
- Owner relationship/bond
- Ascertain whether the presented bird is actually self-plucking/chewing or whether another bird may be the culprit
- Plucking/chewing pattern, e.g. description of plucking activity, timing (in day, when owner present/absent), period of plucking, initial area affected and any progression
- Any other previous or current medical problems and treatments.

## CLINICAL EXAMINATION

A full clinical examination should be performed when any bird is examined (unless restraint will result in undue stress).

- Observe the bird's behaviour and demeanour during the history taking part of the consultation
- General examination (see Birds – an introduction)
- Dermatological assessment:
  - Skin: colour, scale, lesions (e.g. wounds or tears), masses, erythema, folliculitis
  - Feathers: general feather condition, powder down, currently moulting, blood feathers, colour, dystrophy, damage, feather or follicle loss, ectoparasites.

### CLINICAL TIPS

Restraint of a medium-sized parrot:
- Prepare all potential equipment and sampling materials beforehand to minimize the period of restraint.
- Use a soft towel to handle the bird (restraint with bare hands will result in the bird

associating hands with an unpleasant experience, and future attacks on hands).

- Grasp the bird's head from caudally, with the thumb and first finger in a C-shape around the neck supporting the mandible.
- Wrap the towel loosely around the bird's body to control the wings.
- It is useful for the restraining assistant to grasp the bird's distal limbs to prevent the bird grasping the clinician during examination of the body.

## INVESTIGATIONS

Anaesthesia was induced and maintained with isoflurane administered via a facemask. As a short procedure time was predicted (<15 minutes), the bird was not intubated (although an endotracheal tube was on hand).

### Blood sample

Haematology and clinical chemistries were performed. The results were generally unremarkable. A mild relative heterophilia was noted ($15.0 \times 10^9$/l, reference range $1.55–12.07 \times 10^9$/l), without toxic changes on smear examination.

### CLINICAL TIPS

#### Phlebotomy

- Phlebotomy was performed from the right jugular vein (Fig. 13.2).
- The bird weighed 400 g and so its blood volume (5–13% of a normal bird's body weight) was approximately 40 ml.
- In a healthy bird, up to 8% of the blood volume may be sampled. In this case, a sample of 2.5 ml was sufficient for the testing required.

### Feather pulp analysis

Cytology revealed heterophils with Gram-positive cocci. Bacteriology cultured a moderate growth of *Staphylococcus* sp, sensitive to several antibiotics.

### Other investigations that may be indicated

- Dermatological investigations:
  - Microscopy on skin scrape, acetate strip, or feather digest

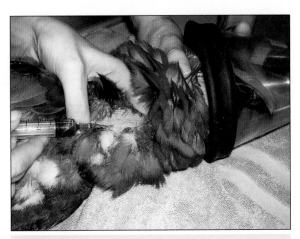

**Figure 13.2** Phlebotomy from the right jugular vein in a green-winged macaw (*Ara chloroptera*).

- Skin biopsy for histopathology
- Intradermal skin testing
- Other blood tests: zinc level, viral tests (e.g. circovirus (PBFD) and polyomavirus)
- Sexing (by blood, feather pulp, or coelioscopy)
- Faecal analysis for endoparasites: wet preparation and Gram-stain
- Skin and feather pulp cytology
- Radiography: body (e.g. include liver) and focal area where feather loss is present
- Skin biopsy
- Coelioscopy
- Trial therapy (e.g. antibiotics, simplified organic diet)
- If husbandry, clinical examination and laboratory tests are all normal, behavioural problems should be considered. History details may allude to behavioural issues.

## DIAGNOSIS

Bacterial folliculitis associated with *Staphylococcus* sp. The infection was suspected to be associated with malnutrition, and stress due to the change in routine.

## ANATOMY AND PHYSIOLOGY REFRESHER

Avian skin is very thin, and lightly attached to underlying muscle but strongly attached to bone. Birds do not have sweat glands. The epidermis is thicker around the beak and on the feet. The dermis comprises connective tissue, feather follicles, nerves and blood vessels. Loose connective tissue and adipose tissue make up the subcutaneous

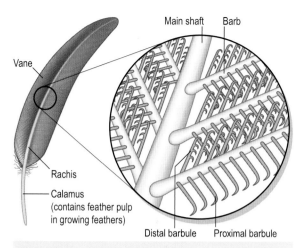

Main shaft  Barb

Vane

Rachis

Calamus
(contains feather pulp
in growing feathers)

Distal barbule  Proximal barbule

**Figure 13.3** Anatomy of a feather.

layer; this layer is thin and hence the skin is very inelastic.

Feathers (Fig. 13.3) are derived from follicles in the dermis, and are composed of keratinized epidermis. The feather follicle is a tubular invagination of the epidermis, with a dermal papilla that produces the feathers. The blood supply to the growing follicle degenerates when the feather matures. Immature 'blood' feathers will haemorrhage if broken. Feathers are set into feather tracts, the pterylae. Feather types vary, with the main contour feather having a hollow shaft and a feather vane of stiff filaments (barbs, with finer barbules) that interlock. Preening realigns the barbules, zipping them together.

Feathers are replaced at each moult. Triggers for moulting include nutrition (low-protein diets inhibit moulting), reproduction, season, temperature and photoperiod. Newly emerging feathers are highly vascular. Most species gradually lose their feathers so they are never unable to fly. (Ducks and geese are temporarily flightless, as they lose all contour feathers simultaneously.)

## AETIOPATHOGENESIS OF FEATHER PLUCKING

As evidenced in the differential diagnosis box above, there are many causes of feather plucking in birds. In some cases, the aetiology is multifactorial. There may be several inciting causes, or an initial medical cause may progress to 'habit'. For this reason, a standardized and methodical approach is required to the investigation of feather plucking. Medical causes are investigated and obvious husbandry problems corrected initially; if no causes can be found or no improvement is seen on treatment, behavioural disease is then assessed. In some cases, normal preening may become prolonged and exaggerated, resulting in feather mutilation.

## EPIDEMIOLOGY

Many psittacines are affected by feather plucking. Grey parrots, cockatoos and Hahn's macaws appear to be over-represented. Since other aetiologies include husbandry factors, captive birds with an inappropriate environment and diet are predisposed to the problem.

## TREATMENT

The bacteria isolated from feather pulp in this case were sensitive to several antibiotics, including amoxicillin clavulanate. The bird received a 3 week course of amoxicillin clavulanate (125 mg/kg q12hr BID).

Some changes were made to the parrot's environment. The owner was advised to clean food and water bowls daily using a mild disinfectant, rinsing well afterwards. The bird was sprayed daily with water to encourage normal preening. The parrot's food was gradually changed to a more balanced diet (consisting of a proprietary extruded pellet diet supplemented with fresh fruit and vegetables). The owner instigated a regular training regime, teaching basic commands such as 'step up' and 'step down'.

### CLINICAL TIPS

**Dietary changes in parrots**
- Do any changes gradually, over a period of several weeks.
- Owner compliance and patience is paramount to dietary change.
- Gradually introduce new foods. In the first instance, they may not be recognized by the bird as food.
- It may help to pass through a transition diet, e.g. from sunflower seed to soaked and sprouted sunflower seed to soaked and sprouted pulses.
- Eat (or pretend to eat) the food in the bird's presence. This is more effective if the parrot is trained or bonded to the owner.

- Offer the new food solely in the morning, giving a later feed of the previous diet. As the bird accepts the new diet, increase the morning feed and phase out the second feed.
- Do not starve the parrot. If the bird does not recognize the new food, it may eat nothing in preference.
- Be patient and persistent.

## TREATMENT OPTIONS AND MANAGEMENT

If a specific problem is diagnosed, treatment of this is the clinician's first prong of attack against feather plucking. Unfortunately, it is common that another aetiology is also present, and the case should be regularly re-evaluated to monitor: (a) owner compliance with prescribed medications and husbandry changes and (b) patient progress. Difficulties with making an accurate diagnosis should be discussed with the owner at the outset, as otherwise they may become disheartened and husbandry changes or treatment will lapse.

If the owner does not wish to pursue investigation, it is reasonable to trial therapy against common causes of feather plucking; these commonly involve husbandry optimization. If investigation does not reveal any specific medical aetiology or if no response is seen with therapy, behavioural causes should be considered. If the condition recurs, it is beneficial to re-evaluate the case.

Husbandry inadequacies often predispose to avian pathology. Even if the feather plucking is not due to malnutrition, it will be beneficial for the bird to improve the diet. The veterinary clinician should therefore seize the opportunity of the consultation to advise the client on good husbandry conditions. In the best-case scenario, this will result in the bird having better living conditions, being healthier, and the owner becoming committed to preventative healthcare.

Alternative therapies that have been suggested include herbal therapy or aromatherapy, acupuncture, nutraceuticals (e.g. aloe vera, and omega-3 fatty acids) and antioxidant therapy (oligomeric proanthocyanidins such as grape seed extract, Pycnogenol, bilberry and citrus bioflavonoids).

## TREATMENT OF OTHER CAUSES OF FEATHER PLUCKING

Feather picking associated with reproductive problems is usually treated with a combination of pharmacological treatment, behaviour counselling, and environmental changes (aimed at reducing reproductive drive and hormone levels). Note that some of these birds initially moult heavily when treated.

If a behavioural problem is diagnosed (or suspected), the bird's living situation and routine should be completely evaluated. The parrot's relationship with its owner(s) is particularly important. Most companion birds benefit from some basic training. Rotation of toys and other stimulation in the environment (e.g. human company, radio or TV, or a companion bird in some instances) are useful in improving the animal's condition.

Several texts are available on training and behavioural modification in birds. In some cases, it can be beneficial to use a drug to modify the bird's behaviour during this training period. The author does not advocate long-term use of behavioural modification drugs, as many have adverse side-effects. Similarly, buster collars may be useful in the short term to prevent self-trauma, but should not be seen as a cure for the problem. Behavioural modification drugs are best used during the period of environmental and behavioural changes (Table 13.1).

**Table 13.1** Some behavioural modification drugs (to be used in conjunction with behavioural training)

| Drug | Dose | Side-effects |
|---|---|---|
| Clomipramine | 0.5–1.0 mg/kg q8–24hr | Regurgitation, drowsiness, transient ataxia, arrhythmias |
| Diazepam | 0.5 mg/kg q8–12hr | Sedation, chronic hepatic damage |
| Fluoxetine | 1 mg/kg q24hr | None reported |
| Haloperidol | 0.15–0.20 mg/kg q12hr | Anorexia, depression or excitability/agitation |
| Leuprolide acetate* | 0.25–0.75 mg/kg q month | No reported side-effects |
| Medroxyprogesterone acetate* | 5–25 mg/kg q4–6weeks | Hepatic damage, diabetes mellitus, obesity |

* For reproductive aetiologies.

## FOLLOW-UP

The parrot's self-trauma reduced after a period of 2 weeks. At the following moult, feathers grew without dystrophy.

Initially, the Amazon refused the pelleted bird food, but gradually started to accept the new food after 1 month. It continues to be selective about which fruit and vegetables will be eaten.

## PREVENTION

Good husbandry and biosecurity will prevent access to most infectious and non-infectious aetiologies for feather plucking. Appropriate socialization and owner interaction will reduce the risk of behavioural causes.

## PROGNOSIS

The prognosis for this case was good, although in many cases of feather plucking, prolonged or intermittent therapy is required to control the disease. Chronic cases often respond poorly even when the inciting cause is treated.

# Stomatitis in a Harris' hawk

## INITIAL PRESENTATION

Reduced appetite and oral lesions in a Harris' hawk.

## INTRODUCTION

Clinical signs are often not pathognomonic in veterinary medicine, with similar signs often emanating from several aetiologies. This case highlights the need for laboratory investigation to make a diagnosis before treatment can proceed.

### CASE PRESENTING SIGNS

The 4-year-old female Harris' hawk (*Parabuteo unicinctus*) presented with reduced appetite, which was suspected to be due to oral lesions that the owner had seen.

## HUSBANDRY

The Harris' hawk was tethered on a bow perch outdoors during the day, and housed in a bay overnight. A sand substrate was provided; this was spot-cleaned daily and replaced twice yearly. The bow perch was covered with leather padding. A shallow water bowl was provided for drinking and bathing. The bird was moved to an aviary during moulting. The aviary had solid timber walls, and was part-covered with netting across part of the roof and along one side; a sheltered area was included at one end. Branches were present for perching in the aviary.

The bird was flown on 5 days each week. She was weighed daily. The diet consisted mainly of day-old chicks, with occasional quail and rabbit. The quantity fed once daily varied depending on the morning weight, keeping the bird slightly lighter during the flying season and allowing her to put on body condition in preparation for moulting. Adult female Harris' hawks usually weigh 825–1200 g (see Harris' hawk ecology in Ch. 11).

## CASE HISTORY

The Harris' hawk had been flying well through the season, and her appetite was usually good. The owner had noticed some changes over the previous week:
- Appetite reduced; willing to eat, but slower and not finishing the food offered
- Seen flicking head while eating, which was thought to suggest oral discomfort
- Weight reduction which the owner thought correlated with the reduced appetite
- Cream/yellow material had been seen in the oral cavity
- Still willing to fly
- Normal appearance to mutes (droppings) and casting (regurgitated indigestible part of diet).

## CLINICAL EXAMINATION

After observation of the bird on the owner's fist, the Harris' hawk was cast with a towel for examination. Clinical findings were as follows:
- Moderate body condition, keel palpable but not prominent, weight 950 g
- No oculo-nasal discharges externally
- Oral examination revealed caseous off-white material covering the tongue, extending to the oral mucous membranes. The material appeared to be restricting movement of the tongue
- Integument and feathers unremarkable
- Auscultation dorsally and ventrally unremarkable
- Coelomic palpation unremarkable
- No lameness noted when perching on the fist, and no limb laxities or fractures palpated
- No bumblefoot lesions present.

The differentials for *white/cream caseous oropharyngeal lesions* in a raptor were:

- Candidiasis (*Candida albicans*): often pinpoint lesions
- Trichomoniasis (*Trichomonas* spp): usually causes a diphtheritic membrane covering the oropharynx (called 'canker' by pigeon owners and 'frounce' by falconers)
- Capillariasis (*Capillaria* spp)
- Bacterial stomatitis, e.g. *Pseudomonas* spp, *Pasteurella* spp
- Viral infection, e.g. avian pox virus (wet version, particularly seen at the commissures of the beak), owl herpesvirus
- Fungal infection, e.g. *Aspergillus*
- Hypovitaminosis A, may predispose to other conditions: for example abscesses particularly in parrots, candidiasis, and trichomoniasis
- Infection may be secondary to trauma
- Insectivorous birds may suffer from infection with the *Syngamus trachea* nematode
- Visceral gout
- Neoplasia
- Exudate from sinusitis (e.g. due to mycoplasma infection).

## CASE WORK-UP

### Examination under general anaesthesia

This allowed a comprehensive assessment of the oral cavity (Fig. 14.1a) including the base of the tongue, as well as permitting sample collection for further tests. Anaesthesia was induced via a close-fitting facemask. The hawk was not intubated for two reasons: the procedure was rapid, and there was a risk of introducing infection into the lower respiratory tract if an endotracheal tube was passed via the oral cavity. The lesions extended over the tongue, making it slightly rigid, and laterally in the oropharynx (Fig. 14.1b). Lesions did not extend into the oesophagus.

**NURSING ASPECT**

### Fasting before anaesthesia

- Raptors should be fasted before general anaesthesia, to reduce the risk of regurgitation and aspiration.
- In general it is safe to anaesthetize after the bird has passed casting material (usually about 12 hours after eating).
- Alternatively, food without casting (e.g. muscle only with feathers and bones removed from carcase) can be given; this will pass through the gastrointestinal tract more rapidly.

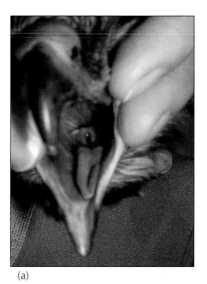
(a)

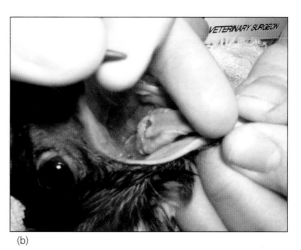
(b)

**Figure 14.1** (a) Normal raptor oral cavity (in a common buzzard, *Buteo buteo*). (b) Harris' hawk (*Parabuteo unicinctus*) with oral lesions, predominantly over the tongue.

## Sample collection

Swabs from the oral lesions were taken for cytology and bacteriology. Microscopy was performed on both a fresh wet preparation (to look for the motile protozoa *Trichomonas*) and Gram-staining (to assess for bacteria and yeast). Gout crystals are also identifiable using light microscopy. In cases of hypovitaminosis A, squamous metaplasia of epithelial cells is seen.

In this case, large numbers of round and budding cells that stained purple-blue with Gram-stain were seen on microscopy – diagnosing yeast infection. *Candida* sp was also cultured (on Sabouraud's agar at 37°C for 48 hours), producing typical shiny white round colonies 3–5 mm in diameter. In some candidiasis infections, pseudohyphae can form on tissue.

## POSSIBLE FURTHER INVESTIGATIONS

### Polymerase chain reaction

This will be necessary to diagnose viral infection such as poxvirus.

### Cytology

Further investigation of the gastrointestinal tract for infection would include cytology of faeces, casts, and swabs from the upper tract (e.g. from the oesophagus/crop).

### Haematology and biochemistry

One would expect to see hyperuricaemia in cases of gout. Haematological deviations (such as lymphocytosis with toxic change seen in white blood cells) may be present with other infections, particularly if the disease has become systemic.

### Radiography

If deep necrotic lesions are present in the oral cavity, bone infiltration may occur (especially with *Trichomonas* spp). Skull radiography may be indicated to assess the extent of pathology.

### Endoscopy

Rigid endoscopy may be indicated to assess the extent of lesions in the gastrointestinal tract. Examination should include the choanal slit, cervical and thoracic oesophagus, crop and proventriculus.

## DIAGNOSIS

Oral candidiasis.

## ANATOMY AND PHYSIOLOGY REFRESHER

The hard palate is split by the choane, linking the nasal cavity to the oropharynx. The raptor tongue is relatively long and triangular in shape. The healthy raptor grasps food with its feet and tears sections off with its beak for swallowing. The salivary glands produce sticky mucus for lubrication of food. Tongue/palate papillae and rostro-caudal movement of the tongue, followed by raising of the head, result in swallowing. Once in the oesophagus, peristalsis propels the food down the gastrointestinal tract.

The oesophagus lies on the right side of the neck. It is thin-walled with longitudinal folds. Mucous glands are present. Oesophageal muscle is all smooth muscle. The crop (ingluvies) is a dilation of the oesophagus at the base of the neck, just cranial to the thoracic inlet. The crop stores food when the stomach is full. Owls do not possess a crop.

The stomach consists of the proventriculus and ventriculus. There is little difference in the two compartments in carnivorous birds. Intestinal reflux (egestion or casting) enables Falconiformes (diurnal birds of prey) and Strigiformes (owls) to void indigestible food from the ventriculus, occurring approximately 12 hours after feeding. Strigiformes egest bone as well as feathers and fur. Falconiformes will hold food for longer (since they have a crop) and digest bones, so the casting contains only feathers and fur.

Small intestines in raptors comprise the duodenum, ileum and jejunum. These are all similar, being thin walled and narrow. The large intestines comprise a short colorectum. Raptors do not possess caeca. The cloaca consists of the coprodeum (into which the rectum empties), urodeum (ureters and genital ducts empty into this) and proctodeum (which empties into the vent).

## AETIOPATHOGENESIS OF CANDIDIASIS

*Candida albicans* is the most common species of *Candida* implicated in candidiasis. Other species that may cause disease include *C. parapsilosis*, *C. krusei* and *C. tropicalis*.

*Candida albicans* is commonly found as a commensal in the upper gastrointestinal tract (including the oral cavity) in raptors. In the healthy bird, host defence mechanisms and bacterial flora control the number of *Candida*. The yeast is an opportunistic pathogen, resulting in disease in cases where prolonged antibiotics or nutritional deficiencies result in an imbalance of normal gut flora. Thus, the source of infection is endogenous, with pathology being secondary to stress, immunosuppression, malnutrition, poor hygiene, debilitation or in birds treatment, with antibiotics. Infection may also originate from foodstuffs. Food storage and preparation should be evaluated, especially for hand-reared chicks. Candidiasis is common in pigeons, so such prey should be checked for signs of disease before feeding to raptors.

Candidiasis affects the gastrointestinal mucosa and muco-cutaneous parts of the body. Pathology particularly occurs in the oropharynx, oesophagus and crop. Plaque-like lesions are common on the mucosa of the tongue, pharynx and crop. A deeper infection of the gastrointestinal tract (where pseudohyphae have penetrated the wall) may occur alone or in conjunction with upper tract lesions. Malabsorption occurs if candidiasis extends along the gastrointestinal tract.

Pathologically, lesions start as thickened mucosa with increased mucous and pseudomembranous patches. A diphtheritic membrane of mycelial growth may develop in the oropharynx, and the choanae may abscessate. White/cream plaques may develop under the tongue, and in the oral cavity and crop. The disease progresses to stomatitis and palpable ingluvitis (crop thickening).

Clinical signs include reduced appetite, dysphagia (reluctance to swallow), oropharyngeal swelling, vomiting, regurgitation, weight loss and lethargy. Regurgitation is seen particularly when ingluvitis (crop inflammation) is present. Delayed crop emptying or complete crop stasis may also occur. Food is poorly digested if the more distal gastrointestinal tract is affected, resulting in abnormal mutes.

Candidiasis often results in the gastrointestinal wall, commonly the crop, becoming thickened with white material (like a Turkish towel). The disease is also known as 'soor' or 'thrush' by falconers in the UK.

## EPIDEMIOLOGY

Candidiasis is most common in immunosuppressed birds. Young raptors (above all in the first few weeks of life) with comparatively naive immune systems are very vulnerable to candidiasis.

## TREATMENT

### Debridement

The oral lesions were gently debrided using cotton buds. Candidiasis lesions are usually easily removed (in contrast to *Trichomonas* and *Capillaria* lesions that typically

haemorrhage). The owner continued to clean the oral cavity with dilute disinfectant (chlorhexidine) daily using cotton buds.

### Antifungal

Nystatin was administered (at 300000 IU/kg orally q12hr) for 7 days. This antifungal is not absorbed from the gastrointestinal tract, making it an excellent choice for infections localized to the gut. The drug is fungistatic, and must contact the organism (so it is ineffective if administered by gavage tube past the oral lesions). For lesions localized to the oral cavity, topical application of the drug may well be effective.

Oral discomfort was suspected due to the bird's reduced appetite. Thus, a 3 day course of non-steroidal anti-inflammatory drug (NSAID, meloxicam at 0.1 mg/kg orally once daily) was also prescribed. The owner was advised to hand-feed the hawk with small pieces of food.

> ### CLINICAL TIPS
>
> #### NSAIDs in birds
>
> - Avian species are susceptible to side-effects including reduced renal perfusion resulting in renal failure.
> - Ensure birds are well hydrated when using NSAIDs.
> - It is also important to calculate the dose based on an accurate body weight.

## OTHER TREATMENT OPTIONS

### Antifungals

Other antifungals that may be used to treat candidiasis include itraconazole (10 mg/kg orally q12hr for 5 days), or topical miconazole gel. Fluconazole (5–15 mg/kg orally q12hr) or ketoconazole (10–30 mg/kg orally q12hr) are recommended in systemic cases.

> ### CLINICAL TIP
>
> Resistance may be present or develop to antifungal therapy. It may therefore become necessary to alter the drug used.

### Probiotics

These may be helpful in re-establishing a normal gastrointestinal microflora.

## Other treatments

Oral chlorhexidine (2.5–5 ml/litre) in drinking water for 3 weeks is useful for control in flock situations, but does not eliminate infections. Apple cider vinegar may also be added to drinking water; this acidifier may be sufficient to treat mild cases of candidiasis.

## Other conditions

If predisposing conditions exist, including husbandry and nutrition problems, these should be identified and corrected.

### NURSING ASPECTS

#### Gavage-feeding

- If a raptor is unable to feed, it can readily be gavage-fed.
- The bird is cast using a towel, and restrained by an assistant who also grasps the legs to control the feet.
- The head is grasped and the beak opened. A gag is placed in the mouth (or a finger at the commissure) before a feeding tube is passed laterally down the oesophagus to the level of the crop. If a metal crop tube is used, a gag is not always required, but the oropharynx should be visualized to ensure that the larynx is not entered. Check positioning by palpating the trachea and tube separately in the neck.
- A total of 30–60 ml/kg per day of food or fluid is administered, usually divided into two or three doses.
- Nutritional support can be provided for raptors using convalescent canine/feline diets. If the bird is dehydrated or has been anorectic for some time, fluids (e.g. water or electrolyte solutions) should be administered in the first instance. In cases with severe dehydration, rehydration should be provided via the subcutaneous, intravenous or intraosseous routes.
- Care should be taken if oral infections are present, as the gavage tube could transfer them mechanically into the more distal gastrointestinal tract.
- While most birds have a dilation in the oesophagus (the crop) for temporary storage of food, certain species including owls do not.

## FOLLOW-UP

A verbal report was obtained from the owner 3 days after the initial consultation. By that stage, the hawk was eating relatively well when hand-fed, and maintaining her body weight.

The Harris' hawk was re-examined after 1 week. Although the oral cavity was not completely healed, the cream material on the tongue and oral mucous membranes had cleared. The bird was self-feeding and had slowly started to increase in weight.

## PREVENTION

Optimization of husbandry conditions, including diet and hygiene, are the principal factors to consider for prevention of candidiasis.

## PROGNOSIS

Candidiasis generally responds well to antifungal medication, although resistance may develop. Supportive care is vital if the patient is severely debilitated at presentation due to chronic and/or systemic infection. Underlying factors need to be addressed to aid treatment and prevent future recurrences.

SECTION 3

# REPTILES

# 15 Reptiles – an introduction

Reptiles are among some of the more unusual pets seen in veterinary practice (Fig. 15.1). An approach similar to that for other pets may be taken with regard to their clinical history and examination, although species-specifics must be known in order to interpret findings pertinent to husbandry conditions. The metabolic rate is in general slower with these ectothermic animals than with mammals, and hence disease processes tend to be more prolonged with reptiles. Investigative techniques and some basic husbandry requirements for selected species will be outlined in this chapter.

## TAXONOMY

Taxonomic classification of reptiles with some examples of those that may be seen as pets are given in Table 15.1.

## BIOLOGY

It is impossible to detail husbandry requirements for the huge range of reptile species that may be seen by the veterinary clinician in practice. The reader is referred to other texts for further information. Husbandry advice for some common species is listed below.

Unless housed outdoors with access to sufficient sunlight, most species will require supplemental UV-B light to synthesize vitamin D, which is necessary for calcium metabolism. Carnivorous species can obtain minerals from digestion of bone in their diet.

As reptiles are ectothermic (relying on environmental temperature to control their body temperature), most require supplemental heating in their captivity enclosure. A temperature range should be provided across the enclosure, to allow the animal to select an appropriate temperature. This preferred optimum temperature range (POTR) varies between species. Many heating sources can be thermostatically controlled, but the environmental temperature should still be monitored using a digital maximum–minimum thermometer (strip and dial thermometers may be inaccurate). Heaters should be protected to prevent accidental burns. In species that hibernate, care should also be taken to control and monitor the environmental temperature during this period.

Most reptiles carry potentially zoonotic pathogens, such as *Salmonella* spp, in their gastrointestinal tract. Although these rarely cause disease in humans, general hygiene precautions should be observed when handling reptiles or cleaning their enclosure, in particular ensuring that transmission does not occur via the faeco-oral route. Enclosures should be spot-cleaned daily, and intermittently disinfection should be carried out and the substrate changed.

Sexing of reptiles depends on the species concerned. In general, adult male tortoises have a longer tail than females; males may also have a concave plastron. Male terrapins may have longer claws on their fore-feet. Some lizards are sexually dimorphic, with males having more prominent pre-femoral pores (such as bearded dragons) or various facial adaptations (such as crests or horns in chameleons, or the dewlap in green iguanas). Few snakes are sexually dimorphic. Where obvious external characteristics do not enable gender identification, probing the hemipenes *in situ* caudal to the cloaca may be used to sex lizards and snakes. An alternative is coelioscopy or coeliotomy to visualize the internal gonads.

### Chelonia

This group is divided into tortoises (terrestrial species), turtles (aquatic marine species) and terrapins (aquatic freshwater species). Owing to space restrictions, smaller species are most commonly kept as pets. Most chelonian species prefer to be solitary, but same-sex individuals may be housed together if accommodation is large enough with several hide areas.

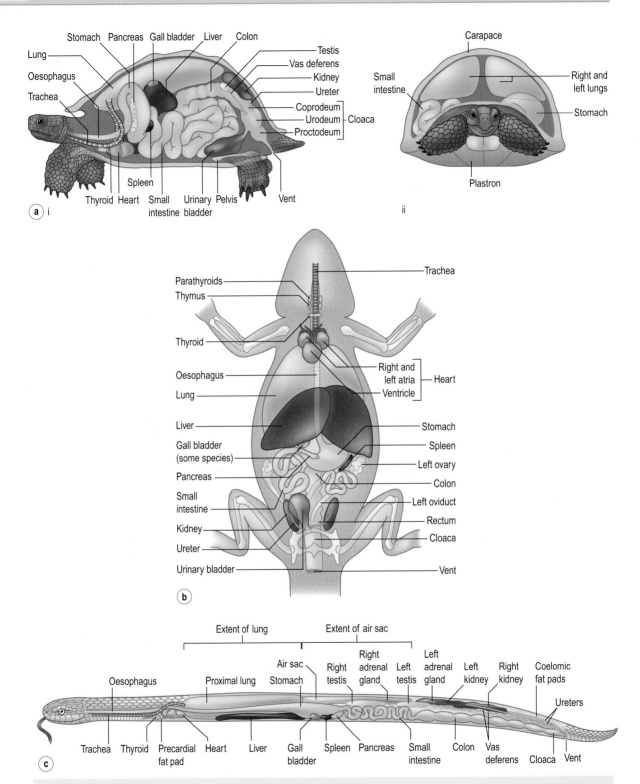

**Figure 15.1** Basic internal anatomy for (a) chelonia, (b) lizards, (c) snakes.

**Table 15.1** Taxonomic classification of reptiles, with some examples of those that may be seen as pets or in collections

| Order | Suborder | Family | Selected species |
|---|---|---|---|
| Testudines (Chelonia, Testudinata) | Cryptodira (hidden-necked) | Chelydridae (snapping turtles) | Snapping turtle (*Chelydra serpentina*) |
| | | Platysternidae (big-headed turtle) | – |
| | | Cheloniidae (sea turtles) | – |
| | | Dermochelyidae (leatherback sea turtle) | – |
| | | Carettochelyidae (pig-nosed turtle) | Pig-nosed turtle (*Carettochelys insculpta*) |
| | | Trionychidae (softshell turtles) | Spiny softshell (*Apalone spinifera*) |
| | | Dermatemydidae (Central American river turtle) | – |
| | | Kinosternidae (American mud and musk turtles) | – |
| | | Emydidae (pond turtles) | Map turtles (*Graptemys* spp), pondsliders (*Trachemys scripta* spp) |
| | | Geoemydidae (Eurasian pond and river turtles, neotropical wood turtles) | Three-striped box turtle (*Cuora trifasciata*) |
| | | Testudinidae (tortoises) | Hinge-backed tortoise (genus *Kinixys*), Hermann's tortoise (*Testudo hermanni*), Spur-thighed tortoise (*Testudo graeca*) |
| | Pleurodira (side-necked) | Chelidae (American side-necked turtles) | Mata-mata (*Chelus fimbriatus*) |
| | | Pelomedusidae (African side-necked turtles) | – |
| | | Podocnemididae (American side-necked river turtles and Madagascan big-headed turtle) | – |
| Squamata | Lizards | Iguanidae (iguanas) | Green iguana (*Iguana iguana*) |
| | | Agamidae (chisel-teeth lizards) | Australian frilled lizard (*Chlamydosaurus kingii*), Egyptian spiny-tailed lizard (*Uromastyx aegyptius*) |
| | | Chamaeleonidae (chameleons) | Jackson's chameleon (*Chamaeleo jacksonii*), veiled chameleon (*C. calyptratus*) |
| | | Eublepharidae (eyelid geckos) | Leopard gecko (*Eublepharis macularius*) |
| | | Gekkonidae (geckos) | Day geckos (genus *Phelsuma*), tokay (*Gekko gecko*) |
| | | Diplodactylidae (Southwest Pacific geckos) | – |
| | | Pygopodidae (flap-footed lizards) | – |
| | | Dibamidae (blind lizards) | Mexican blind lizard (*Anelytropsis papillosus*) |
| | | Xantusiidae (night lizards) | – |
| | | Lacertidae (wall and sand lizards) | European green lizard (*Lacerta viridis*) |
| | | Teiidae (whiptails and racerunners) | Common tegu (*Tupinambis teguixin*) |
| | | Gymnophthalmidae (microteiid lizards) | – |
| | | Scincidae (skinks) | Blue-tongued skinks (genus *Tiliqua*), Solomon Islands prehensile-tailed skink (*Corucia zebrata*) |
| | | Cordylidae (girdled lizards) | – |
| | | Gerrhosauridae (plated lizards) | Dwarf plated lizard (*Cordylosaurus subtessellatus*) |
| | | Anguidae (anguids) | Scheltopusik (*Ophisaurus apodus*), slowworm (*Anguis fragilis*) |
| | | Xenosauridae (xenosaurs) | – |
| | | Helodermatidae (beaded lizards) | Gila monster (*Heloderma suspectum*), Mexican beaded lizard (*H. horridum*); the only venomous lizards |
| | | Lanthanotidae (Bornean earless monitor) | – |
| | | Varanidae (monitor lizards) | Nile monitor (*Varanus niloticus*) |

**Table 15.1** Taxonomic classification of reptiles, with some examples of those that may be seen as pets or in collections   *continued*

| Order | Suborder | Family | Selected species |
|---|---|---|---|
| | Worm-lizards | Amphisbaenidae | – |
| | | Trogonophidae | – |
| | | Bipedidae | – |
| | | Rhineuridae | – |
| | Snakes | Blindsnakes (Scolecophidians): | |
| | | Anomalepididae (early blindsnakes) | – |
| | | Typhlopidae (blindsnakes) | – |
| | | Leptotyphlopidae (threadsnakes or wormsnakes) | – |
| | | 'True snakes' (Althinophidians): | |
| | | Anomochilidae (dwarf pipesnakes) | – |
| | | Uropeltidae (shield-tailed snakes) | – |
| | | Cylindrophiidae (Asian pipesnakes) | – |
| | | Aniliidae (red pipesnake) | – |
| | | Xenopeltidae (Asian sunbeam snakes) | – |
| | | Loxocemidae (neotropical sunbeam snake) | – |
| | | Pythonidae (pythons) | Indian or Burmese python (*Python molurus*), reticulated python (*P. reticulatus*) |
| | | Boidae (boas) | Boa constrictor (*Boa constrictor*) |
| | | Bolyeriidae (Mascarene or split-jawed boas) | – |
| | | Tropidophiidae (dwarf boas) | – |
| | | Advanced snakes (Caenophidians) | |
| | | Acrochordidae (filesnakes) | – |
| | | Viperidae (vipers and pitvipers) | Diamond-backed rattlesnakes (*Crotalus adamanteus, C. atrox*), European adder (*Vipera berus*), Gaboon viper (*Bitis gabonica*), puff adder (*B. arietans*) |
| | | Atractaspididae (stiletto snakes and their allies) | – |
| | | Colubridae (colubrids) | American gartersnakes (*Thamnophis* spp), grass snake (*Natrix natrix*), milksnake (*Lampropeltis triangulum*) |
| | | Elapidae (cobras and their allies) | Spitting cobras (*Naja nigricollis, N. mossambica, Hemachatus haemachatus*), black mamba (*Dendroaspis polylepis*), king cobra (*Ophiophagus hannah*) |
| Rhynchocephalia | | Sphenodontidae | Tuatara (*Sphenodon punctatus, S. guntheri*) |
| Crocodylia | | Alligatoridae (alligators) | Dwarf caiman (*Paleosuchus palpebrosus*) |
| | | Crocodylidae (crocodiles) | Dwarf crocodile (*Osteolaemus tetraspis*) |
| | | Gavialidae (gharial) | – |

Although low numbers of some endoparasites appear to assist with digestion, large numbers are usually associated with disease. Faeces should be examined for parasites annually.

**Hibernation** Many species of chelonia (and some other reptiles) will hibernate in the wild for varying periods of time (Box 15.1). In captivity, it is usually advisable to keep this period to a maximum of 12 weeks, otherwise, metabolic reserves will become dangerously low during hibernation and it may be difficult for the tortoise to eat sufficiently during the warmer months in preparation for hibernation. Tortoises should be fasted for 1 month before hibernation to allow the gastrointestinal tract to empty; otherwise continued fermentation may lead to gas build-up and pressure on the lungs, resulting in dyspnoea. During this pre-hibernation time, the tortoise should be bathed to encourage drinking. Water is stored in the urinary bladder for reabsorption during hibernation.

Traditional hibernaculums include boxes insulated with straw, but these are susceptible to environmental temperature changes. Some animals housed in gardens may dig into soil as their free-ranging counterparts do, but monitoring is nigh on impossible in this situation. Often, owners do not actually know where the tortoise has buried itself, and owners digging in gardens during spring have caused traumatic injuries to hidden pets. A safer alternative is to build an indoor insulated terrarium with thermostatically controlled heating coils underneath protective matting, covered with soil to permit digging. A reasonably constant temperature can be maintained using a refrigerator. It can be helpful to have bowls of water in the fridge to ensure the air does not become excessively dry.

Hibernation is induced below 15°C, and maintained between 2 and 9°C. Temperatures below 0°C will result in pathology such as blindness. The environmental temperature should be measured constantly, for example using a maximum–minimum digital thermometer. Tortoises should be checked daily and weighed weekly during hibernation. If a tortoise urinates during hibernation, it should be awakened and 'over-wintered' (i.e. kept awake and maintained in conditions similar to the warmer months). Similarly if a tortoise loses >5–10% of its body weight during hibernation (or >1% in a week), it should be awakened.

Tortoises should begin eating within a couple of days of wakening from hibernation. Bathing in shallow warm water will encourage the tortoise to drink and urinate.

Often they will pass a large amount of urates at this stage. If they do not start to eat within a week, tortoises are deemed to have 'post-hibernation anorexia', and veterinary investigation and treatment should be instigated.

During excessively hot dry periods of summer, some tortoises (such as free-ranging desert tortoises, *Gopherus agassizii*) may undergo a metabolic change similar to hibernation, called aestivation.

> ### BOX 15.1   IMPORTANT NOTE
>
> *Geochelone* species such as the leopard tortoise (*Geochelone pardalis*) and African spurred tortoise (*Geochelone sulcata*) do not hibernate. They should be over-wintered, ensuring sufficient environmental temperatures are maintained despite outdoor temperatures dropping.

### *Hermann's tortoise (*Testudo hermanni*)*

This species hails from the Mediterranean region, and specimens can grow up to 30 cm in length. Their diet should mostly consist of weeds such as dandelions (both leaves and flowers), plantain, sow thistle and sedum. They will also favour flowers such as hibiscus, nasturtium and honeysuckle. Salad leaves may form a small part of the diet. Mineral supplementation in the form of a proprietary powder is usually added two or three times weekly. Food is placed onto a smooth surface (e.g. a piece of slate) to reduce the risk of ingestion of substrate material and resulting gastrointestinal impaction. Water should be provided in a shallow container (deep enough to submerge their beak to drink), with weekly bathing in shallow warm water to encourage further drinking and excretion of waste products.

Hermann's tortoises require a large (e.g. 90 × 30 cm for a small juvenile) well-ventilated pen with solid sides, usually made of wood or plastic. A background heat source may be provided with a tubular heater or heat mat (against a wall of the enclosure, not underneath). The environmental temperature should be measured using a digital maximum–minimum thermometer aiming for a daytime range of 20–30°C, dropping by 15°C overnight. A basking area (with a temperature up to 40°C) with a spot bulb should be positioned near the feeding area. UV-B lighting should be provided, either via a strip light or mercury vapour lamp (the latter also produces heat). These should be positioned approximately 30 cm above the tortoise to ensure sufficient UV reaches the animal. UV lights usually require changing every 6–12 months as UV output declines (note that output of visual light remains for considerably longer). In appropriate environments, tortoises may have outdoor access in pens.

Hides should be provided, for example a cardboard box, plant pot, or hollow log. A suitable substrate would be a soil/sand mix, along with an area of large pebbles or stones. Tortoises are usually solitary, except during the breeding season (when sexually active males will pursue females).

### Horsfields tortoise (Testudo horsfieldi)

These tortoises come from Eastern Europe, growing up to 20 cm in length. Their husbandry requirements are similar to the Hermann's tortoise.

### Red-foot tortoise (Geochelone carbonaria) and yellow-foot tortoise (G. denticulata)

These South American species do not hibernate. Their natural habitat is dense humid forests, and this should be emulated in captivity. Despite the need for high humidity, ventilation should not be neglected. It can be useful to provide hide chambers with damp substrate, resulting in focal areas of elevated humidity. The daytime temperature should be 25–27°C. Red-foots grow up to 45 cm in length, and yellow-foots up to 70 cm. Large enclosures (4 × 4 m for a pair) are therefore required.

Red- and yellow-foot tortoises are omnivorous. They will eat ripe fruits (40–70%), flowers and green leaves (20%), as well as a small amount (one meal per week) of animal protein (moist low-fat cat food).

### Red-eared terrapin (Trachemys scripta elegans)

This species is semi-aquatic and can grow up to 20 cm in length. They are found in freshwater in South and Central America. Their enclosure should include an aquatic area for swimming, as well as a land area for basking and resting. Plants (both real and plastic) can provide hide areas. Water filtration is useful to maintain water quality, which should be checked regularly. Water changes and tank disinfection should also be performed regularly. Water temperature should be maintained at 24–26°C (>20°C overnight), usually requiring a water heater. A spot bulb should provide a basking temperature of 32°C. UV-B should be provided as for tortoises.

These animals are omnivorous. Captive diets should be 70–80% animal matter (e.g. low-fat dried cat, dog or trout pellets, bloodworms, earthworms, small fish,

and commercial terrapin diets), and 20–30% leafy green vegetables and aquatic plants. Vitamin and mineral supplements are added. They are usually fed in a separate tank to the main enclosure to reduce water soiling.

### Spur-thighed tortoises (Testudo graeca subspecies, T. ibera)

These hail from the Mediterranean, Asia and North Africa. Some subspecies do not hibernate. As with other Testudo species, the diet is predominantly weeds and flowers. The enclosure and environmental requirements are also similar to those for Hermann's tortoises.

### Leopard tortoise (Geochelone pardalis)

These large tortoises, growing to over 70 cm in length and weighing up to 20 kg, are from the grasslands of sub-Saharan Africa. The enclosure should reflect the size of the tortoise. Heating should result in a background temperature over 25°C (>22°C overnight), with a basking spot of 40°C. As with other Geochelone species, leopard tortoises do not hibernate, and it is particularly important to consider heating provision over the winter months. UV lighting should be provided.

This species eats mostly grasses and hay, along with some weeds and flowers. Vitamin and mineral supplementation is particularly important for large tortoise species.

### African spurred tortoise (Geochelone sulcata)

These originate from sub-Saharan Africa, in arid savannahs and acacia scrublands. They may reach 83 cm in length and 105 kg body weight. Captivity requirements are similar to those for leopard tortoises, with a high-fibre diet and facilities for over-wintering.

## Lizards

Lizards are common pets, with many species frequently seen in veterinary practice. The clinician should be conversant with husbandry requirements for each species in question. Enclosure design, and temperature and humidity requirements will vary between species. In general, supplemental heating and UV-B light is necessary. The substrate for most lizards may be newspaper, artificial turf or other proprietary substrate material. Wood chip substrates are commonly associated with gastrointestinal impactions in lizards, and should be avoided. For insectivores, insects should be fed salad or fruit, and gut-loaded with a proprietary product (high calcium content) for 24 hours prior to being fed to the lizard. Insects, and vegetation for herbivorous species, should be dusted with mineral supplement before being offered to the reptile.

## Leopard gecko (Eublepharis macularius)

These geckos are common pets, originating from north-west India, south-west Afghanistan, eastern Iran and Pakistan. They can reach up to 25 cm in length. Leopard geckos are usually housed alone, although adults may be paired. Vivaria are usually wooden or fibreglass, with a glass aspect for viewing. A visual barrier at the lizard's ground level will reduce stress. Ideally, the vivarium should be 0.6 m wide × 1.2 m long × 0.6 m deep. Ventilation should be provided. The cool end should be 25°C, with a hot spot at the other end of 32°C. Although this species is predominantly nocturnal, a low-output UV-B light is usually provided. A shallow water bowl should be provided. It is important to provide hides, and one should contain a damp substrate (e.g. moss or absorbent kitchen paper) to increase humidity and assist ecdysis.

Leopard geckos are insectivorous, and are fed on crickets and locusts in captivity. Although they will also take waxworms and mealworms, these invertebrates should be fed in limited quantities only.

## Green iguana (Iguana iguana)

This lizard comes from tropical rainforests in Central and South America, and grows up to 2 m in length. As an arboreal species, their enclosure should be vertically oriented, usually with a base at least 2 × 2 m square and 1.5 m high, with branches for climbing and basking. Background heating is provided, with a lower daytime temperature of 25°C and a basking spot of 40°C. The humidity should be high (80–90%), maintained by regular spraying or misting and placement of the water bowl at the warmer end of the vivarium. A UV-B light should be provided over a basking branch. Iguanas are territorial (particularly uncastrated adult males) and should be housed alone.

Green iguanas are herbivorous, with their diet comprising 90% vegetables (mostly leafy greens) and 10% fruits. They will also eat flowers. Food should be supplemented with a vitamin and mineral powder twice a week. A large container of water will allow the iguana to drink and also to submerge completely.

## Bearded dragon (Pogona vitticeps)

This eastern Australian species grows up to 50 cm long. The vivarium should be at least 0.6 × 1.2 × 0.6 m. The temperature gradient is similar to that for green iguanas.

Although omnivorous, dietary preferences change with age. Juveniles eat a high proportion of invertebrates (such as crickets and locusts). Leafy green vegetables form the main part of the diet in adults. All food should be supplemented with a calcium powder. The water bowl should be large enough for the animal to submerge.

Coccidiosis (usually *Isospora amphibolurus*) is common in bearded dragons, especially juveniles; other coccidian species may be more common in other reptiles. Along with gastrointestinal disease, the infection may also predispose the bearded dragon to other infections. Transmission is faeco-oral, and may occur via fomites, so good hygiene is required to reduce spread.

## Veiled chameleon (Chamaeleo calyptratus)

This chameleon is also known as the Yemen chameleon, and originates from Yemen and Saudi Arabia. Free-ranging animals are mostly arboreal, and captive specimens should be provided with plenty of climbing and perching facilities. A large vivarium is required for this species, at least 1 m long × 1 m wide × 1.5 m high. Mesh-sided enclosures are preferable, as chameleons may become stressed and attack their reflection in glass. For this reason, chameleons are usually housed alone. Mesh provides visual security and good ventilation. A basking temperature of 35°C should be provided at one end of the enclosure, with a cool temperature of 24°C at the other end. UV-B light should be provided.

An omnivorous species, chameleons should receive approximately 80% insects (such as crickets and locusts) and 20% plants in their diet. Live food should be gut-loaded and all food supplemented with a high-calcium (8%) product. Chameleons drink predominantly from water droplets on plants, usually obtained by regular spraying or by an artificial dripper system. Humidity in the enclosure should be 50–60%.

## Water dragons (Physignathus spp)

The most common species in captivity is *Physignathus cocincinus* (the Chinese, Thai or green water dragon). They may reach 100 cm in length. Like leopard geckos and green iguanas, this species can undergo autotomy (tail shedding) as a defence mechanism. A large vivarium, usually constructed of wood or fibreglass, should be provided (at least 2 m long × 1 m wide × 2 m high). The cool end should be maintained at 29°C, with a basking area of 35°C at the other end. A high humidity (80–90%), hides, branches for climbing, and UV-B lighting should be provided.

Free-ranging water dragons consume insects and small prey; captive animals are predominantly fed on crickets and locusts (gut-loaded and dusted with a calcium supplement). The water container should be deep enough for the lizard to submerge completely.

## Snakes

Snakes make interesting pets. It is vital to design a snake enclosure that is secure, preventing escape. However, snakes are susceptible to respiratory disease and ventilation is important with housing, and should not be compromised while providing secure accommodation. Hides will provide security for the animal. As with lizards, non-ingestable substrates should be used. Snake vivaria should be cleaned and regularly disinfected. Quarantine checks should include assessment for ectoparasites such as mites (*Ophionyssus natricis*). As snakes obtain most minerals from their diet, UV may not be an absolute requirement; however, a low-output UV-B light is often provided.

### Corn snake (Elaphe guttata)

This species originate from North America, and can reach up to 1.5 m in length. The vivarium should be 0.6 × 1.2 m (× 0.6 m high). The cool end should be 25°C, with a basking area of 32°C.

As with most snakes, they are carnivorous. Young corn snakes are fed on pinkies (newborn mice without any fur) and fuzzies (mice with some fur), progressing to adult mice and large rats when fully grown. Adults are usually fed once weekly. Food should be thoroughly defrosted and warmed (to approximately 37°C) before feeding. A water bowl should be provided, deep enough to permit submerging.

### Garter snake (Thamnophis spp)

These species also come from North America, residing in the vicinity of woodlands, marshes and rivers. They will grow up to 1.3 m long. The vivarium should be 0.6 m in length × 0.3 m × 0.3 m. Provision of hide areas for snakes will reduce stress. The temperature should range from a cool of 25°C to a basking hot spot of 32°C.

The free-ranging diet will consist of fish (they are good swimmers), amphibians, and invertebrates, with occasional young birds or mammals. Captive diets are predominantly freshwater fish and earthworms. Frozen fish may be deficient in vitamin B1 (resulting in neurological disease in the garter snake), and a supplement should be added. Water for drinking should be deep enough for the snake to submerge.

### Hognose snake (Heterodon nasicus)

Western hognose snakes originate from North America and Mexico, and may reach 75 cm in length. Housing and diet is similar to that required for the corn snake.

### Royal python (Python regius)

This snake is from Central and Western Africa, and may reach 1.5 m in length. Diet and husbandry requirements are similar to corn snakes, although royal pythons require a slightly warmer basking spot of 35°C.

## HISTORY

The most important component of reptile history taking is their husbandry (Box 15.2). Since most reptilian pets will be maintained in a climate different from their normal environmental range, the owner needs to simulate normal conditions. This will usually involve supplemental heating and lighting. It is vital that conditions are monitored, for example that a thermometer is used to measure temperature rather than relying on a thermostat attached to a heater, and preferably that records are kept of these conditions. Poor husbandry conditions result in stress, and this often contributes to invasion by secondary infectious agents.

It is extremely useful if owners also maintain records of the reptile's appetite, faecal production, and shedding. The frequencies of these along with any problems or changes noted offer a valuable resource for assessment of animal health. The source and storage conditions of food should be ascertained. It is preferable to feed some species such as terrapins outside their normal enclosure, owing to the potential for food remnants to deteriorate water quality.

> ### BOX 15.2    SUGGESTED TOPICS TO COVER DURING HISTORY TAKING FOR REPTILES
>
> - Species
> - Age
> - Gender
> - Source, e.g. petshop or breeder, imported, captive-bred or wild-caught, relevant paperwork (e.g. CITES)
> - Period in owner's possession (if this is relatively short, husbandry details from the previous carer may be important)
> - Reproductive history
> - Housing: size, construction materials, location, substrate, cleaning regime

- Supplemental heating source, method of maintenance (e.g. thermostat) and monitoring (e.g. digital thermometer) of environmental temperature in enclosure. Temperature range in enclosure during day and night
- UV-B provision, including when bulbs were last changed and day to night cycle. (UV meters may be used to assess UV output in older bulbs or tubes, as visible light is still produced when UV production has waned.)
- Relative humidity in enclosure, including method of monitoring
- Presence of hides or shelters (particularly for outdoor animals), and other enclosure furniture (e.g. branches for arboreal species)
- Hibernation history (in appropriate species): including details of period of time, description of hibernaculum, monitoring during hibernation, any period of post-hibernation anorexia
- Diet: what food is offered (including supplements) and what is eaten, frequency of feeding. For insectivorous species, whether insects are fed or gut-loaded before offering to the reptile.
- Water provision: including for drinking, bathing (particularly in tortoises that prefer to drink when they have access to shallow water), and swimming (in aquatic or semi-aquatic species). Water quality checks for aquatic or semi-aquatic species
- Ecdysis: frequency, date of last shed, any dysecdysis noted
- Handling frequency and periods, including periods the reptile spends outside the enclosure
- Previous medical history (including any treatments)
- Current problem: time period, outline of clinical signs and progression noted by owner
- Current physiology: appetite, thirst, faecal, urine and urates output (including number/size, frequency/volume, and description)
- Question owner further about the pet's current health: any other clinical signs of disease or changes in behaviour (these may be subtle)
- Companion animals in same enclosure/airspace/indirect contact: any health problems (current or previous).

It is useful to ascertain direct or indirect contact with other reptiles owing to the risk of disease transmission. Many infectious agents can be spread between animals and collections in this way. Some agents may have a long incubation period, or may remain dormant within animals until immune compromise results in a susceptible animal. It can be extremely difficult to clear some infections from a collection, with some (in particular viral infections such as ophidian paramyxovirus (OPMV)) requiring culling of animals to clear a collection.

Biosecurity measures are therefore vital, as prevention of an agent entering a collection is much preferred to dealing with the condition. It is advisable to instigate a quarantine policy (for example 90 days for snakes, and at least 30 days for other reptile species) for new stock in a collection, with appropriate testing performed during this period. Testing may include faecal parasitology for all reptiles, and other infectious agent testing dependent on the species (such as herpesvirus and mycoplasma for chelonia, and OPMV and inclusion body disease for susceptible snake species). Herpetologists may have difficulty in selling animals if they have a history of certain diseases in their collection.

## CLINICAL EXAMINATION

### Handling/restraint

Chelonia and lizards are usually transported to the veterinary clinic in a rigid box. It is important to have a secure lid on containers with active animals, for example small geckos. Snakes and some lizards are best transported in cloth bags (e.g. a pillow-case or duvet cover) with a knot tied to contain them. Reptiles should be kept warm during transport, for example by placing a warm water bottle within or under the container (ensuring it is not so hot as to cause burns). Insulated boxes, for example polystyrene, are useful for long journeys.

Examination gloves should be worn when handling reptiles. The risks of transferring bacterial infections such as *Salmonella* spp from animal to human are low, particularly when good hygiene procedures are followed (i.e. hand-washing). Other zoonotic risks include pentastomiasis and mycobacterial infections. The risk of transferring viral infections between reptiles via the handler's hands is high. It is simpler to change examination gloves than to thoroughly disinfect your hands after each patient.

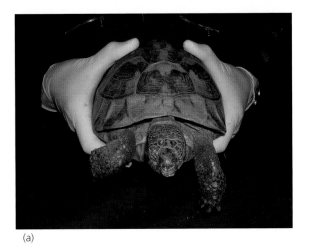

(a)

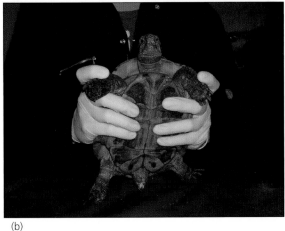

(b)

**Figure 15.2** (a) The 'hamburger' grip can be used to pick up most tortoises. (b) Gently restrain the forelimbs for examination of the head.

## Chelonia

Most terrestrial chelonia (tortoises) are not aggressive, and are easily handled. However, care should be taken not to allow the handler's fingers to become trapped in the shell if an animal draws its limbs in or closes functional hinges in the shell. In general, the 'hamburger' grip is used to pick up tortoises, gripping both plastron and carapace securely (Fig. 15.2). More than one handler may be required for larger specimens. For more aggressive species, such as many terrapins and turtles, the caudal carapace should be grasped to minimize the risk of being bitten.

Larger or very strong animals may require sedation to enable examination to be performed. In these circumstances, ketamine or ketamine combinations are commonly injected intramuscularly (for example into the cranial muscle mass of the forelimbs when they are withdrawn).

## Lizards

Care should be taken in species that undergo autotomy (e.g. iguanas and leopard geckos). The tail should not be grabbed. Sudden grasping movements should be avoided, as this may also initiate loss of the tail. It is useful to warn owners that autotomy may occur during handling of such species, particularly if an animal is not habituated to restraint. Tail regrowth takes several months and the new tail is visibly different, usually with smaller scales and different colouration (Fig. 22.1). The new section contains cartilage rather than bony vertebrae.

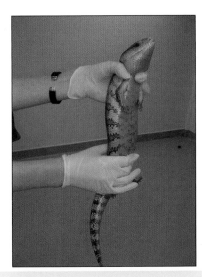

**Figure 15.3** Restraint of a lizard, holding the forelimbs and hindlimbs close to the body.

For most lizards, one hand is used to restrain the forelimbs by holding around the pectoral girdle, and the other hand restrains the hindlimbs by holding around the pelvic girdle (Fig. 15.3).

Small lizards are held in one hand, gently but securely. Many geckos have fragile skin that tears easily. It may be advisable to observe these species in a clear container before catching and restraining in a small net for examination.

Large lizards such as monitors and iguanas may inflict damage to their captor by scratching with their claws and whipping their tail. Rarely, lizards may bite. It is beneficial to restrain larger animals using a towel wrapped over the reptile, moving the towel to enable a gradual examination.

The only venomous species of lizard belong to the family Helodermatidae. The venom from these species (*Heloderma horridum*, the beaded lizard, and *Heloderma suspectum*, the Gila monster) flows in grooves along the teeth, and is transmitted to the victim by chewing. Only experienced handlers should restrain these species, and safety protocols should be in place in case of envenomation.

### Snakes

The head is usually grasped from outside the transport bag before the rest of the body is unwrapped. If the snake is in a box, a towel can be used to restrain it for capture. Snakes have only a single occiput, and dislocation of the head from the neck is possible with inappropriate restraint. The neck is held with three fingers and the thumb, while the first finger rests on top of the head to stabilize the joint. The body of the snake is supported halfway along (Fig. 15.4). Most snakes will move around somewhat when restrained, and this should be allowed providing the head is secure.

Multiple handlers may be required to restrain larger specimens (>2 m long), particularly constrictors that may pose a personal risk to a single human.

Herpetologists may keep venomous species (national legislation, such as the Dangerous Wild Animals Act

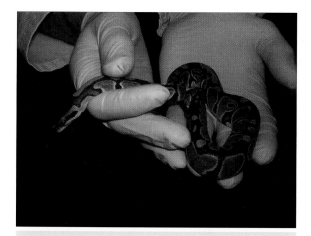

**Figure 15.4** Restraint of a snake, demonstrating support of the head and the body.

1976 in the UK, may restrict keeping of such species). As with the heloderm lizards, handlers should be experienced and safety protocols in place before dealing with these species. Snake hooks and tongs, and plastic tubes are useful for restraint of aggressive or venomous species. Hooks are particularly useful for capture and restraint of agile or dangerous (aggressive or venomous) individuals. Tongs are used to hold the snake before it can be grasped behind the head. Plastic tubes can be designed with holes along the length for access to inject sedative or anaesthetic agents. The tube should not be wide enough to permit the snake to turn. The snake is encouraged to enter the tube partway, so its caudal body can be held along with the tube.

### Crocodilians

Small individuals are restrained as for lizards. Animals may bite, scratch, or writhe with their tail. Care should be taken to hold or tape the mouth closed.

## Examination

If possible, the animal is initially observed within its normal enclosure or the transport container, to gauge locomotion and demeanour. Any obvious external abnormalities can be noted for further evaluation during restraint (Box 15.3). Chelonia and lizards should be able to hold their body above ground level, particularly during locomotion. Respiratory movements can be observed and any obvious noises should be noted.

Reptiles do not possess a diaphragm as found in mammals, resulting in significantly different internal anatomy. The lungs lie in a cranio-dorsal position. Chelonia have a fibrous septum horizontal (a pleuroperitoneal membrane) below the lungs, connected to the limbs which thus effect breathing movements when moved in and out of the shell. Crocodilia have a muscular septum that is similar to the mammalian diaphragm. In chelonia and most lizards, the heart lies in the midline quite cranially near the thoracic inlet; in monitor lizards the heart is more caudally situated. The serpentine heart is approximately a third of the way along the body. In Crocodilia the heart lies caudal to the forelimbs by approximately 11 scale rows, in the ventral midline.

Auscultation is limited in reptiles due to the difficulty with sound transmission between the scales and stethoscope. In chelonia, a damp towel may be placed between the stethoscope and shell, but normal lung sounds are usually not heard. Doppler blood flow monitors are useful to monitor reptilian hearts.

## BOX 15.3   CHECKLIST FOR CLINICAL EXAMINATION

- Confirm species/breed and sex: many chelonia and lizards are sexually dimorphic when mature, some snakes are but many require probing of the hemipenes to determine the gender
- Weigh (using digital scales)
- Assess body condition (see below for details)
- Measure: total length, snout-to-vent length (SVL) in lizards/snakes/crocodilians, straight carapace length (SCL) in chelonia
- Head: eyes, ears (tuatara do not have external ears), nares, heat sensor pits (present in some snakes such as vipers), rostrum (abrasions are common in stressed lizards) or beak (overgrowth may be seen in tortoises with a variety of conditions), oral cavity (including assessment for stomatitis and periodontitis), observe and palpate for symmetry
- Cranial coelomic cavity: auscultate lungs and heart, ± percuss (to assess for fluid presence) or compress thoracic cavity (to assess compliance)
- Caudal coelomic cavity:
  - Gastrointestinal tract: palpate
  - Urinary tract: palpate (e.g. for bladder stones)
  - Reproductive tract: palpate for pregnancy (eggs or fetuses) or abnormalities
- Reproductive system: prolapses, discharges, swellings, wounds
- Skin: palpate for masses, assess for lesions (e.g. alopecia, crusts, wounds) or discharges, ectoparasites (commonly in skin folds around the eyes and mouth), evidence of dysecdysis (e.g. retained shed especially around toes/ eyes/mouth, partial digit loss due to avascular necrosis)
- Musculoskeletal: observe locomotion, palpate and examine limbs, assess muscles for tone and tetany (commonly seen with nutritional or metabolic disease, or toxins), assess strength in snakes by testing whether it can support part of the body
- Nervous system: observe demeanour, perform further neurological tests if warranted (e.g. if head tilt, facial asymmetry or ataxia present), check if righting reflex present.

The coelomic cavity can be relatively easily palpated in lizards and snakes. In snakes, palpation is performed ventrally between the ribs. In chelonia, the pre-femoral fossae are used as 'windows' through which limited palpation may be possible. These fossae are also useful for ultrasound probe placement to assess coelomic organs. Transillumination may be useful in small individuals of lizards such as leopard geckos and snakes such as albino animals. The cloaca may be carefully probed digitally in larger animals.

### Body condition assessment

Thin chelonia will feel light for their size, feel empty on palpation of the coelomic cavity via the pre-femoral fossa, and will often have reduced muscle mass of their limbs. The 'Jackson's ratio' may be useful for some species (such as Mediterranean spur-thighed, *Testudo graeca*, and Hermann's, *Testudo hermanni*, tortoises).

Some geckos store fat in their tail (e.g. the leopard gecko, *Eublepharis macularius*), and body condition is readily noted by observing the diameter of the tail near the base. Many lizards store fat in bilateral intracoelomic fat pads, resulting in a distended coelomic cavity in obese individuals.

Thin snakes appear triangular in cross-section, with prominent ribs and spinal processes. Overweight snakes deposit fat in the caudal third of the coelomic cavity, resulting in an enlarged body region cranial to the cloaca.

### Sexing

**Chelonia** The males have concave plastrons and longer tails in many species of tortoise. Females are larger than males in many species (such as the spur-thighed and Hermann's tortoises, and red-eared sliders, *Trachemys scripta elegans*), while females are smaller in African spurred tortoises (*Geochelone sulcata*). Some aquatic species (such as the red-eared slider) have longer nails on the forefeet of males.

**Lizards** Sexual dimorphism exists in some species (Fig. 17.1). For example, secretory glands on the ventral thigh or precloacal region are larger in the males of many lizards (iguanids and agamids), male Jackson's chameleons (*Chamaeleo jacksonii*) have horns on their head. Hemipenes may be detected using ultrasound, for example in monitors (*Varanus* spp) and inland bearded dragons (*Pogona vitticeps*). Some species can be probed, for example green iguanas (*Iguana iguana*).

**Snakes** Sexual dimorphism is subtler in snakes, with many having broader and longer tails (due to the presence of the hemipenes at the base). The spurs that remain as hindlimb vestiges near the vent are larger in male boids (pythons and boas). Most commonly, snakes are sexed by probing the hemipenes (a lubricated probe is gently passed into the vent and directed caudally, passing six to ten scale lengths into males and two to six in females). The hemipenes may be everted either side of the vent by rolling cranially; however, this procedure may damage the organs.

Coelioscopy may be used to sex reptiles.

---

### BOX 15.4  PROBING SNAKES AND LIZARDS TO DETERMINE SEX

- Lubricate a blunt-ended probe (using a non-spermicidal lubricant).
- Insert the probe into the cloaca. Direct it caudally in the region of a hemipene (i.e. at the lateral edges of the cloaca, as there are two hemipenes).
- In males, the probe will be able to pass further caudally (e.g. eight scale lengths in many snakes) than in females.
- If only a short distance is probed, check the other side as hemipenal plugs may form from time to time and restrict passage of the probe.

---

## INVESTIGATION

### Phlebotomy

Sedation or general anaesthesia may be necessary for phlebotomy in some reptiles (Table 15.2), but in most individuals venepuncture can be performed using conscious restraint. The skin should be prepared as for a surgical procedure, particularly at contaminated sites such as the tail. A surgical cut-down is usually required for placement of an intravenous catheter.

Haematology is performed on a sample preserved in anticoagulant, usually calcium EDTA (although this may haemolyse blood from some species, including many chelonians, in which lithium heparin is the preferred anticoagulant). A freshly prepared blood smear is useful to assess erythrocyte and leucocyte morphology, and to check for haemoparasites. Biochemical analyses are performed on either plasma or serum samples. In very small animals, a basic profile including estimated total and differential white cell count, packed-cell volume (PCV) and total solids can be performed on a blood smear and haematocrit tube sample. Samples containing lymph will be diluted, affecting test results.

Blood results vary greatly between species, between sexes, and seasonally. The reader is referred to other texts and specialist laboratories for reference ranges.

### Radiography

It is often possible to radiograph lizards and chelonia without chemical restraint, although adhesive tape is useful to extend limbs. Chelonia may be balanced on an upside down mug or bowl to prevent significant movement during horizontal beam radiography (Fig. 15.5). Small- to medium-sized lizards often respond well to the vago-vagal response, using bandage over cotton wool balls to put pressure over the eyes. Larger, livelier animals may require some sedation to aid positioning. Similarly, chelonia often require sedation to allow positioning for radiography of the limbs. Perspex tubes are useful restraint tools for snakes, although sedation is often required to permit positioning for two orthogonal views.

The main difference between radiography of mammals and reptiles relates to their anatomy. Owing to the lack of diaphragm, lateral views should be taken with a horizontal X-ray beam (otherwise the organs fall onto the lungs and give an abnormal and non-diagnostic appearance). For lizards and snakes, a dorso-ventral view (using a vertical X-ray beam) and lateral view (using a horizontal beam) are taken routinely. For chelonia, these are supplemented with a cranio-caudal view (using the horizontal beam again). For localized assessments views may vary, but the aim is always to have two orthogonal views of the site.

Markers (e.g. metal strips on the film corresponding to tape on the animal) should be used to identify the location along the length of a snake's body for film interpretation after processing.

### Other imaging modalities

*Ultrasonography* is particularly useful for assessing the coelomic cavity in reptiles. Coupling gel should be applied several minutes before the procedure is performed, to increase contact time and reduce air pockets that will affect the quality of the ultrasound image.

Reproductive assessment is easily performed using ultrasound, enabling visualization of ovaries, follicles, eggs, and fetuses within the reproductive tract. Ultrasound-guided fine needle aspirates may be performed to obtain samples from abnormal structures for cytology

**Table 15.2** Preferred sites for phlebotomy in reptiles

| Site | Comment | Species |
|---|---|---|
| Brachial plexus | At flexor surface of elbow | Larger chelonia; some lizards |
| Cardiocentesis | Locate heart and steady with gentle pressure cranially and caudally. Insert needle into ventricular region. Avoid multiple needle sticks, as this increases the risk of detrimental cardiac damage | Snakes |
| Cephalic vein | Cut-down procedure required, can place in-dwelling catheter | Larger lizards |
| Dorsal coccygeal vein | Often contaminated by urates and faecal material | Chelonia |
| Jugular vein | Extend neck of chelonia and raise vein with pressure at base of neck. Cut-down procedure in lizards and snakes; can place in-dwelling catheter | Chelonia, lizards, snakes |
| Palatine vein | Medial surface of palatine dental arcade; anaesthetized animals | Large snakes |
| Sub-carapacial sinus | Useful where jugular venepuncture not possible (e.g. in small specimens or larger ones); sample may be contaminated by lymph. Midline below cranial carapace; use a long needle | Chelonia |
| Ventral abdominal vein | A surgical approach may be required (risk severe haemorrhage if lacerate vein and cannot compress); can place in-dwelling catheter (though difficult to maintain as ventrum contacts substrate) | Lizards |
| Ventral coccygeal vein* | Can be difficult to get sample from small snakes. Ventral midline or lateral approach in lizards; long needle required | Lizards, snakes |

*Samples from small Crocodilia are obtained as from lizards.

or culture. Some echocardiography has been performed in reptiles; however, reference values are still limited. Masses on peripheral body parts may also be beneficially examined by ultrasound.

Computed tomography (CT) and magnetic resonance imaging (MRI) may be used in reptiles. Chemical immobilization is required to prevent excessive movement during the procedure. The interpretation of images from reptiles is in its infancy, but the application of general anatomical and medical knowledge aids in understanding.

## Sampling

Many samples from reptiles may usefully be analysed. As for blood samples, it is advisable to use a laboratory that specializes in exotic pets; they are more likely to have appropriate reference ranges and be accustomed to working with reptilian samples.

Faecal analysis is routinely performed on new stock and periodically on current animals. Parasitology may detect protozoa, parasitic ova and larvae. Other information may be gained from the sample, for example the presence of bacterial overgrowth, fungi, or inflammatory cells. Urine may be examined, although the sample is usually mixed with gastrointestinal excretions due to the common chamber (the cloaca) between the renal and gastrointestinal tracts.

Cytology may be performed on impression smears or scrapes obtained from lesions, or from fine needle aspirates. Cavity washes (e.g. cloacal, gastric, tracheal or lung washes) may also be examined microscopically or cultured; usually sterile isotonic fluid is utilized. Bone marrow or cerebrospinal fluid samples may be obtained for analysis. Tissue biopsy samples are analysed fresh or frozen for culture or PCR, or preserved in formalin for histological assessment. Other samples may be analysed for suspected toxins or infectious agents; the specialist laboratory should be contacted to obtain details of the best sample and storage conditions for the suspected condition.

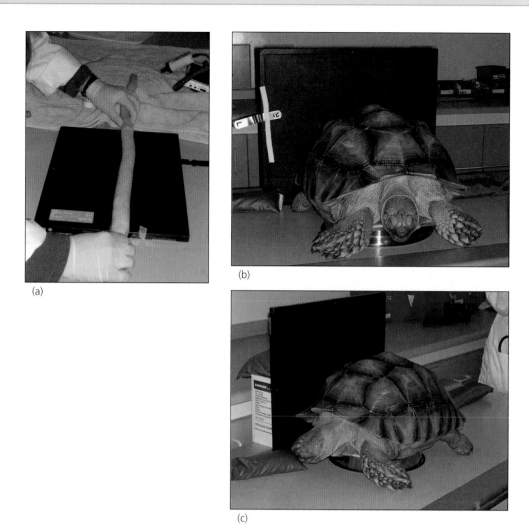

**Figure 15.5** (a–c) Reptiles positioned for radiography, including horizontal beam positioning of a tortoise (b, c).

## TREATMENT

### Basic procedures

#### Drug administration

*Topical* medication may be applied to treat ocular or skin disease.

*Oral* administration is relatively easy in most reptiles. It is useful to utilize a mouth gag to prevent damage to the oral structures and to the syringe or tube being used for administration. Gavage is commonly used to administer fluids and nutritional supplementation, as well as medications. The tube should be pre-measured to the level of the stomach. Bathing reptiles in shallow warm liquids (mostly water) will encourage drinking and also

passage of urine/urates/faeces. Pharyngostomy tubes are placed under general anaesthesia, and allow ease of long-term treatments.

Reptilian skin is relatively inelastic, and only small volumes may be injected *subcutaneously*. This route is contraindicated in lizard species such as geckos that have thin, fragile skin.

The *intramuscular* route is often employed to administer medications such as antibiotics and anaesthetics. In chelonia and lizards the triceps or quadriceps muscle groups are utilized. In snakes and larger lizards the epaxial muscles may also be used.

As described above, *intravenous* access may be difficult (particularly for prolonged administrations). This route is commonly used for administration of anaesthetics, and placement of a catheter permits pro-longed administration of fluids and other medications.

The *intracoelomic* route is useful predominantly for fluid administration. Where large volumes are injected, it is important to ensure they are pre-warmed to the animal's POTR. In chelonia, the pre-femoral fossa is accessed after tilting the body away from the site. A ventro-caudal lateral approach is used for lizards. In snakes the left caudal flank is used. In all species caudo-ventral placement of needles should reduce the risk of lung or air sac penetration, although positioning should be checked by withdrawing the syringe plunger before injection to ensure other coelomic organs have not been entered.

In tortoises, the *epicoelomic* route may be used for relatively rapid absorption. This site is approached crani-ally near the shoulder joint.

*Intraosseous* access is possible in chelonia and lizards. In chelonia, the cannula is placed in the cancel-lous bone of the caudal plastro-carapacial pillar. In lizards the distal humerus, proximal tibia or distal femur are used.

*Nebulization* is a technique frequently used in cases with respiratory tract disease. Saline will reduce viscous secretions and moisten the airways. Antimicrobial agents can be targeted to the respiratory tract.

*Other routes* of medication include intra-lesional, intra-articular and sub-spectacular injections, cloacal and nasal flushing. Antibiotic-impregnated polymethylmeth-acrylate beads may be implanted into lesions.

### Assist-feeding

Any nutritional support should be appropriate for the species. In the short-term, human baby foods may be used, but most reptiles require long-term support and diets more closely allied to their natural diet should be given. Proprietary convalescent herbivore and carnivore diets are available.

Although some reptiles become habituated, most (particularly snakes) are secretive feeders and do not respond well to *hand-feeding*. It can be helpful to warm prey items for carnivores and move it to simulate a live animal; this may stimulate a strike response and swal-lowing by an ill patient. Debilitated tortoises may take food willingly from human carers. *Syringe-feeding* into the oral cavity is generally not well tolerated.

*Gavage* is typically easy to perform on reptiles. Pre-measure the gavage tube to mid-way along the body, and pre-warm food to body temperature. A gag should be placed in the oral cavity (taking care not to damage any teeth). For more chronic conditions, food or medication is better administered via an *oesophagos-tomy tube*.

## Anaesthesia

### Pre-anaesthesia

Before sedation or anaesthesia, the reptile should be clinically assessed. This includes assessment of the ani-mal's husbandry, to identify any factors that may increase the risk of disease or debilitation, as well as a clinical examination to assess for current pathology. The patient should be weighed on digital scales, in order to permit accurate drug dosing.

Severely debilitated animals should be stabilized before induction of anaesthesia. This may include fluid administration, nutritional support, or basic husbandry provision. All reptiles should be housed appropriately during their stay at the veterinary clinic. This usually involves provision of a secure enclosure with supplemen-tal heating, often with UV-B lighting. The environmental temperature should be assessed using a digital ther-mometer, maintaining the temperature within the species' POTR.

Carnivorous species such as snakes should be fasted before elective procedures to reduce the risk of regurgi-tation. The period of fast depends on the normal gas-trointestinal transit time.

### Pre-medication

Commonly used pre-medicants in reptiles are given in Table 15.3.

### Inhalation agents

Volatile agents are often used to induce anaesthesia in lizards (using an induction chamber or closely fitting facemask), usually after pre-medication to reduce breath holding.

Anaesthesia is generally maintained using volatile agents once the patient is intubated. Apnoea is common, and IPPV is performed at 2–4 breaths/minute during anaesthesia.

### Injectable agents

#### Chelonia

Injectable agents (Table 15.4) are used to induce anaes-thesia. Options include propofol, alfaxalone, ketamine, or ketamine with medetomidine. Intravenous access is commonly via the jugular vein.

**Table 15.3** Commonly used pre-medicants in reptiles

| Drug | Dose (mg/kg) | Route | Comment |
|---|---|---|---|
| Buprenorphine | 0.02–0.20 | SC, IM | Analgesic, may cause sedation |
| Butorphanol | 0.4–2.0 | SC, IM, IV | Analgesic, may cause sedation in some lizard species |
| Midazolam | 2 | IM | Minimal sedation if used alone |
| Ketamine | 5–20<br>5–10 | IM | Dose-dependent sedative effects, pre-medication doses<br>Chelonia<br>Lizards, snakes |
| Acepromazine | 0.05–0.50 | IM | Can be used with ketamine |
| Butorphanol + midazolam | 0.4 + 2.0 | IM | – |
| Tiletamine + zolazepam | 4–10 | IM | Sedation for non-invasive procedures |

IM, intramuscular; IV, intravenous; SC, subcutaneous.

**Table 15.4** Commonly used injectable anaesthetic protocols in reptiles

| Drug | Dose (mg/kg) | Comment | Route | Species |
|---|---|---|---|---|
| Alphaxalone | 10–15<br>10 | – | IV | Chelonia<br>Lizards |
| Ketamine | <90<br><60 | Anaesthesia<br>Deep sedation | IM | Chelonia<br>Snakes |
| Ketamine + medetomidine | 5 + 0.05–0.10 | Supplement oxygen; assist ventilation | IM/IV | Chelonia |
| Propofol | 3–15<br>3–5<br>5–10 | <10 mg/kg if not pre-medicated | IV | Chelonia<br>Lizards<br>Snakes |

### Lizards

Similar injectable agents (Table 15.4) are used as in chelonia, including propofol or alfaxalone. The most easily accessible vein is usually the ventral coccygeal; care should be taken in species that may autotomize their tail if this vein is accessed for induction. Pre-medications may include butorphanol or ketamine.

### Snakes

Intravenous access is difficult in snakes, but if the ventral coccygeal vein is accessible propofol is the induction agent of choice (Table 15.4). Alternatively, ketamine can be used to sedate before volatile agents are used to induce anaesthesia, or higher doses of ketamine administered to induce anaesthesia outright. In some snakes (not venomous species!), conscious intubation may be performed and IPPV with a volatile agent used to induce anaesthesia.

### Monitoring anaesthesia

Voluntary respiratory efforts may be observed by watching the movement of the animal's thoracic cavity or of the reservoir bag on the anaesthetic circuit. Since most reptiles will be manually ventilated, this rate should also be recorded on the anaesthetic sheet (preferably using a different symbol from voluntary breaths).

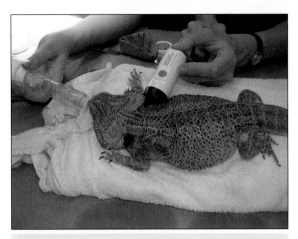

**Figure 15.6** Doppler probe used to monitor pulse on carotid artery.

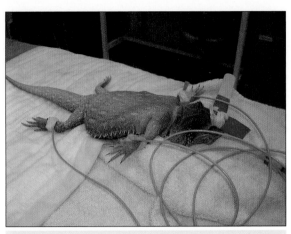

**Figure 15.7** ECG attached to a bearded dragon (*Pogona vitticeps*).

The heart rate is usually monitored using a Doppler probe over the heart or a large artery such as the carotid (Fig. 15.6). An oesophageal stethoscope may be used in larger animals. In snakes, the heartbeat may be visible. ECG leads (Fig. 15.7) may be attached to the patient, although reptilian skin has poor conductivity and contact is better if ECG clips are attached to needles inserted through the animal's skin.

Reflexes to monitor include the toe or tail pinch, and jaw tone. In snakes, muscle tone in the tail is lost last when anaesthesia is induced, and regained first before cranial musculature on recovery.

### Peri-anaesthetic care

During anaesthesia, provision of supplemental heating is necessary (within the species' POTR).

As low oxygen levels stimulate reptile respiration, oxygen should not be supplemented excessively during recovery. In general, the patient is disconnected from oxygen but kept intubated until voluntary breathing movements are seen. IPPV can be continued using a manual resuscitator.

Fluids are usually administered peri-anaesthetically. This is particularly important when procedures under anaesthesia are prolonged, and/or when injectable agents are used that may be renally excreted.

## Surgery

To aid healing, skin incisions should be made between scales where possible. Access to the coelomic cavity is usually via a paramedian incision (avoiding the ventral midline abdominal vein) in lizards, ventrolaterally (between the first two rows of scales on the side) in snakes, and via a plastronotomy in chelonia (although a pre-femoral approach may be used in larger specimens).

The coelomic membrane and body wall are typically thin with little suture-holding strength, and wound closure relies on skin sutures. Reptiles uncommonly interfere with wounds. A major difference with reptilian surgery is the requirement to use an everting suture pattern (e.g. horizontal or vertical mattress sutures) when closing skin wounds. If an appositional pattern is used as in other species, the wound edges will invert. Wound healing is prolonged, requiring 4–6 weeks for skin healing in most cases; hence non-absorbable suture materials (e.g. polypropylene, nylon, or skin staples) are utilized. Catgut is contraindicated, causing severe granulomatous reactions or acting as a permanent foreign body. The owner should be warned that dysecdysis is likely at the wound site, although this should resolve after a few sheds.

Bone incisions may take a year to heal. Where chelonia undergo shell repair, healing may take years to complete. Plastronotomies in chelonia are commonly closed using fibreglass sheets and resin.

A good anatomical knowledge is necessary for coeliotomies, particularly in snakes where the internal organs are arranged in a predominantly linear fashion. Multiple incisions may be required, for example to perform surgery on a female snake's reproductive tract. Internal organs in reptiles are delicate, and manipulation is often easiest using stay sutures. Stainless steel surgical clips are preferred by many surgeons for internal sutures and ligatures, alternatives include rapidly absorbed materials like poliglecaprone 25.

Analgesia should be provided for any animal undergoing a painful procedure.

## Euthanasia

Where possible, pentobarbitone is injected into the circulation via a vein (or intracardiac in snakes). In some animals, this will not be possible, and the intracoelomic or intrahepatic routes are used. It may be useful to sedate or anaesthetize the patient prior to injection. Death is confirmed by checking for a heartbeat using a Doppler probe or an ECG.

# 16 Gastrointestinal foreign body in a tortoise

## INITIAL PRESENTATION

Inappetence, reduced faecal output, hindlimb paresis in a Hermann's tortoise.

## INTRODUCTION

Pet chelonia often roam in large outdoor areas, which include access to various substrates. Ingestion of foreign material may or may not lead to gastrointestinal obstruction. A major concern in chelonia is the decision over whether medical therapy will result in a cure, or if surgical intervention (usually necessitating a trans-plastron coeliotomy) is required.

## CASE PRESENTING SIGNS

A 7-year-old male Hermann's tortoise (*Testudo hermanni*) was presented with inappetence, reduced faecal output and hindlimb paresis.

## HUSBANDRY

This captive-bred tortoise had been in the current owner's possession since approximately 1 year old. He was housed on his own for most of the year in an indoor enclosure, with supplemental heating (bulb) and lighting (including UV-B), although he did roam one of the rooms periodically. During the summer months, he was permitted outdoor access in the owner's garden – usually supervised. His diet comprised various weeds and vegetables (including clover, dandelions, cabbage, and sweetcorn), dusted with mineral supplement (Nutrobal®, Vetark, Winchester, UK; and cuttlefish). He had grown from 150 g to 1.28 kg over 6 years, and had never been hibernated.

## CASE HISTORY

During one of the tortoise's outdoor excursions, 4 weeks prior to presentation at the veterinary practice, the owner temporarily left him unattended and returned to find him consuming pieces of gravel. Clinical signs were noted for a few days before presentation:

- Greatly reduced faecal output, but no straining reported
- Inappetence
- Reduced use of hindlimbs.

## CLINICAL EXAMINATION

As tortoise clinical examinations are restricted due to anatomical constraints, findings were brief:

- Not raising plastron above ground when walking
- Body condition good, weighing 1.28 kg. Muscle mass good, with no generalized weakness noted
- Carapace showed mild pyramiding of carapacial scutes, consistent with rapid growth seen in many pet tortoises with excessive nutritional intake
- Oral mucous membranes were pink and moist (no sign of dehydration)
- No masses or foreign bodies were detected in the coelomic cavity via palpation in the pre-femoral region.

## DIFFERENTIAL DIAGNOSES

Inappetence is a common presenting sign for many illnesses in reptiles, and further investigations are required to determine the disease process(es) occurring.

The differentials for *reduced faecal output* were:

- Secondary to reduced food intake (gastrointestinal transit time may be <20 days in chelonia)
- Systemic illness, e.g. dehydration, hypocalcaemia
- Obstruction in gastrointestinal tract, e.g. cloacolith/faecolith (often associated with dehydration), intussusception (possibly secondary to other disease, e.g. foreign body), foreign body, endoparasitism (e.g. ascarids such as *Augusticaecum* sp), neoplasia, volvulus
- Space-occupying lesion compressing gastrointestinal tract, e.g. cystic calculi, reproduction in female (gravidity, dystocia, pre- or post-ovulatory stasis), organomegaly (e.g. renomegaly, hepatomegaly), pelvic fracture, neoplasia, granuloma
- Poor husbandry, e.g. low environmental temperature

The differentials for *hindlimb paresis* were:

- Inappropriate husbandry, particularly inadequate environmental temperature
- Nutritional or renal secondary hyperparathyroidism (also known as metabolic bone disease, MBD), hypocalcaemia
- Systemic illness may result in generalized paresis, e.g. septicaemia, organ failure, end-stage starvation
- Renomegaly
- Articular gout/pseudogout
- Toxicity, e.g. ivermectin, pesticides
- Infection, e.g. abscess, cellulitis, or osteomyelitis (usually bacterial)
- Cystic calculi
- In a female, egg retention or after oviposition
- Neoplasia, in nervous or musculoskeletal systems
- Neurological, e.g. infection (bacterial, fungal, parasitic), spinal cord lesion (trauma, pathological after vertebral body collapse in MBD)
- Musculoskeletal disease (common in males if they fall off the female's carapace after mating): tendon or ligament damage, fracture (traumatic or pathological) – less likely in this case as bilateral paresis noted
- Less commonly, flaccid paresis may result from: shock, drowning, hyperthermia or bloat.

## CASE WORK-UP

### Radiography

Three views were taken of the conscious tortoise – dorso-ventral (Fig. 16.1) using a vertical beam, and cranio-caudal and lateral using a horizontal beam. These orthogonal views outlined the presence of foreign material within the gastrointestinal tract. The object was less dense than bone but more radiodense than soft tissue, and its shape was consistent with a piece of gravel. The absence of gas near the mass suggested that it was not completely obstructing the gastrointestinal tract. No musculoskeletal pathology was detected on the radiographs.

### Haematology and biochemistry

Financial consideration may preclude blood analysis in practice, and the clinician should be aware that analysis is not sensitive in reptiles. In this case, results showed mild dehydration (haematocrit and total protein were slightly elevated). There was no evidence of systemic infection (total white cell count normal, and no 'toxic' or 'reactive' white blood cells were seen on microscopy). Biochemical parameters (including renal parameters (uric acid), hepatic enzymes (AST, LDH, CK), and ionized calcium, and calcium to phosphorus ratio (1.85)) were within reported ranges – reducing the likelihood of metabolic bone disease or other metabolic derangement (Table 16.1).

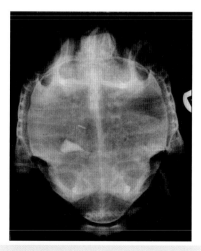

**Figure 16.1** Dorso-ventral radiograph of the tortoise, showing radiodense foreign body within the gastrointestinal tract. (Lateral and cranio-caudal views were also taken, using a horizontal beam.)

**Table 16.1** Hermann tortoise blood results (with reference ranges for comparison)

| Parameter | Unit | Result | Reference range |
|---|---|---|---|
| Total protein | g/l | 53.6* | 23–44 |
| Albumin | g/l | 15 | 13–16 |
| Globulin | g/l | 19.8 | 14–29 |
| Glucose | mmol/l | 2.33* | 4.3–10.7 |
| Calcium | mmol/l | 2.87 | 1.65–3.3 |
| Ionized calcium | mmol/l | 2.01 | >1.0 |
| Phosphorus | mmol/l | 1.55 | 0.48–1.81 |
| AST | U/l | 70 | 0–210 |
| CK | U/l | 100 | 0–620 |
| Uric acid | µmol/l | 250 | 124–466 |
| LDH | U/l | 197 | 0–300 |
| Sodium | mmol/l | 139.3 | 123–145 |
| Potassium | mmol/l | 8.18 | 3.6–5.3 |
| Haemoglobin | g/dl | 11.6 | 3.9–12.6 |
| Haematocrit | l/l | 0.45* | 0.15–0.43 |
| Red blood cells | $\times 10^{12}$/l | 1.02 | 0.35–1.11 |
| MCV | fl | 358.2 | 357.5–436.4 |
| MCHC | g/dl | 32.2 | 25.7–33.3 |
| MCH | $\times 10^9$/l | 113.7 | 94.3–140.2 |
| White blood cells | $\times 10^9$/l | 0.8 | 0.1–3.1 |
| Heterophils | $\times 10^9$/l | 0.30 | 0.00–1.91 |
| Monocytes | $\times 10^9$/l | 0.02 | 0.00–0.10 |
| Basophils | $\times 10^9$/l | 0.03 | 0.00–0.09 |
| Thrombocytes | $\times 10^9$/l | 8* | 1–5 |

* Abnormal values outside reference range.
AST = aspartate aminotransferase; CK = creatinine kinase; LDH = lactate dehydrogenase; MCV = mean corpuscular volume; MCHC = mean corpuscular haemoglobin concentration; MCH = mean corpuscular haemoglobin

## Other diagnostic tests which could have been performed

Cloacal swabs or wash for microscopy/culture (for endoparasites, enteric infection), ultrasound, coelioscopy.

The history was suggestive of a gastrointestinal foreign body, although other pathological processes could also be concurrent. The diagnosis was supported by the positive radiographic findings.

## DIAGNOSIS

The diagnosis in this case was that of gastrointestinal foreign body. The clinical signs of inappetence and hindlimb paresis were attributed to intestinal discomfort. Dehydration likely developed with the reduced appetite.

Radiodense foreign bodies are relatively easy to detect on radiography. Obstruction is often accompanied by an enlargement of the intestinal diameter. Obstructive ileus presents as gas-distended portions of intestine, which can usually be seen on both the dorso-ventral and lateral (impinging the lung region dorsally) radiographs. Contrast studies (e.g. barium sulphate, water-soluble iodinated media, or barium-impregnated polyethylene spheres, BIPS) may be required to outline a non-radiodense object. Other imaging techniques may be useful, for example ultrasound and MRI.

## ANATOMY AND PHYSIOLOGY REFRESHER

### Gastrointestinal tract

The chelonian oesophagus passes on the left-hand side of the neck (Fig. 16.2). The stomach is simple and fusiform, positioned caudal to the liver on the left with the pylorus centrally or to the right. Thick folds at the cardia in *Testudo* spp act like a sphincter; there may be a muscular sphincter at the pylorus. The small intestine is not well divided into sections, and lies caudally in the coelom. There is a muscular valve between the duodenum and caecum, caudally on the right. The large intestine consists of ascending, transverse and descending colon. The colon empties into the coprodeum of the cloaca, and thence material is voided via the vent. Various membranes and ligaments suspend the intestines, restricting movement of some parts of the gastrointestinal tract and permitting others to move more freely (e.g. the transverse colon can move dorso-ventrally, and heavy ingested material commonly becomes trapped in this region owing to gravity).

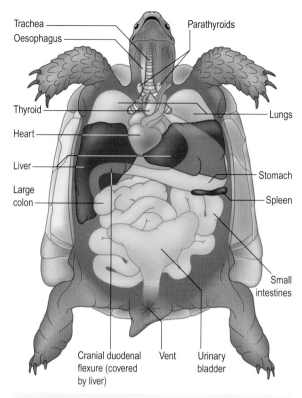

Trachea
Oesophagus
Parathyroids
Thyroid
Heart
Liver
Large colon
Lungs
Stomach
Spleen
Small intestines
Cranial duodenal flexure (covered by liver)
Vent
Urinary bladder

**Figure 16.2** The ventral view of viscera within the chelonian coelomic cavity.

## Nutrition

Mediterranean tortoises such as this Hermann's require a diet high in slowly digestable carbohydrate and fibre, along with appropriate vitamins and minerals. The energy density in the diet of free-ranging animals is fairly low, and they are browsers of herbaceous plants. It can be difficult to mimic this diet in captivity, and deficiencies or excesses may lead to disease in the gastrointestinal tract as well as systemically (e.g. in bone growth and shell formation).

Free-ranging animals have been reported to ingest bones and soil, presumably for dietary supplementation, e.g. of calcium and sodium. Some animals appear predisposed to this activity, possibly relating to nutritional imbalances.

## AETIOPATHOGENESIS AND EPIDEMIOLOGY

Predisposing factors include:
- Access to inappropriate substrate, particularly if liable to be ingested along with food during normal feeding.
- Inadequate provision for calcium metabolism (including dietary calcium deficiency and lack of UV-B light). Animals with husbandry inadequacies such as inappropriate nutrition with mineral deficiencies may be predisposed to pica. Although female chelonia are more likely to require higher levels of minerals such as calcium (for reproduction), no sex predilection for ingestion of foreign items has been reported.
- Dehydration due to lack of water source/bathing or low environmental humidity.

Common foreign bodies ingested are small stones/gravel, pieces of metal, pottery, woody material, and coal. Where metal objects are detected, blood should be assayed for toxic heavy metals such as lead and zinc. Sand impaction after substrate ingestion has been reported in Aldabran (*Dipsochelys elephantina*) and Galapagos (*Chelonoidis nigra*) tortoises. Female tortoises may be more likely to ingest white material during folliculogenesis (e.g. bone or broken pottery). Semi-aquatic animals appear predisposed to ingestion of gravel substrate, e.g. red-eared sliders (*Trachemys scripta*). An intussusception may form after foreign body obstruction in the intestinal tract, and in some cases this may slough and be passed. It should be remembered that a small amount of intestinal foreign material may be an incidental finding on radiography.

Intestinal intussusception results in some cases, and volvulus has also been reported with foreign material in the intestines.

Clinical signs with intestinal obstruction are often vague, including anorexia and listlessness. Other signs that may be seen include regurgitation, dyschezia (with the animal extending the hindlegs and elevating the plastron caudally) and haematochezia. Dehydration, weight loss, cachexia and generalized debility worsen with chronicity. Anaemia and leucocytosis may be present on haematology; hepatic and muscle enzymes may be elevated, and electrolyte abnormalities seen on serum biochemistry – although none of these changes were present in this case.

Metal or mineral materials are easily visualized on plain radiographs. Contrast studies may be required to outline rubber or plastic materials – repeating exposures over several days or weeks to follow passage of contrast through the slow gastrointestinal transit time. Other imaging modalities such as ultrasound, CT and MRI may be useful.

## TREATMENT

The tortoise was in good body condition, and reacted normally to examination. After discussing options with the owner, medical therapy was embarked upon.

### Fluids

Several routes of fluid administration are used in tortoises, and systemic and oral rehydration is advocated in cases of intestinal obstruction. Intracoelomic fluids were administered (Box 16.1), at a rate of 15 ml/kg of warmed Jarchow's solution (this is an isotonic solution, comprising a 1 : 1 : 1 mix of sterile saline, water for injection, and Hartmann's solution). Nutritional support was given in the form of a dextrose/amino acid solution (Critical Care Formula®, Vetark, Winchester) at 15 ml/kg via gavage tube (Box 16.2).

> **BOX 16.1   TECHNIQUE: INTRACOELOMIC INJECTION IN A TORTOISE**
>
> - Patient restrained in dorsal recumbency with right side slightly elevated – allowing viscera to drop away from the body wall under gravity. Right hindlimb pulled caudally
> - Skin in right prefemoral fossa is surgically prepared
> - Needle is inserted at 30–45° angle, and aspirated to check not in intestinal lumen (ventrally) or lung (dorsally)
> - Fluids should always be warmed before administration.
>
> **Advantages**
>
> - Rapid absorption of fluids.
>
> **Disadvantages**
>
> - Risk of accidental visceral penetration and subsequent adhesion (or drowning if lung punctured).

The owner bathed the tortoise once daily for 10–20 minutes in shallow tepid water, to stimulate drinking and defaecation, and possibly peristalsis. This also allows water absorption via the cloaca. Any faeces passed were examined for the presence of the foreign body.

### Prokinetics

Metoclopramide was administered (1 mg/kg PO q24hr) to stimulate gastrointestinal motility (although the effectiveness of motility agents in tortoises is not proven).

> **BOX 16.2   TECHNIQUE: GAVAGE FEEDING A TORTOISE**
>
> - An assistant holds the patient, restraining the forelimbs (Fig. 15.2b).
> - Hold the head bilaterally caudal to the skull.
> - Use a finger (or wooden gag) to depress the mandible. A finger from the hand restraining the head can be placed into the caudal angle of the jaw to keep the mouth open.
> - Pre-measure the length of the rubber tubing (metal crop tubes may also be used) (Fig. 16.3) to mid-way along the plastron (i.e. at the level of the stomach), and lubricate the tip. Insert the tube laterally into the mouth and pass smoothly into the oesophagus to the appropriate distance.
> - Inject the contents of the syringe steadily, stopping if regurgitation is seen.
> - Hold the tortoise upright for 30–60 seconds after the procedure to minimize regurgitation.
> - Always pre-warm fluids (e.g. water, electrolyte solution, puréed food) before administration.
> - <15 ml/kg can be administered at a time.
>
> **Advantages**
>
> - Large volumes can be administered rapidly, including nutritionally rich fluids.
> - Some owners may be able to perform this technique for nursing at home.
> - Good technique for rehydration in mild–moderate illness.
>
> **Disadvantages**
>
> - Require functioning gastrointestinal tract for absorption. Insufficient as sole method of rehydration in debilitated animals.
> - Usually not possible in un-sedated large animals, or in certain species (e.g. sulcata or leopard tortoises) that are resistant to oral examination.
> - Risk of mandibular or maxillary damage in animals with metabolic bone disease.

### Other aspects of management

It is important to address underlying causes and optimize husbandry conditions in sick reptiles. In this case, the owner was advised to keep the tortoise within the vivarium, where the environmental temperature could be controlled and maintained at the species' preferred optimal temperature range (POTR). This was particularly important as gastrointestinal motility is greatly affected by temperature. Appropriate nutrition of high fibre content and low energy density (predominantly weeds such as dandelions, clover, vetch and plantain) was advised, to stimulate normal gastrointestinal function. The tortoise was no longer permitted access to gravel substrate.

## NURSING ASPECTS

Supportive care of this tortoise was the cornerstone of successful treatment. Although the owner was able to administer some medication, gavage feeding was not easy in this strong animal. Some patients may benefit from a period of hospitalization for this, or placement of an oesophagostomy feeding tube (Box 16.3) to permit easier administration of fluids and medication.

## CLINICAL TIPS

- The owner should be made aware at the outset that treatment of reptiles is often prolonged. Alteration of the patient's condition may necessitate a change of treatment. It is advisable to explain this and to discuss possible treatments and outcomes at the initial consultation, and to impress on the owner the requirement for regular monitoring.
- Involve the owner in nursing care if possible. Many are able to gavage-feed tortoises (particularly placid species such as *Testudo* species) once the technique has been demonstrated. Daily bathing in shallow tepid water is an excellent method of rehydration, as tortoises will absorb water via their cloaca.

## OTHER TREATMENT OPTIONS

### Analgesia

If discomfort is suspected, some cases respond well to analgesia. However, little work on analgesics in chelonia has been reported. Opioids such as butorphanol (0.2–1.0 mg/kg IM q12hr) may be useful. NSAIDs have also

### BOX 16.3   TECHNIQUE: OESOPHAGOSTOMY TUBE PLACEMENT IN A TORTOISE

- Deep sedation (e.g. medetomidine, ± ketamine) or brief general anaesthesia (e.g. propofol, alfaxalone) is usually required, unless the animal is severely debilitated, along with appropriate analgesia (e.g. local anaesthetic injected at the skin incision site).
- Pre-measure and mark a soft, long feeding tube from the neck to the stomach (half-way down the plastron), and pre-fill with water (noting the volume required for future flushing).
- Aseptically prepare the skin on the lateral neck.
- Introduce long curved haemostat forceps into the oral cavity, and use to tent the oesophagus to the skin on the caudo-lateral neck. Make a small incision through both skin and oesophagus to allow the tip of the forceps to exit.
- Grasp the tip of the feeding tube and pull it out of the oral cavity.
- Re-position the forceps grasp, and redirect the tube into the oesophagus towards the stomach. Advance the tube to the pre-measured mark.
- Use a finger-trap suture to attach the tube to the skin on the neck (Fig. 16.4).
- Visualizing with an auroscope or rigid endoscope in the proximal oesophagus can check positioning proximally, and a radiograph can ascertain whether the tip of the tube lies in the distal oesophagus.

#### Advantages

- Ease of administration of oral fluids and medications, making nursing much easier and less stressful for the patient.
- Can be left *in situ* for several weeks.
- Patient can eat around tube.

#### Disadvantages

- Risk of abscess formation at skin incision site (rare).

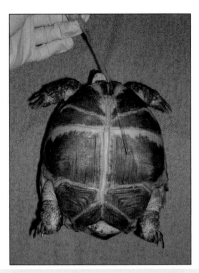

**Figure 16.3** Measurement of the tube to the location of the stomach before gavage in a tortoise.

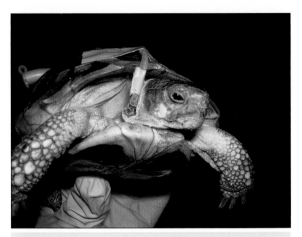

**Figure 16.4** Oesophagostomy tube placed in a tortoise.

been anecdotally reported (e.g. carprofen 2–4 mg/kg IM/SC/PO q24–72hr, meloxicam 0.2 mg/kg PO/SC q24hr), but, as in other species, care should be taken in cases of gastrointestinal disease since ulceration may be induced.

## Gastric protectants

Although their effects are not proven in reptiles, an antacid such as cimetidine (4 mg/kg PO/IM q8–12hr) or protective barrier such as sucralfate (0.5–1.0 g/kg PO q6–12hr) may be helpful if gastrointestinal damage is present.

## Other medication

Enemas (e.g. warm water) may be useful, particularly for obstructions in the distal colon. Lactulose is an orally administered osmotic laxative, and may help. If endoparasites are present (detected on faecal microscopy), they should be treated with appropriate anthelmintics. If faeces are not passed, a cloacal wash can be used to obtain a sample for analysis – cloacal washing with warm water is also a method of rehydration. Oral lactulose (0.5 ml/kg q24hr), administered by gavage or oesophagostomy tube, may assist with rehydration of gastrointestinal contents by osmotic diuresis.

## Endoscopic retrieval

Usually this is only possible if the object(s) is still within the oesophagus or stomach, but more difficult if it is further distal in the gastrointestinal tract.

## Exploratory coeliotomy with enterotomy

Indications for surgery include a poor response to the medical management as described above, or if imaging suggests complete gastrointestinal obstruction (e.g. no change in ileus patterns on radiography after 24 hours). In small- to medium-sized animals, a trans-plastron approach must be used (Box 16.4). Possible complications include bladder rupture and pericardial trauma (during osteotomy), haemorrhage, poor healing (often associated with inappropriate environmental conditions), wound dehiscence (of the enterotomy site as well as the shell), infection (including osteomyelitis of the plastron), postoperative ileus, adhesion formation. In large chelonia, a pre-femoral approach to the coelomic cavity may be possible, through the skin and abdominal musculature, and is associated with fewer complications. Closure of enterotomy incisions is via a routine two-layer continuous suture pattern, and the coelomic cavity is lavaged with warm saline before skin or plastron closure.

Supportive care and nursing is particularly important when surgery is required. Preoperative fluids, antibiotics (e.g. parenteral metronidazole and ceftazidime, or oral aminoglycosides such as neomycin or paromomycin) and analgesia should be administered as required.

## FOLLOW-UP

The tortoise was re-examined periodically over the following few months. He did not lose any weight or body condition, and remained strong and active throughout. His appetite improved but was variable over this time, in part due to seasonal sexual activity. If he did not eat for more than a few days, supportive care with oral and

## BOX 16.4 TECHNIQUE: TRANS-PLASTRON COELIOTOMY

- Patient is anaesthetized, and intubated to allow IPPV. Placed in dorsal recumbency.
- Aseptic preparation of plastron.
- Osteotomy in plastron using oscillating sagittal saw or high-speed circulating disc. Bevelled edges to ensure can lift flap up. Incisions in abdominal scutes: lateral incisions central to lateral (bone is thicker more laterally); caudal incision near caudal margin with femoral scutes; cranial incision just caudal to humeral scutes (heart lies at cross-section of humeral and abdominal scutes).
- Elevate flap caudally, separating abdominal musculature and ventral abdominal veins from plastron. Retain integrity of veins if possible (though often need to ligate one to increase access). Incise coelomic membrane to access coelomic cavity.
- Closure: continuous absorbable suture in coelomic membrane; plastron flap secured with epoxy resin (Fig. 16.5) or acrylic.

### Advantages

- Good access to coelomic cavity.

### Disadvantages

- Coelomic viscera compress lungs when in dorsal recumbency.
- Osteotomy required for access, with risk of vascular damage (to heart and bilateral ventral abdominal veins). Complications may occur with healing of plastron, e.g. associated with infection, or damage to plastron hinges in some species.

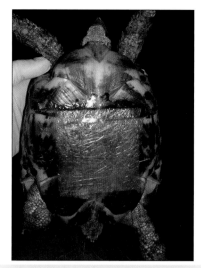

**Figure 16.5** Fibre-glass may be used to close a plastronotomy wound.

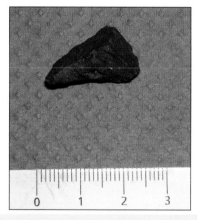

**Figure 16.6** Piece of gravel passed after 5 months (cm scale).

intracoelomic fluids was repeated. Metoclopramide was intermittently administered orally, but was associated with a fall in appetite (probably because of the medication flavour). Repeat radiographs every 4–8 weeks continued to show no evidence of ileus or obstruction. The piece of gravel was passed in normal faeces 5 months after initial presentation (Fig. 16.6).

## PREVENTION

Removing materials that may result in obstruction from tortoise enclosures, along with continuous close super-vision when in an outdoor area that has not been made 'tortoise-safe', can prevent future episodes.

## PROGNOSIS

Where chelonia with gastrointestinal foreign bodies can be medically managed until the object(s) is passed, the prognosis is good. If coeliotomy is required to remove the object(s), this is associated with an increased risk of complications and the prognosis is less good. If metal material is ingested, rapid retrieval is advised if heavy metal toxicity is diagnosed or suspected.

# Bearded dragon with hepatic disease

## INITIAL PRESENTATION

Reduced appetite in a bearded dragon.

## INTRODUCTION

Reptiles often present with vague clinical signs that may have many differential diagnoses, often with multi-factorial aetiologies. As ectotherms, their metabolism is slower than mammals and, as such, progression of disease (and resolution of problems) is more prolonged. This case took several months to resolve, requiring great commitment from the owner.

## CASE PRESENTING SIGNS

A 1-year-old male bearded dragon (*Pogona vitticeps*, Box 17.2) presented with a 2 week history of reduced appetite and dysecdysis, and 1 day of dyschezia.

## HUSBANDRY

The bearded dragon was housed in a large glass vivarium (1.4 × 0.6 × 0.8 m). The substrate was sand, although linoleum was used in the feeding area to reduce the risk of ingestion of sand and resultant gastrointestinal impaction. Cage furniture included a hide area (synthetic material) and wooden branches for climbing (sited near the basking lamp).

A ceramic bulb, attached to a thermostat, provided supplemental heating. A digital thermometer was used to monitor temperature variations, and showed an ambient temperature in the enclosure of 21°C with a basking temperature under the bulb of 35–41°C. A UV striplight was provided (Box 17.1), positioned approxi-

mately 30 cm above the substrate. The light cycle was routinely 12 hours/day.

The bearded dragon was fed on invertebrates (locusts and silk worms) and fresh vegetables (kale, butternut squash and spring greens). Invertebrates were fed on fruit and vegetables, and dusted with a calcium supplement daily. Vitamin supplements were added to food twice weekly. A shallow water bowl was provided but the animal was not seen drinking from it.

## CASE HISTORY

The owner acquired the bearded dragon from a pet-shop at approximately 1 month of age. Ecdysis occurred roughly every 10 weeks. Urine/urates/faeces were regularly passed every other day. Endoparasites (oxyurids) had previously been detected and treated (with fenbendazole) in the individual. There had been no recent changes in husbandry.

The current presenting complaints were:
- Reduced appetite for 2 weeks
- Dysecdysis, with intermittent shedding (skin lost piecemeal)
- Straining to pass faeces for 24 hours.

## CLINICAL EXAMINATION

Initial examination on presentation revealed:
- Good body condition (weight 540 g)
- Abdominal palpation: no abnormalities palpated, bilateral abdominal fat pads present (normal)
- Oral examination: no abnormalities detected
- No current dysecdysis.

## BOX 17.1 UV LIGHTING FOR REPTILES

- Most reptiles require access to ultraviolet light in the UV-B range, specifically 290–315 nm wavelength, for vitamin D synthesis. (Carnivorous species obtain vitamin D and calcium from the bones in their prey, and some herbivores may also absorb vitamin D from their diet.)
- Artificial UV lights for captive reptiles are usually in the form of a striplight or bulb, some of which also produce heat. These lights produce both visible light and light in the UV range.
- UV production wanes with the age of artificial lights, and it is recommended to replace most every 6–12 months. More accurately, a UV meter can be utilized to gauge UV output and determine when replacement is necessary.
- The lights are usually positioned approximately 12 inches (30 cm) above the reptile. Further away will greatly reduce the quantity of UV reaching the animal's skin and any closer may result in ocular damage.

## BOX 17.2 ECOLOGY OF BEARDED DRAGONS

- Central bearded dragons originate from Central Australia.
- Their native habitat is semi-arid or arid woodland, and rocky desert.
- They are mostly arboreal, and spend a large amount of time basking on branches or rocks.
- Head bobbing and colour change of the 'beard' (throat frill) are used for communication.
- Free-ranging bearded dragons are omnivorous. They mainly eat invertebrates, but may also consume small vertebrates. As they mature, they eat more plant material (e.g. green leaves, fruits, vegetables and flowers).
- Most water intake is via their food.
- Sexual maturity is reached at approximately 18 months of age. The female lays 5–30 eggs per clutch. Males develop prominent pre-femoral pores and bilateral swellings over the hemipenes caudal to the cloaca (Fig. 17.1).

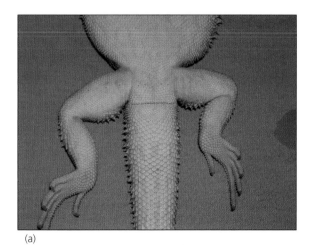

(a)

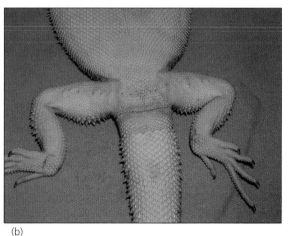

(b)

**Figure 17.1** (a) Cloacal region of a female bearded dragon. (b) Male bearded dragon with prominent pre-femoral pores and hemipenal bulges.

## DIFFERENTIAL DIAGNOSES

The differentials for *reduced appetite* are varied, but may commonly include the following in reptiles:

- Husbandry problems, e.g. inappropriate temperature (too hot or too cool), light or relative humidity
- Gastrointestinal obstruction, endoparasites, or enteritis
- Stomatitis, dental disease (common in captive bearded dragons), or other lesions resulting in oral discomfort
- Offering an inappropriate diet, e.g. herbivorous diet to a carnivore, feeding terrestrial species in a high location
- Hepatic disease, e.g. hepatic lipidosis
- Nutritional disease, e.g. hypocalcaemia, hypovitaminosis A
- Urogenital disease, e.g. renal failure, follicular stasis or egg retention
- Physiologically normal anorexia, e.g. males of certain species in the breeding season, gravid females, hibernation or aestivation, snakes during shedding
- Post-hibernation anorexia (chelonia)
- Respiratory disease, e.g. upper respiratory tract infection, rhinitis/sinusitis, pneumonia
- Metabolic disease
- Intra- or inter-specific aggression
- Viral infections, e.g. herpesvirus (chelonia), paramyxovirus (snakes)
- Sensual deprivation, e.g. blind (e.g. cataracts, corneal lipidosis), loss of smell (e.g. upper respiratory tract [URT] infection)
- Postoperative or post-traumatic 'stress'
- Psychological, e.g. excess noise, excessive handling (particularly shy specimens), disruptive light patterns, maladaption syndrome in wild-caught individuals, lack of a hide box for visual security
- Terminal neoplasia.

### The differentials for *dysecdysis* are

- Husbandry problems affecting the process of ecdysis
  - Excessive environmental temperature
  - Low relative humidity
  - Lack of rough surfaces to abrade skin

- Poor conditions such as overcrowding may result in immunosuppression, predisposing individuals to infection
- Dehydration
- Ectoparasites, e.g. mites, ticks
- Malnutrition, e.g. hypovitaminosis A (chameleons)
- Dermatitis, bacterial or fungal infection
- Scarring, e.g. from burns or other wounds.

### The differentials for *dyschezia* are

- Constipation (cloacolith or faecolith): owing to reduced gastrointestinal motility in association with hypocalcaemia (husbandry causes), dehydration, or an inappropriate diet
- Enteritis, e.g. endoparasitism, bacterial enteritis
- Poor husbandry, e.g. chronic low environmental temperature
- Gastrointestinal obstruction: foreign body (often substrate ingestion) or gastrolith, intussusception
- Cystic calculi
- Dystocia (females)
- Organomegaly resulting in a space-occupying lesion in the coelomic cavity, e.g. renomegaly with nephritis, abscess(es), neoplasia
- Narrow pelvic canal after trauma or MBD (metabolic bone disease)
- Lethargy.

## CASE WORK-UP

### Radiographs

Two projections were taken, a dorso-ventral view using a vertical beam and a lateral view using a horizontal beam (Fig. 17.2). Gas was present within the gastrointestinal tract, but there was no evidence of foreign bodies or other obstruction. There was a suspicion of respiratory disease, with patchy lung fields present (although no respiratory signs had been noted). Increased abdominal volume suggested the presence of faeces, a mass lesion or effusion. A lack of serosal detail precluded a clear picture of the gastrointestinal tract, and may have reflected the presence of fluid or inflammation.

### Blood sampling

The most reliable site for phlebotomy in most lizards is the ventral coccygeal vein (Fig. 17.3). Serial blood

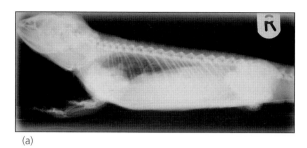

(a)

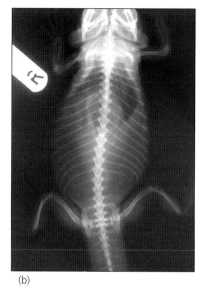

(b)

**Figure 17.2** (a) Lateral and (b) dorso-ventral radiographs of the bearded dragon. In the mid-coelomic cavity, the gas-filled stomach is visible, also seen as a gas-filled dome on the lateral view. The fat bodies appear hazy and further coelomic structures cannot be easily identified. The lung fields appear mildly patchy with uneven borders and the size of the lung fields appears reduced.

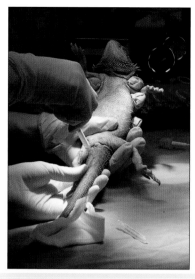

**Figure 17.3** Venepuncture in the ventral coccygeal vein in a bearded dragon, in this case to inject anaesthetic agent.

samples were taken to aid in making a diagnosis and to monitor the disease process (Table 17.1).

Many *enzymes* found in reptilian livers are found in other tissues, including ALP, ALT, AST, GGT and LDH. These are thus non-specific assays for hepatic damage. Simultaneously elevated CK usually indicates the alterations are due to muscular damage. GLDH (glutamate dehydrogenase) is a specific test for hepatic disease, but is not sensitive. As little hepatocellular damage occurs in hepatic lipidosis, the enzyme levels often remain normal in this condition. Bile acids may be a useful indicator of liver function, but the major bile acid varies with reptile taxonomic order and normal values are not reported for most species. Cholesterol and triglycerides may be elevated in hepatic lipidosis; both

may also be physiologically increased during normal vitellogenesis (females) and pre-hibernation (chelonia).

In this bearded dragon, CK was elevated on one occasion, likely associated with the trauma of restraint and phlebotomy. LDH was elevated when CK was within the normal range over a prolonged period, suggesting the presence of hepatic disease. An improvement was seen over time during treatment, although a normal level was not recorded (suggesting there was still some degree of hepatic change even over 1 year after treatment commenced).

Total *protein* levels often decrease with chronic hepatic disease (and other diseases). In this case, the values remained within the reference range except on one occasion, where dehydration likely resulted in hyperproteinaemia. Similarly, one would expect hypoalbuminaemia with chronic hepatic disease, but hyperalbuminaemia will be seen with dehydration.

*Potassium* fluctuated in the early course of treatment. Hyperkalaemia is usually the result of decreased renal secretion (e.g. where dehydration is present), but can be due to excessive dietary potassium intake or severe acidosis. Hypokalaemia is seen with inadequate dietary intake (e.g. with anorexia) or excessive gastrointestinal loss (e.g. with diarrhoea), but can be associated with severe alkalosis.

Changes in the *haematological* picture, including elevations in the haematocrit, likely relate to dehydration (considered in conjunction with the protein changes listed above). Red blood cells and haemoglobin levels

**Table 17.1** Serial blood sample results. (Not all parameters were tested at each time point).

| Parameter | Units | Reference range | Initial presentation | 1 month | 2 months | 3 months | 6 months | 9 months | 1 year 9 months |
|---|---|---|---|---|---|---|---|---|---|
| Total protein | g/l | 31–85 | 63.3 | 62.7 | 68.4 | 62.2 | 67.0 | – | 87.8* |
| Albumin | g/l | 13–46 | 41.0 | 40.1 | 48.1* | 47.7* | 49.4* | – | 54.2* |
| Globulin | g/l | 10–44 | 22.3 | 22.6 | 20.3 | 14.5 | 17.6 | – | 33.6 |
| Glucose | mmol/l | 6.5–23.1 | – | 8.26 | 8.25 | 9.69 | – | – | 10.12 |
| Calcium (total) | mmol/l | 1.78–14.00 | 3.11 | 3.24 | 3.74 | 3.29 | 3.97 | – | 4.67 |
| Phosphorus | mmol/l | 0.87–4.88 | 1.22 | 1.23 | 1.97 | 1.24 | 1.73 | – | 2.39 |
| Uric acid | μmol/l | 0–684 | 446 | 248 | 283 | 125 | 470 | – | 89 |
| Sodium | mmol/l | 137–186 | – | 148.8 | 149.6 | 151.8 | – | – | 159.5 |
| Potassium | mmol/l | 1.3–6.3 | – | 7.64* | 0.63* | 5.39 | – | – | 0.45* |
| Amylase | U/l | | – | – | – | – | – | – | 1170 |
| CK (creatinine kinase) | U/l | 59–7000 | 8220* | 1701 | 906 | 2000 | 1488 | – | 217 |
| ALP (alkaline phosphatase) | U/l | 15–447 | – | – | – | 795* | – | – | – |
| ALT (alanine aminotransferase) | U/l | 4–20 | – | – | – | 9 | – | – | – |
| AST (aspartate amino- transferase) | U/l | 0–92 | 56 | 52 | 36 | 35 | 50 | – | 17 |

**Table 17.1** Serial blood sample results. *continued*

| Parameter | Units | Reference range | Initial presentation | 1 month | 2 months | 3 months | 6 months | 9 months | 1 year 9 months |
|---|---|---|---|---|---|---|---|---|---|
| GGT (γ-glutamyl-transferase) | U/l | 0–81 | – | – | – | – | – | – | 1 |
| LDH (lactate dehydrogenase) | U/l | 35–628 | – | 2063* | 1691* | 1542* | – | 1859* | 925* |
| Bile acids | μmol/l | <60 | – | – | – | 3 | – | – | – |
| Cholesterol | mmol/l | 4.14–23.31 | – | – | – | 5.74 | – | – | – |
| Total bilirubin | μmol/l | 0–63 | – | – | – | 2.2 | – | – | – |
| Triglycerides | mmol/l | 1.05–5.19 | – | – | – | 0.42* | – | – | – |
| Comment on sample | | | Icteric | Icteric | Icteric | Icteric | Icteric | Icteric | Icteric |
| Haemoglobin | g/dl | 6.7–12.0 | 12.8* | 12.8* | 12.6* | 12.8* | 14.0* | – | 15.1* |
| Haematocrit | l/l | 0.19–0.40 | 0.37 | 0.37 | 0.42* | 0.39 | 0.40 | – | 0.47* |
| Red blood cells | ×10$^{12}$/l | 0.68–1.21 | 1.44* | 1.42* | 1.35* | 1.36* | 1.55* | – | 1.61* |
| MCV (mean corpuscular volume) | fl | 236.4–397.1 | 256.9 | 260.6 | 311.1 | 286.8 | 258.1 | – | 291.9 |
| MCHC (mean cell haemoglobin concentration) | g/dl | 23.9–44.7 | 34.6 | 34.6 | 30.0 | 32.8 | 35.0 | – | 32.1 |
| MCH (mean corpuscular haemoglobin) | pg | 80.6–139.7 | 88.9 | 90.1 | 93.3 | 94.1 | 90.3 | – | 93.8 |

**Table 17.1** Serial blood sample results. *continued*

| Parameter | Units | Reference range | Initial presentation | 1 month | 2 months | 3 months | 6 months | 9 months | 1 year 9 months |
|---|---|---|---|---|---|---|---|---|---|
| White blood cells (WBC) | ×10⁹/l | 2.0–23.0 | 3.0 | 5.3 | 7.5 | 2.3 | 2.0 | – | 5.1 |
| Heterophils | ×10⁹/l | 0.35–4.99 | 1.5 | 1.54 | 1.13 | 0.32* | 0.40 | – | 1.84 |
| Lymphocytes | ×10⁹/l | 0.57–17.00 | 0.12* | 3.18 | 4.95 | 1.24 | 1.34 | – | 1.63 |
| Eosinophils | ×10⁹/l | 0.06–0.27 | 0.21 | 0.00 | 0.08 | 0.00* | 0.02* | – | 0.05* |
| Monocytes | ×10⁹/l | 0.03–2.72 | 0.09 | 0.00 | 0.15 | 0.00* | 0.00* | – | 0.26 |
| Azurophils | ×10⁹/l | 0.04–1.84 | 0.63 | 0.21 | 0.53 | 0.05 | 0.02* | – | 0.77 |
| Basophils | ×10⁹/l | 0.05–1.01 | 0.45 | 0.37 | 0.68 | 0.69 | 0.22 | – | 0.56 |
| Thrombocytes | ×10⁹/l | | 13 | 28 | 17 | 8 | 6 | – | 19 |
| Comment on blood smear | | | Red cells appear normal. Slight lymphopenia. Some heterophils partially degranulated | Approximately 75% red cells contain inclusion (similar to Pirhemocyton/iridovirus/degenerate organelle), otherwise they appear normal. WBC morphology appears normal | Approximately 90% red cells contain inclusions, otherwise they appear normal. Heterophils show part degranulation | Approximately 50% red cells contain inclusions, otherwise they appear normal. WBC morphology appears normal | Red cells slight degree of polychromasia. Approximately 90% red ells show inclusions. WBC morphology appears normal | – | Approximately 50% red cells contain inclusions, otherwise they appear normal. WBC morphology appears normal |

* Values outside the reference range.
ALP = alkaline phosphatase; ALT = alanine aminotransferase; AST = aspartate aminotransferase; GGT = γ-glutamyl transferase (or gamma-glutamyl transferase); LDH = lactate dehydrogenase; CK = creatinine kinase; GLDH = glutamate dehydrogenase.

usually decrease with chronic disease. Anaemia in chronic hepatopathy may mask fluid deficits. Hyperuricaemia may be seen during severe dehydration, but production in the liver is reduced with hepatic disease; these factors probably cancelled each other out and resulted in a normal uric acid level in this case.

A heterophilia and monocytosis (including azurophilia) are usually present if acute hepatic inflammation or necrosis exists. However, chronic cases may show minimal changes in the haematological parameters; the latter is likely in this case. Some heterophil degranulation was noted at the start of treatment but this resolved over time, suggesting that any inflammation or necrosis was settling. Although the total white cell count remained within the normal range, relative reductions were seen periodically with individual cell lines (i.e. heteropenia, lymphopenia, eosinopenia, and monocytopenia); these may have related to immunosuppression associated with chronic disease.

## Ultrasound

The abdominal region was initially scanned with the patient conscious. The liver was enlarged and hyperechoic. Tubular structures within the liver parenchyma did not show flow on Doppler examination, and were thought to be distended intrahepatic bile ducts. The gall bladder was enlarged with hyperechoic margins and had a tortuous neck; this suggested some biliary tract stasis was present. The stomach was mainly empty and its continuation into the duodenum could be demonstrated. A rounded, fluid-filled structure was visible superficially in the cranial abdomen; this may have been an accumulation of abdominal fluid between the liver lobes.

A repeat examination was performed later in the day after the bearded dragon had passed faeces. The gall bladder was hardly visible, but some of the hyperechoic material remained. Administration of propofol (15 mg/kg IV, into the ventral coccygeal vein) produced sufficient sedation to enable a fine needle aspirate (FNA) to be taken of the liver. Aspiration of the abdominal fluid was not possible under the sedation.

### Cytology of liver FNA

Medium-sized hepatocytes had moderate amounts of basophilic cytoplasm containing multiple small vacuoles, considered an excessive amount. The hepatocytes had indistinct cell boundaries and a central to eccentric nucleus with smooth chromatin. The background contained numerous variably sized fat globules throughout, as well as moderate numbers of red blood cells, nude nuclei cells and cell debris. There were also small numbers

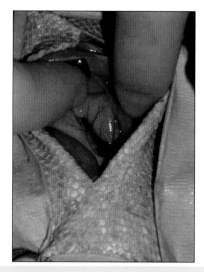

**Figure 17.4** Yellow appearance to liver seen at exploratory coeliotomy in a bearded dragon. This is suggestive of hepatic lipidosis (but histology is required to confirm the diagnosis).

of segmented heterophils and scattered groups of normal-looking thrombocytes.

Based on the cytology, a diagnosis was made of moderate hepatic lipidosis. A liver biopsy was suggested to determine the severity of the disease (but the owner declined) (Fig. 17.4).

## OTHER POSSIBLE INVESTIGATIONS

Contrast radiographs can be taken (after barium or iodine-based contrast has been administered by gavage) to assess the gastrointestinal tract more fully. Coelioscopy or exploratory coeliotomy may be indicated after non-invasive imaging modalities. These techniques will enable direct visualization of organs, and sampling for further tests such as histology and culture.

Urinalysis may be useful, although normal ranges for most parameters have not been reported for many reptiles.

The respiratory tract can be further assessed using endoscopy and/or performing a lung wash (obtaining samples for cytology and culture).

If dysecdysis is considered a major problem, investigation should include a full assessment of husbandry conditions. The integument should be thoroughly checked for ectoparasites. Any moist lesions should be cultured. Virology testing, using histology and molecular techniques, may be appropriate as some viruses cause dermal lesions.

## DIAGNOSIS

- Hepatic lipidosis
- Gastrointestinal malabsorption may have been present secondary to the previous endoparasitism noted, or associated with the hepatic disease.

## ANATOMY AND PHYSIOLOGY REFRESHER

Lizards do not have a diaphragm, although the positioning of organs is quite similar to that in mammals. For this reason, lateral radiographs should be taken using a horizontal X-ray beam (local radiological safety requirements permitting), as tilting the lizard on its side will alter the anatomical positioning of the internal organs.

The lungs lie dorsally and in the cranial portion of the coelomic cavity. The heart in most lizards is situated quite cranially near the thoracic inlet (it is more caudal in monitor lizards).

The liver is ventro-caudal to the lungs, and the rest of the intestinal tract lies caudal to the liver. Reptile livers are similar to mammalian organs, usually with a gall bladder present. Hepatic functions are also similar, including fat, protein and glycogen metabolism, and production of uric acid and clotting factors. The gastrointestinal tract of omnivorous reptiles is relatively simple. The oesophagus enters the tubular stomach on the left of the body, and the gastrointestinal tract proceeds into the short small intestine and large intestine. Bearded dragons have bilateral intracoelomic fat bodies as an energy store.

The kidneys are found dorsally in the coelomic space (Fig. 17.5), and in many species are intra-pelvic. Many reptiles do not possess a urinary bladder.

### CLINICAL TIP

The skin and mucous membranes of bearded dragons are normally yellow-orange in colour. However, prehepatic or hepatic icterus may result in jaundice, with further yellowing of the membranes.

## AETIOPATHOGENESIS OF HEPATIC LIPIDOSIS

Hepatic lipidosis is a metabolic derangement, associated with a variety of factors (Boxes 17.3 and 17.4). It is often associated with an excessively fatty diet (e.g. waxworm-based), or in animals that become obese due to inactivity. The disease is usually chronic, and onset of clinical signs is usually gradual (although signs may appear acute in onset associated with periods of high metabolic demand such as breeding). Other disease problems, such as dietary imbalances, toxins, or any causes of anorexia may secondarily lead to hepatic lipidosis.

### BOX 17.3 CAUSES OF HEPATIC LIPIDOSIS IN REPTILES

- Obesity
  - Excessively fatty diet
  - Inactivity
  - Non-breeding females
- Secondary to other illness, e.g. dietary imbalance (impaired metabolism of carbohydrate and volatile fatty acids), toxins, anorexia.

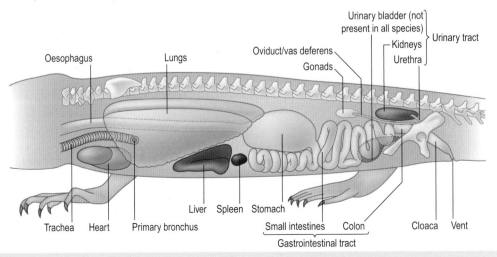

**Figure 17.5** Lateral view of lizard anatomy (coelomic cavity) – compare with lateral radiograph on page 141.

It is very useful for owners to monitor and record their pet reptile's dietary intake and weight. Gradual changes may otherwise be missed until the animal is severely ill.

The liver is usually swollen with rounded edges. Other organ changes may be seen on imaging the coelomic cavity, potentially those with pathologies that predisposed the hepatic lipidosis.

Blood analysis may be useful in diagnosing hepatic disease, but is currently insensitive and non-specific. Radiography may permit crude assessment of liver size and shape, but ultrasound is more accurate (e.g. detecting a generalized hyperechoic appearance in severe cases of hepatic lipidosis). Other modalities that can be used to image the liver include endoscopy, computed tomography (CT) and magnetic resonance imaging (MRI). Liver biopsy (performed under ultrasound guidance, coelioscopy, or coeliotomy) provides the best tool for diagnosing and monitoring hepatic disease, permitting histology and culture of liver tissue.

## BOX 17.4    DEFINITION OF HEPATIC LIPIDOSIS

- Small fat droplets that are normally found in cytoplasm are associated with 'fatty change', and are not necessarily hepatic lipidosis *per se*.
- Hepatic lipidosis is defined as 'excessive accumulation of lipid within hepatocytes'.

## EPIDEMIOLOGY

Hepatic disease, particularly hepatic lipidosis, is common in captive reptiles. Adult to aged non-breeding females appear to be predisposed, presumably associated with obesity in captivity due to a lack of breeding after cycles of lipogenesis.

## TREATMENT

### Supportive care

Any ill reptile should be maintained in an appropriate environment. Therefore any husbandry inadequacies should be corrected. It is particularly important to ensure that the species-specific preferred optimum temperature

range (POTR) is provided, enabling the animal to select a preferred body temperature (PBT). During hospitalization, the reptile was housed in a vivarium with supplemental heating at the species' POTR and UV-B lighting. For bearded dragons the background temperature should be 24–29°C during the day, and maintained above 13°C overnight. A daytime basking spot of 35–41°C should be provided.

The bearded dragon was bathed in shallow warm water for 10–15 minutes twice daily; this encourages reptiles to drink and to void urine/urates/faeces. Electrolyte solutions may be used for this bath, although care should be taken to rinse solution from the animal afterwards, so as not to encourage superficial growth of pathogens.

### Nutritional support

This involved administration of vegetable baby food (organic and dairy-free) and crushed invertebrates (a total of 10 ml/kg was administered by gavage tube q8hr). Gavage-feeding was demonstrated to the owner, who continued this at home for a period of weeks. The bearded dragon was also offered various fresh chopped vegetables and live foods to tempt him to self-feed.

Do not leave live invertebrates in the vivarium unsupervised with debilitated reptiles. The invertebrates may attack the reptile, resulting in skin lesions.

### Gavage-feeding lizards

- Commercial tubes are available, or a piece of giving set tubing may be used. A soft tube can be used providing a gag is employed to prevent the animal biting through the tube. Lubricate the tube, particularly in dehydrated animals.
- Use a wooden tongue depressor wrapped in non-adhesive elastic wrap as a mouth gag. This enables the mouth to be held open without damaging the teeth.
- Pre-measure the tube to the mid-body level.
- Pass the tube laterally in the oropharynx to avoid the glottis that lies midline at the base of the tongue.
- If resistance is felt, withdraw the tube, re-lubricate, and re-insert.

## Medication

An anabolic steroid injection was administered (nandrolone, see below), as an appetite and metabolic stimulant. Hepatic support was given over a period of months in the form of a nutritional supplement containing S-adenosylmethionine (SAMe) and vitamin K1 (at the same dose as that used for cats), and lactulose (0.5 ml/kg PO q24h). Metoclopramide (0.05 mg/kg PO q24hr) was given as a gastrointestinal prokinetic until faecal frequency and consistency were more normal. Antibiotics were also dispensed: enrofloxacin (5 mg/kg PO q24hr for 6 weeks) and metronidazole (40 mg/kg PO q24hr for 1 week).

## Husbandry

Optimization of husbandry conditions, including the environment and diet, are important constituents of treatment for this condition. This should also reduce recurrence of problems. Temperature ranges were monitored closely and recorded. Invertebrates containing higher levels of fat (e.g. mealworms) were avoided in the diet.

## TREATMENT OPTIONS AND MANAGEMENT

### Fluid therapy

The route of fluid administration depends on how ill the animal is. Oral fluids can be utilized for mild to moderate cases of dehydration that are in good body condition. Intravenous, intracoelomic or intraosseous fluids should be given in severe cases. Avoid solutions containing lactate.

### Nutritional support

Administration of convalescent diets may be done via gavage-feeding in the short term. For longer term nutritional support, use of an oesophagostomy tube should be considered.

### Other medications

Carnitine is thought to improve hepatic metabolism of fat. Some references suggest dosing 250 mg/kg carnitine daily when assist-feeding reptiles.

Choline is thought to promote conversion of hepatic fat to phospholipids, which are rapidly transferred into blood, and is also involved in lipoprotein synthesis. Methionine is a precursor of choline. Some reports suggest adding choline at 40–50 mg/kg to feeds daily.

Thyroxine (20 mg/kg PO q48hr) and the anabolic steroid nandrolone (0.5–5 mg/kg IM q7–28 days) may improve hepatic metabolism of fat, reduce catabolism, and improve appetite.

### NURSING ASPECTS

- Fluid therapy:
  - Oral fluids may be used in mildly (<5%) dehydrated animals with a functional gastrointestinal tract. Owing to the poor blood supply, absorption from the subcutaneous site is slow.
  - Patients with moderate to severe dehydration should be given fluids intracoelomically, intravenously, or intraosseously.
  - Warm fluids to 30–35°C before administration.
  - Isotonic crystalloids are used to replace fluid loss. Avoid fluid types with lactate in animals with hepatic disease.
- Nutritional support:
  - Consider the animal's energy and nutritional needs.
  - Consider natural dietary preference, e.g. omnivorous.
  - Use natural foods if possible over artificial substitutes, especially for long-term cases.

## FOLLOW-UP

The bearded dragon improved well over a period of 6 months. In the initial few weeks, his appetite, weight and demeanour were extremely variable, and the owner assist-fed him most days. After that period, the animal's appetite improved and he maintained his body condition. At times, the owner was able to administer the nutritional supplements on food.

Blood testing was performed at regular intervals to assess progress, but as discussed above these are not very sensitive or specific in reptiles. It would have been useful to monitor progress using sequential assessment of liver architecture, utilizing cytology on FNAs or histology on biopsy samples. However, the costs associated with the laboratory fees and the risks associated with anaesthesia precluded this option.

## PREVENTION

Avoidance of the risk factors listed above will reduce the occurrence or recurrence of hepatic lipidosis. As with many diseases of pet reptiles, husbandry problems must be corrected to allow a cure to be effected.

## PROGNOSIS

Although the liver is capable of regeneration from quite severe insults, recovery is prolonged. Reptile metabolism is also much slower than that of mammals, and is dependent on environmental temperature, so a return to normal function will take comparatively longer. Treatment should not be stopped too soon.

# 18 Osteomyelitis in a Hermann's tortoise

## INITIAL PRESENTATION

Nail loss in a Hermann's tortoise.

## INTRODUCTION

Reptilian metabolism is slower than that of mammals. Pathological processes therefore usually develop (and heal) much more slowly, resulting in a longer course of the disease and treatment. An accurate diagnosis aids greatly in selection of treatment, which is often of necessity protracted.

## CASE PRESENTING SIGNS

A 53-year-old male Hermann's tortoise (*Testudo hermanni*) (Box 18.1) presented with loss of nails (onychomadesis) from both forefeet.

## HUSBANDRY

The tortoise had been in the owner's family in Scotland for over three decades. During the previous 20 years, he had been housed in an outdoor pen during the day and in a greenhouse overnight. At the time of presentation, he was housed mainly indoors, roaming in the house during the day and returned to a plastic container measuring approximately 1 × 0.25 m overnight. The substrate in the indoor enclosure was a mixture of newspaper and towel. An outdoor pen was used for daytime housing during good weather.

A heat lamp was present, but used only intermittently. The owner did not measure the environmental temperature. No supplemental UV lighting was provided.

The tortoise's diet was mainly mixed salad (lettuce, tomatoes and cucumber) and fruit (pears and satsuma oranges), and he also had access to various weeds (e.g. dandelions) in his outdoor pen. Water was provided in a shallow bowl, and the tortoise was bathed weekly to encourage drinking.

The tortoise had previously been hibernated, but not during recent years.

## CASE HISTORY

Two years prior to presentation, the tortoise had sustained trauma to both forefeet from rough substrate, resulting in small abrasions that were treated with topical antiseptic solution (povidone–iodine) and appeared to resolve.

More recently, the tortoise had lost some nails from the forefeet. The owner did not notice any other abnormalities. No changes were noted in appetite or activity.

## CLINICAL EXAMINATION

Mediterranean species of tortoise are relatively easy to examine conscious, and the tortoise received a full clinical examination. Findings were as follows:
- Bright, alert and reactive
- Good body condition with well-muscled limbs and no evidence of oedema. Weight 1.95 kg, with a straight carapacial length (SCL) of 18 cm
- No ocular, nasal or oral lesions. Mucous membranes pink, with no evidence of stomatitis
- Carapace and plastron unremarkable

## BOX 18.1 ECOLOGY OF HERMANN'S TORTOISES

- Hermann's tortoises have a wide distribution throughout the Mediterranean and Eastern Europe.
- They are generally solitary, except during the breeding season.
- The IUCN has identified Hermann's tortoises as Lower Risk/Near Threatened, although the Western subspecies *Testudo hermanni* ssp *hermanni* is classed as Endangered. Hermann's are listed with other Testudinae on CITES Appendix I, restricting their trade.
- They live in evergreen Mediterranean oak forest (though this habitat is now rare), coarse arid scrub and hillsides.
- In captivity, the species tolerates an arid to moderately damp environment, but requires plenty of warmth and sun. Heating and UV-B lighting should be supplemented in more temperate climes.
- Their free-ranging diet is herbaceous and succulent plants.
- Captive individuals should be fed a wide range of weeds and green vegetation. Edible plants include: dandelion, sow thistle, plantains, vetch, mallows, clovers, grapevine leaves, succulents (e.g. *Sedum* spp and *Aloe vera* spp), *Hibiscus* spp, *Rubus* spp (raspberry and blackberry), dead-nettles and bindweeds. When available, edible flowers from the above plants as well as honeysuckle are appreciated. Although fruits are well accepted, only small quantities (<5% of the diet) should be allowed. Salads are a poor substitute for the free-ranging diet. Animal protein (e.g. dog/cat food) should not be fed.
- Tortoises may live up to 100 years.

- Limb examination:
  - No obvious lameness
  - Forelimbs: firm swellings of both feet, loss of all nails, skin smoothed with some scale loss, some inflammation and erythema ventrally on distal limbs, feet swollen and firm
  - Hindlimbs: obvious stifles, possibly abnormally swollen. Nails present and no swellings on feet.

## DIFFERENTIAL DIAGNOSES

The differentials for *limb swelling* were:
- Infection – abscess or osteomyelitis, aetiological agents may include bacteria (including mycobacteria) and fungi
- Granuloma
- Intra-articular gout
- Trauma, e.g. fracture, dislocation, soft tissue injury
- Haematoma
- Parasitic cysts
- Neoplasia (may be associated with pathological fracture)
- Scar tissue.

## INITIAL CASE WORK-UP

### Blood sample

Since two limbs were affected and systemic disease is common in ageing tortoises, haematology and biochemistry tests were performed as a general health check (Box 18.2). The sample also gave information regarding some of the differential diagnoses listed above (Table 18.1):
- One would expect to see changes in the white cell picture if local or systemic infection were present.
- Hyperuricaemia would be present in cases of gout.
- Elevated creatinine kinase may be seen in cases of trauma, although possibly not in chronic disease.

Hyperproteinaemia (in particular hyperalbuminaemia) is often seen in dehydrated tortoises (usually in association with haematological changes such as elevated haematocrit), or in females associated with normal reproductive activity (e.g. vitellogenesis). Hyperglobulinaemia may reflect chronic inflammatory activity. The mild hypoglycaemia may have reflected a reduction in food intake during the autumn months (the sample was taken in October). Other reasons for reduced blood glucose include anorexia, malnutrition, septicaemia and hepatopathy. The hyperkalaemia is commonly artefactual in samples posted to external laboratories for analysis, associated with haemolysis during the delay in processing. Elevations in potassium may be seen in cases with renal failure (usually with concurrent hyperuricaemia).

Red cells showed marked anisocytosis, poikilocytosis, polychromasia and hypochromia. Several red cells also showed multiple inclusions that may have been atypical

## BOX 18.2   PHLEBOTOMY IN TORTOISES: JUGULAR VEIN

- The jugular vein should be accessed if possible (Fig. 18.1). It is less likely to be diluted by lymph than other commonly used sites such as the dorsal coccygeal vein (which is difficult to obtain a large sample from) and the sub-carapacial (or subvertebral) venous sinus, and a sufficiently large volume should be readily obtainable.
- An assistant holds the tortoise, including gentle restraint on the forelimbs to keep them away from the neck area during the procedure.
- The phlebotomist grasps the head – the author prefers to extend the neck by grasping behind the head laterally (caudal to the tympanic membranes), but then holds the head dorsally and ventrally during venepuncture.
- The skin on the lateral neck is surgically prepared.
- The assistant puts pressure at the base of the neck to raise the vein.
- The vein runs superficially in a line from the tympanic membrane to the base of the neck.
- A 23–25 gauge hypodermic needle is inserted at a shallow angle. A 2 ml syringe is sufficient for most tortoises, although care should be taken not to collapse the vein with excess suction.
- Pressure is applied to the site for a few minutes after sampling to reduce the risk of haematoma formation. If the tortoise is strong and the neck cannot be extended for this period of time, use a large ball of cotton wool inserted between the neck and limb to provide pressure.

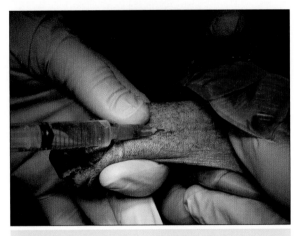

**Figure 18.1** Venous access to the jugular vein in a tortoise (here, to induce general anaesthesia using alfaxalone).

**Table 18.1** Hermann's tortoise blood results (with reference ranges for comparison)

| Parameter | Unit | Result | Reference range |
|---|---|---|---|
| **Biochemistry** | | | |
| Total protein | g/l | 55.8* | 23–44 |
| Albumin | g/l | 23.2* | 13–16 |
| Globulin | g/l | 32.6* | 14–29 |
| Glucose | mmol/l | 2.7* | 4.3–10.7 |
| Calcium | mmol/l | 2.45 | 1.65–3.3 |
| Phosphorus | mmol/l | 1.81 | 0.48–1.81 |
| AST | U/l | 78 | 0–210 |
| CK | U/l | 18 | 0–620 |
| Uric acid | μmol/l | 428 | 124–466 |
| LDH | U/l | 471 | 0–300 |
| Sodium | mmol/l | 133.7 | 123–145 |
| Potassium | mmol/l | 8.8* | 3.6–5.3 |
| **Haematology** | | | |
| Haemoglobin | g/dl | 8.8 | 3.9–12.6 |
| Haematocrit | l/l | 0.30 | 0.15–0.43 |
| Red blood cells | ×10$^{12}$/l | 1.00 | 0.35–1.11 |
| MCV | fl | 300* | 357.5–436.4 |
| MCHC | g/dl | 29.3 | 25.7–33.3 |
| MCH | ×10$^9$/l | 88* | 94.3–140.2 |
| White blood cells | ×10$^9$/l | 3.6* | 0.1–3.1 |
| Heterophils | ×10$^9$/l | 2.38* | 0.00–1.91 |
| Lymphocytes | ×10$^9$/l | 1.08 | 0.01–1.45 |
| Monocytes | ×10$^9$/l | 0 | 0.00–0.10 |
| Azurophils | ×10$^9$/l | 0.07 | – |
| Basophils | ×10$^9$/l | 0 | 0.00–0.09 |
| Thrombocytes | ×10$^9$/l | 2 | 1–5 |

* Abnormal values outside reference range.

basophilic stippling. Although anaemia was not present, these red cell changes suggest chronicity in the disease with a regenerative response (which occurs slower in reptiles (up to 4 months) than in birds or mammals (within 1 week)). Leucocytosis with heterophilia commonly suggests infection or inflammation, although the smear report did not show the presence of any toxic changes in white blood cells. Other differentials for heterophilia are trauma, stress and neoplasia.

## Radiography

The tortoise was amenable to positioning and the sites of interest on the limbs were distal, so radiography was performed conscious. Initially dorso-ventral radiographs were taken of the distal limbs (Fig. 18.5a,b).

At the time of initial presentation, severe bone lysis was present in both forefeet. Both showed a focal moth-eaten appearance of the digits, metacarpal and carpal bones. There was also destruction of the left distal ulna. The destruction was more extensive in the left foot, with almost complete loss of the digits, radial aspect of the carpal bones and distal ulna. In the right foot, the destruction mainly affected digits II–V, and some focal lesions were visible in the carpal bones. Despite concerns over stifle swellings, no obvious destructive changes were identified on radiographs of the hindlimbs. Bone density in the tortoise was good (i.e. there was no evidence of metabolic bone disease).

## Fine needle aspirate (FNA)

After surgical preparation of the skin, an FNA was taken from the left foot of the tortoise. A small amount of haemorrhagic material was obtained, and sent for culture (aerobic and anaerobic bacteriology, and fungal culture). The owner was warned that this small sample may not be representative of the lesion, and that more invasive procedures may be required under general anaesthesia.

## Culture

No bacteria were grown from the FNA sample, and only fungal saprophytes were cultured.

## INITIAL TREATMENT

Initial blood analysis suggested dehydration may be present, and the owner was advised to bathe the tortoise in shallow warm water daily for 10 minutes to encourage drinking. The owner was also advised regarding suitable nutrition, encouraging the tortoise to feed, and to monitor his appetite closely to avoid any further deterioration in glucose levels. The owner moved the tortoise indoors, but despite advice to do so did not supply constant supplemental heating (over central heating in the owner's house) or UV light for the tortoise.

---

**NURSING ASPECT**

### UV-B and heating for tortoises

- Unless tortoises are maintained in an appropriately warm environmental temperature, their metabolism will slow. This affects all body processes, including muscular activity, gastrointestinal activity and the immune system.
- UV lighting is necessary for calcium metabolism and also is beneficial in stimulating chelonian appetite.

---

**NURSING ASPECTS**

### Bathing tortoises

- It is useful to bathe tortoises in shallow warm water to encourage them to drink, and also to void urine/urates/faeces.
- Electrolyte solutions can be used to bathe tortoises, but the animal should be rinsed off afterwards to remove any substances that may promote bacterial or fungal growth on the skin and shell.
- The water should be sufficiently warm to prevent cooling of the animal when it is removed from its enclosure's preferred optimum temperature range (POTR). If possible, the bath should be placed within the enclosure to prevent rapid cooling of the water, or a heated plant propagator may be used.
- The water should be deep enough for the tortoise to drink. To do this, they partially immerse their head and suck water through the sides of their mouth. Thus, the water is usually up to the level of the plastron–carapace junction.
- Debilitated animals should be monitored continuously during bathing to prevent drowning.

## FURTHER INVESTIGATION AND TREATMENT

A diagnosis had not yet been reached, and the owner agreed to further investigation of the lesions. The tortoise was anaesthetized (see below) for the following procedures.

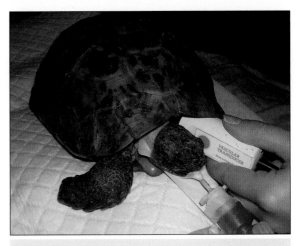

**Figure 18.2** Intubated tortoise, showing tape to secure the endotracheal tube and wooden tongue depressor to stabilize the tube and connector to the anaesthetic circuit. The heart rate is being monitored using a Doppler probe.

a combination of blunt dissection and a biopsy punch (Fig. 18.3a).

As the tissue appeared to be bony and decalcification thought necessary, impression smears were prepared for cytology as well as samples preserved in formalin for histology.

### Bead implantation

Although it is preferable to await culture results before choosing an antibiotic, it was considered worthwhile to implant antibiotic-impregnated methylmethacrylate beads at the time of the procedure (in case the owner declined a further anaesthetic). Tobramycin beads were inserted into the biopsy site before closure (Fig. 18.3b). Systemic antibiotics were not administered at this time due to their unlikely penetration of the lesion.

The skin was closed using polydioxanone in a horizontal mattress pattern. (The sutures were removed 6 weeks after placement, allowing time for the skin to heal.)

### Surgical biopsy

Although the skin changes and most prominent swelling were on the ventral surface of the limb, it was considered prudent to approach from dorsally to reduce the risk of wound dehiscence due to trauma postoperatively. Initial attempts to obtain a larger FNA using a 14 gauge needle were unsuccessful, as the tissue within the lesion was extremely hard. A small incision was made dorsally over the carpal joint, and tissue samples obtained using

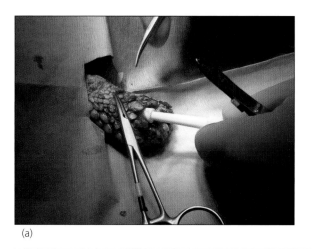

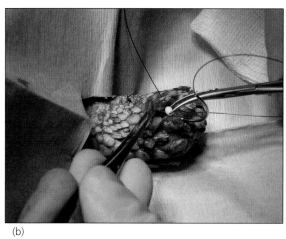

(a)                                                        (b)

**Figure 18.3** (a) Intraoperative photograph showing biopsy of tissue. (b) Implanting an antibiotic bead.

- The implantation of antibiotic-impregnated beads is the preferred treatment by some clinicians for osteomyelitis or septic arthritis.
- There is good drug delivery locally and a low risk of systemic toxicity.
- It is preferable for antibiotic choice to be based on culture and sensitivity, and that devitalized or infected tissue (including bone) is removed before insertion of the beads. Aminoglycosides and clindamycin are common choices of antibiotic.
- The beads are prepared in a sterile manner, or can be gas-sterilized.
- Small beads have a greater surface area to volume ratio, and will thus release antibiotic more rapidly than larger beads.
- If placed in a joint, the beads should be removed (to limit further degenerative joint disease) when a cure is detected radiographically. There is no need to remove beads placed in bone.

stains the polysaccharide-laden wall of most fungal organisms), Ziehl–Neelsen (an acid-fast stain, for mycobacteria) and Gram (to identify bacteria). These stains were negative for fungi and mycobacteria. Small numbers of Gram-positive coccobacilli were seen.

## Culture

Bacterial and fungal culture were performed, and demonstrated mixed bacterial growth. As acid-fast (Ziehl–Neelsen) staining was negative, mycobacterial culture was not performed.

---

**CLINICAL TIPS**

**Sample collection for culture**

- To enhance positive culture results, it is important to sample from the inner lining of any fibrous abscess capsule present.
- Samples from the centre of the lesions are often negative, as this region has outgrown the blood supply.

---

## Pathology

The cytology samples were non-diagnostic, with only red blood cells present. Chronic pyogranulomatous inflammation was demonstrated on histology, probably due to an infectious organism.

Special stains were used in an attempt to identify the causal agent, including periodic acid–Schiff (PAS, which

## OTHER INVESTIGATIONS POSSIBLE

### Other radiographs

It is advisable to take radiographs from two views, to fully assess lesions present. This was not performed in this case as sedation would have been required to obtain the orthogonal views (e.g. oblique or cranio-caudal), and sufficient information was gained from the dorso-ventral views to proceed with other investigations.

It would be useful to take full body radiographs to assess for any other signs of illness. Usually three views are taken: dorso-ventral using a vertical X-ray beam, and cranio-caudal and lateral using a horizontal X-ray beam.

### Other imaging techniques

CT and MRI may have been useful to image the extent of the lesions more fully.

### DIAGNOSIS

Bilateral forelimb osteomyelitis.

### ANATOMY AND PHYSIOLOGY REFRESHER

Limb anatomy (Fig. 18.4) in chelonia is similar to that of mammals. Limb girdles are modified, and lie inside the ribs.

The skin of terrestrial tortoises is thick and scaled, having evolved to resist abrasions and arid climates. There is an outer epidermis, which forms scales, and a deeper dermis, which supports and nourishes the

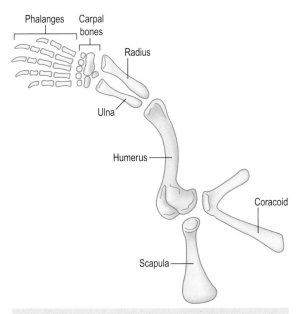

**Figure 18.4** Normal anatomy of the forelimb of a tortoise.

epidermis. Skin shedding (ecdysis) is uncoordinated and continues through life; often only skin from the neck and proximal limbs is shed.

Although fabled as slow, chelonian locomotion can be surprisingly rapid. Tortoises use their forelimbs to ambulate, in respiratory movements, and to steady food while tearing portions to swallow.

### AETIOPATHOGENESIS OF OSTEOMYELITIS IN TORTOISES

Heterophils function differently to mammalian white blood cells and reptile pus is caseous and relatively impenetrable to antibiotics. Many abscesses are lamellar, solid, and well encapsulated. Inciting causes include bacteria, fungi, parasites and foreign bodies. Agents enter the body via the skin, gastrointestinal tract or lungs. Although trauma, bites and scratches commonly permit entry of agents, immunocompromised animals are more susceptible to disease. Haematogenous spread is possible, resulting in disseminated disease. Osteomyelitis may originate from bacteraemia, for example commonly tail tip necrosis seen in lizards. More often, a local infection occurs and infiltrates bone.

Often osteomyelitis is present in chelonia with a lack of external clinical signs. If the infection originated as an abscess, a mass or swelling may be noticed. Other signs are dependent on the location of the abscess, for example a lung abscess producing respiratory signs. If osteomyelitis results in spinal abscesses, neurological signs will be seen. Haematology and clinical chemistry is often unremarkable, although some animals develop a leucocytosis.

It can be difficult to differentiate osteoarthritis, osteoarthrosis and osteomyelitis radiographically in reptiles. Osteomyelitis is lytic rather than proliferative. The lesion often resembles mammalian bone neoplasia. Local anatomy becomes enlarged and distorted, and corticomedullary definition is lost. After treatment a lytic area may remain without necessarily showing the presence or recurrence of infection or sequestrum formation. In cases of septic arthritis, the joint appears swollen; radiographically articular bone surfaces are lytic and there is an increase in soft tissue density within the joint space.

Histologically, it can also be difficult to differentiate between osteoarthritis and osteomyelitis. Where vertebral osteomyelitis occurs, lesions are usually present in the ribs concomitantly.

In this case, superficial skin lesions on the limbs appeared to have invaded the tissues and resulted in deeper infection. It is extremely difficult to treat infection once it has entered bone, as antibiotic penetration to bone is poor.

Chronic lesions often have associated inflammatory or granulomatous tissue whose presence may result in clinical signs. This tissue will also affect penetration of the host's attack on the infection and of any medication administered parenterally.

Ideally, any infection in reptiles is excised surgically. This is often not possible where bones are involved, but limb amputation is an option. Alternative treatments include the use of antibiotics locally (e.g. using antibiotic-impregnated materials), or long-term (weeks or months) systemically. The latter option may not completely resolve the infection, but may prevent any further progression.

## EPIDEMIOLOGY

There are no age or sex predilections for abscess formation. However, individuals with immune compromise are more susceptible to pathology development. Often, poor husbandry results in immunosuppression.

## TREATMENT

Postoperatively, the tortoise's feet were bathed daily in dilute povidone–iodine solution to reduce local bacterial load.

Husbandry conditions were discussed again with the owner. A UV light was to be purchased now that the tortoise was housed indoors over the winter. The environmental temperature was to be monitored using a digital thermometer. If necessary, supplemental heating was to be obtained so that the tortoise's POTR could be provided in his environment. Supplemental heating is usually in the form of ceramic heat bulbs and heat mats (although mats should be positioned on the side of enclosures and not underneath for tortoises). Dietary modifications suggested included offering more variety of leafy greens, as improved nutritional status would aid immune function.

Systemic antibiosis was considered, but not used due to concern over the likely lack of penetration of the lesions. Although the period of antibiotic release from the beads will be finite (but varies from months to years), they are often left *in situ* without causing any problems.

---

### CLINICAL TIPS

- Amikacin and enrofloxacin are commonly ineffective at treating abscesses in reptiles.
- Chloramphenicol has good penetration of tissues, and is effective in anaerobic and acidic conditions. Use of this drug should be based on culture results, as it has a limited spectrum of activity.
- Systemic antibiotics should be continued for at least 14 days.
- Daily cleaning of postoperative abscesses or wounds should be carried out by the owner.

---

Owing to the suspected infectious aetiology of the condition, it was advised not to hibernate the tortoise as immunosuppression at that time may permit recurrence or progression of the disease. It was also suggested that the tortoise be protected from possible contamination, for example keeping off any soil substrate during the summer when any skin lesions were present.

## OTHER TREATMENT OPTIONS AND MANAGEMENT

### Other surgical options

Debridement of the infected area is advocated. Ideally, if an abscess is present, the surrounding fibrous capsule should be excised; this is difficult when bone is involved in the infection. Necrotic and degenerate material should be removed, including curettage of bone (drills and burrs are useful for this procedure). Open wounds after surgery may require management using dressings.

If a single limb is affected, tortoises do remarkably well after limb amputation. This again removes the infected material. The limb is usually amputated quite proximally, as more distal amputations may result in wound dehiscence due to use of the stump. It is useful to attach a plastic ball (e.g. half a ping pong ball) or toy wheel to the plastron to provide support for the plastron after a limb has been amputated. Although the left forelimb was more severely affected than the right in this case, the potential for the right to progress was a consideration.

Laser ablation of the wound bed after debridement may help sterilize any infective material remaining. If the wound is left open, topical debridement can be performed daily. Iodine-based disinfectants will also be effective against remaining bacteria.

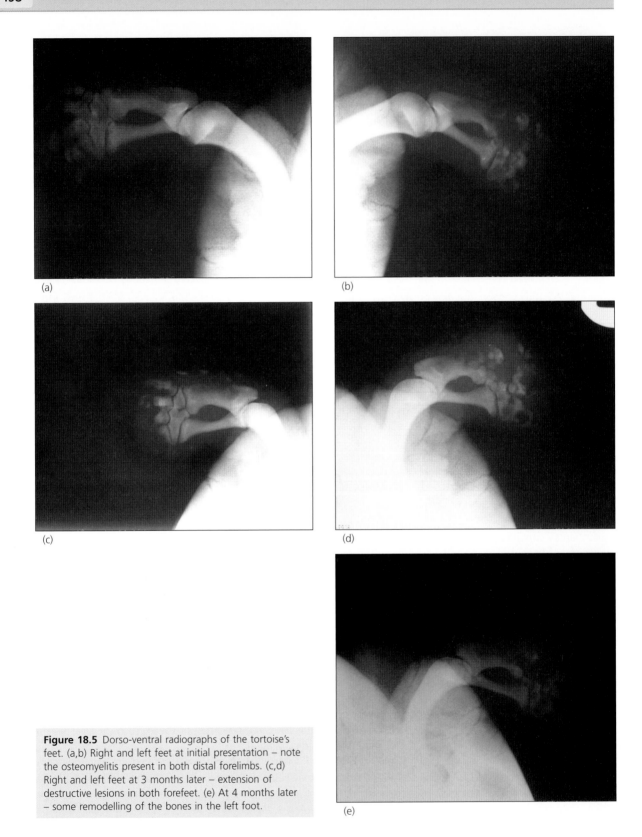

**Figure 18.5** Dorso-ventral radiographs of the tortoise's feet. (a,b) Right and left feet at initial presentation – note the osteomyelitis present in both distal forelimbs. (c,d) Right and left feet at 3 months later – extension of destructive lesions in both forefeet. (e) At 4 months later – some remodelling of the bones in the left foot.

## Supportive care

If a tortoise is anorexic due to any illness, consideration should be given to placement of an oesophagostomy tube for assisted-feeding (see page 135). This also enables easy administration of any medications or supplements required by the patient.

## FOLLOW-UP

The tortoise's appetite and demeanour were generally good, although variable. This is often the case with captive tortoises, which are incredibly susceptible to environmental changes such as temperature variability, or the presence or absence of ultraviolet light.

One of the large skin scales at the biopsy site became necrotic and sloughed. Otherwise, the skin healed well.

## Repeat radiographs

Radiographs were performed 3 months after initial presentation (Fig. 18.5c,d). There was extension of the previous lytic changes in the left forefoot. Destructive changes of the left ulna were more marked and extensive. The radius appeared intact. Similarly, the changes in the right forefoot had extended, affecting mostly the digits and metacarpals. Digits III–V were almost completely lost.

This progression was supportive of the diagnosis of septic osteomyelitis with destructive bone lesions in both forefeet. At this point, no lameness was present and the tortoise was eating well.

Radiographs 4 months later (i.e. 7 months after initial presentation and bead implantation) still showed some bony changes (Fig. 18.5e). The left forefoot lesions had not progressed. There appeared to be some remodelling in the right forefoot, with lytic lesion margins appearing slightly less acute. However, no further progression of the lytic changes was expected unless re-infection or resurgence of infection occurred. Skin on both feet was no longer inflamed, thought to be due to the current substrate of grass and rubber matting. There had been no change in size or firmness of the feet swellings. The tortoise was active and eating well.

In summary, the extensive lytic lesions in the forefeet had initially progressed before becoming static in radiographic appearance. The lysis was suspected to reflect chronic osteomyelitis or osteoarthritis, most likely septic in aetiology. Reptiles show less proliferative reaction to septic bone lesions than mammals. Lack of progression over time indicated removal of the causative agent, which may have been bacterial or fungal infection. Follow-up radiographs were advised, with increased remodelling expected; no further progression of lytic changes was expected unless re-infection occurred.

The condition appeared to have stabilized, and no further treatment was advised at that stage. It was suggested that the owner monitored the tortoise's condition, in particular assessing for any reduction in use of

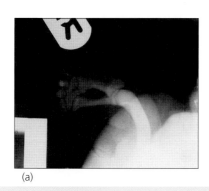
(a)

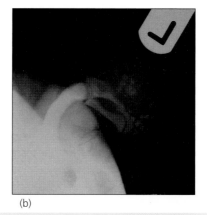
(b)

**Figure 18.6** (a) Radiography of the right forefoot 18 months later – note the large soft tissue mass (abscess) and inactive bone lesions (evidenced by rounding of bone edges). (b) Radiography of the left foot 18 months later – note the presence of spherical antibiotic beads in this foot.

the forelimbs that may be associated with discomfort or any new lesions on the limbs, as well as the animal's general demeanour, appetite and activity. If any deterioration was noted, radiographs would be repeated and consideration given to further surgery (e.g. to debride the lesion and re-implant fresh antibiotic beads).

## PREVENTION

Appropriate selection of substrate for tortoises may help prevent lesions, for example avoidance of sharp stones that may cut into the skin, or exposure to excessively wet habitat that may soften the skin and render it more susceptible to trauma. However, tortoises are adapted to most substrates and it is usually a case of regular examination by owners to detect and treat any minor lesions before deeper infection occurs.

Underlying systemic illness may predispose progression of minor superficial lesions to deeper or systemic infection. Maintenance of a high standard of husbandry should minimize the risks of immunosuppression and systemic illness.

## PROGNOSIS

In the short term, skin wounds (e.g. after surgery) in reptiles heal slowly, generally over 6–8 weeks. Scar tissue usually shrinks over time, although dysecdysis may occur in the meantime.

The long-term prognosis for this case was guarded. In some cases of infection in reptiles, the nidus of infection becomes walled off and no further problems are noted. However, there is the potential for infection to recur locally or for new lesions to develop at distant sites after haematogenous spread, particularly if the animal becomes immunosuppressed (e.g. during hibernation or with other disease).

The tortoise re-presented 18 months later with a large abscess in the distal left forelimb. Radiography (Fig. 18.6) showed the bone lesions to be inactive, but further soft tissue damage had occurred. The owner declined further surgery (e.g. repeated debridement or amputation) and the tortoise was euthanized.

# 19 Dystocia in a snake

**INITIAL PRESENTATION**

Inappetence and condition loss in a corn snake.

## INTRODUCTION

Although many herpetologists keep snakes for breeding, it is not uncommon for owners to retain a single animal of one species. Unlike some other taxonomic groups, female snakes may undergo reproductive activity and produce (infertile) eggs without necessarily contacting a male. Similarly, mating with a fertile male does not always ensure reproductive success. The cues for such activity are often environmental.

**CASE PRESENTING SIGNS**

A 5-year-old corn snake (*Elaphe guttata*) (Box 19.1), suspected to be female – although there was no previous history of reproductive activity – was presented with a month-long history of anorexia, reduced faecal production and condition loss.

## HUSBANDRY

The snake was housed in a vivarium approximately 150 cm long × 60 cm wide × 60 cm high. The vivarium was constructed mostly of wood, with glass doors at the front and a partially meshed ceiling to provide ventilation. The substrate was bark chippings. Background heating was provided by a tubular heater near the top of the rear wall of the vivarium, connected to a thermostat. Although stimulation of reproductive activity was not intended, a period of cooling had occurred over the winter months during some renovations at the owner's premises. A basking spot was present at one end of the vivarium, created by a ceramic bulb. The environmental temperatures were measured using a digital thermometer, and ranged from 27°C to 28°C during the day (dropping to 24°C overnight).

The day length was typically 12 hours although this had been reduced to 8 hours over the winter months; UV lighting was provided by a striplight (changed 4 months prior to presentation). A small hide box was present. The snake was generally handled daily for approximately 5 minutes, although handling had been reduced since signs of illness were noted.

A water bowl large enough for the snake to bathe in was provided, with the water changed daily. The animal was typically fed on two or three whole mice once a week, although, more recently, smaller mice had been offered to tempt the snake to eat.

## CASE HISTORY

Although it is not uncommon for snakes to be inappetent for short periods of time, the owner was concerned about the length of the current period of anorexia combined with weight loss. The owner had been administering fluids and nutritional support by gavage for 2 weeks prior to presentation. Although ecdysis was regular (every 6 weeks), the previous shed contained tears. Clinical signs reported included:

- Anorexia of approximately 2 month's duration
- Condition loss, including a 4% loss in body weight (from 810 g to 776 g)
- Reduced amount of faeces passed (typically weekly, but now only once every 2–3 weeks).

## BOX 19.1   ECOLOGY OF CORN SNAKES

- Belong to Colubridae snake family, in the subfamily Colubrinae. *Elaphe* spp are rat snakes
- Range in the wild covers much of the USA and northern Mexico
- Normal habitat: overgrown fields, wooded groves and forest openings, rocky hillsides, meadowlands, common in disused farm buildings. Readily climb trees. Very secretive
- Usually attain 60 cm in length within the first year of life, and 1.2–1.8 m when fully grown
- Hibernate during the winter in colder regions. In more temperate areas, brumate (during cold periods they shelter in rock crevices and logs, and emerge to heat up in the sun on warm days)
- Free-ranging diet: lizards and tree frogs as young hatchlings, mainly small mammals (mice, rats, birds and bats) when adult. Kill by constriction
- Reproduction: sexual maturity at around 600 days of age. Breeding season March–May. Oviparous: lay 10–30 eggs per clutch, in rotting stumps or piles of decaying vegetation. Gestation of eggs is 60–65 days at around 28°C
- Popular pet, as relatively easy to keep in captivity. Often very colourful (many colour varieties) and frequently bred. Non-venomous. Live 15–20 years (up to 23 in captivity).

## CLINICAL EXAMINATION

Corn snakes are relatively easy to handle, and a complete clinical examination was possible. The findings were:

- Moderate body condition, weighing 776 g. Dorsal spinous processes of vertebrae readily palpated. Moderate muscle strength (no paresis noted)
- No stomatitis or other oral lesions that would result in discomfort and reduced appetite
- No signs of dyspnoea or respiratory secretions
- Some dysecdysis, with patchy/piecemeal shedding. (Snakes should shed their complete skin-including spectacles – in one piece.)
- No apparent dehydration. (It is difficult to clinically assess dehydration in snakes, but severe dehydration will result in a wrinkling of the skin and tacky mucous membranes.)
- Gender determined as female by probing (probe passed to a depth of only three scales caudal to the cloaca).

## DIFFERENTIAL DIAGNOSES

As discussed in other cases, anorexia is a common presenting sign in reptiles, with many possible aetiologies. The main differentials considered for *anorexia* in this case were:

- Systemic disease, e.g. septicaemia.
- Gastrointestinal disease: infections (e.g. bacteria, protozoa (e.g. *Cryptosporidium*), nematodes), neoplasia, constipation (often associated with dehydration), inappropriate diet (e.g. feeding prey items that are too large)
- Metabolic disease, e.g. hypocalcaemia (often due to nutritional secondary hyperparathyroidism) resulting in paresis and delayed gastrointestinal motility
- Urogenital disease, e.g. renal failure
- Hepatic disease, e.g. hepatic lipidosis
- Normal reproductive behaviour: anorexia may be normal in gravid females, although this period is usually only for the final 15–20 days of gestation in corn snakes
- Reproductive disease: dysfunction may result in anorexia (often as a result of the space occupied in the coelomic cavity by the reproductive tract), e.g. follicular stasis or egg retention (due to dystocia or reproductive stasis)
- Respiratory tract disease: snakes with upper or lower respiratory tract infections are often anorexic, although clinical signs of respiratory difficulty are usually present (e.g. nasal discharge or open-mouth breathing)
- Behavioural causes of anorexia: intra- or inter-specific aggression when reptiles are housed together, psychological (e.g. associated with excessive noise or irregular light patterns)
- Neurological, e.g. loss of vision (e.g. due to spectacular abscesses) or smell (e.g. due to rhinitis)
- Other space-occupying lesions, e.g. neoplasia.

## CASE WORK-UP

The history did not suggest obvious husbandry or dietary inadequacies that may have predisposed to disease. Apart from the obvious loss of body condition, the physical examination did not reveal any significant findings.

### Haematology and biochemistry

A blood sample was taken by cardiocentesis to perform a general health profile, investigating for signs of generalized infection or inflammation as well as renal or hepatic disease (Table 19.1). Although a few parameters were outside the normal ranges reported for corn snakes, none were significantly abnormal. A relative heteropenia was present, but the total white cell count was within normal limits and white cell morphology was normal on microscopy. Often poikilocytosis is noted with anorexia, but was not present in this case. Elevations in calcium and phosphorus are sometimes associated with reproductive activity.

### Radiography

The snake was anaesthetized (via conscious intubation and IPPV with isoflurane) in order to facilitate positioning for lateral and dorso-ventral radiographs. The heart, lungs and trachea had a normal appearance. There were no obvious skeletal abnormalities. The radiographs demonstrated at least 13 oval well-defined homogeneous soft tissue opacities roughly midline throughout the caudal third of the coelomic cavity (Fig. 19.1), suspected to be either faecal material within the gastrointestinal tract or eggs within the reproductive tract. A less likely differential was multiple soft tissue tumours.

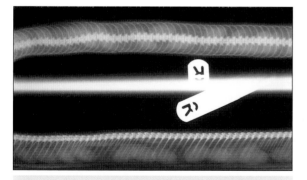

**Figure 19.1** Dorsoventral and lateral radiographs of the snake showing multiple soft tissue density masses within the coelomic cavity.

**Table 19.1** Corn snake blood results (with reference ranges for comparison)

| Parameter | Unit | Result | Reference range |
|---|---|---|---|
| Total protein | g/l | 80 | 46–84 |
| Albumin | g/l | 32.9 | 18–34 |
| Globulin | g/l | 47.1 | 33.57 |
| Glucose | mmol/l | 1.17* | 1.7–4.8 |
| Calcium | mmol/l | 7.5* | 3–4.9 |
| Phosphorus | mmol/l | 2.37* | 0.61–1.94 |
| AST | U/l | 41 | 9–224 |
| CK | U/l | 590 | 77–2460 |
| Uric acid | μmol/l | 557 | 77–1184 |
| LDH | U/l | 331 | 48–444 |
| Sodium | mmol/l | 171.9 | 147–183 |
| Potassium | mmol/l | 2.44 | 1.9–13.2 |
| Haemoglobin | g/dl | 9.6* | 9.7–13.5 |
| Haematocrit | l/l | 0.26 | 0.21–0.52 |
| Red blood cells | ×10$^{12}$/l | 0.91 | 0.62–1.86 |
| MCV | fl | 285.7 | 170.6–403.8 |
| MCHC | g/dl | 36.9 | 32.1–39.8 |
| MCH | ×10$^9$/l | 105.5* | 110.2–143 |
| White blood cells | ×10$^9$/l | 6 | 1.0–31.4 |
| Heterophils | ×10$^9$/l | 0.24 (4%) | 0.14–8.35 |
| Lymphocytes | ×10$^9$/l | 4.86 (81%) | 0.41–22.90 |
| Eosinophils | ×10$^9$/l | 0* | 0.08–0.15 |
| Monocytes | ×10$^9$/l | 0* | 0.04–2.2 |
| Azurophils | ×10$^9$/l | 0.9 | 0.08–5.34 |
| Basophils | ×10$^9$/l | 0* | 0.05–1.44 |
| Thrombocytes | ×10$^9$/l | 17 | – |

* Abnormal values outside reference range.

## Ultrasound

Ultrasonography revealed numerous echodense masses in the coelomic cavity, within a fluid-filled viscus. Each mass was ovoid, approximately 2.5 cm in length, with a thick hyperechoic rim and mottled heterogeneous centre. It was not possible to determine from ultrasound which organ(s) contained the masses, although they did not appear to be free-floating within the coelomic cavity. The structure and location of the masses was consistent with a diagnosis of egg retention.

## OTHER POSSIBLE INVESTIGATIONS

### Faecal analysis

Where gastrointestinal disease is suspected, it is useful to perform faecal analysis to check for endoparasitism or bacterial infection.

### Gastric lavage

If a single mid-body swelling is detected on clinical examination or ultrasonography, gastric hypertrophy due to cryptosporidiosis should be suspected. This organism is difficult to detect, but may be seen by microscopy on a gastric lavage sample. Endoscopy and stomach biopsy for histology provide a more sensitive test.

### Contrast radiography

A barium study after oral administration would outline material within the gastrointestinal tract, helping to differentiate gastrointestinal from reproductive tract disease. However, since the gastrointestinal transit time is slow in reptiles (typically 1 week in a snake of this size), the delay in diagnosis was not deemed appropriate.

### Coelioscopy

Endoscopy is useful to investigate a localized problem, and may enable sample collection from abnormal structures for further analysis, such as culture or histology. However, this is a difficult procedure to perform in snakes, as limited gas dilation and thence visualization of the coelomic cavity is possible in these linear animals.

### Respiratory tract sampling

If lower respiratory tract disease is suspected, a lung wash is routinely performed (using sterile saline) to obtain samples of material in the airways for culture and microscopy. Swabs may be taken from upper respiratory tract lesions.

### Virology

Inclusion body disease (IBD) may be seen in Boidae (boid) species of snakes, and may result in gastrointestinal as well as respiratory disease. Diagnosis is usually based on virus isolation or histopathology of oesophageal tonsils or coelomic organs such as liver, kidney and spleen.

## DIAGNOSIS

Egg retention was diagnosed using a combination of imaging techniques. It is difficult to differentiate between tracts within the coelomic cavity due to the linear anatomy of snakes, and exploratory surgery may be required to identify the exact location of lesions.

## ANATOMY AND PHYSIOLOGY REFRESHER

The reproductive tract (Fig. 19.2) in snakes lies predominantly in the caudal third of the coelomic cavity, with the gonads most cranially (near the spleen, pancreas and gall bladder). The right gonad is more cranial than the left, which is cranial to the kidneys. Male snakes have two hemipenes that may be everted during copulation (only one is required at a time). The right ovary is often larger than the left. The oviducts are thin-walled in snakes.

Sexual dimorphism is not universal in snakes. The easiest method of gender determination in corn snakes is to probe caudally from the cloaca to check for hemipenes (see page 122-123).

Rat snakes are among the species that have 'associated cycles' of reproduction. A cool winter period (4–6 weeks) of dormancy or hibernation is required for breeding activity to occur. Photoperiod and temperature cues are important at the end of hibernation, with a gradual increase in day length on emergence. Secretion of sex hormones and gonadogenesis during the active season stimulate copulation and egg development. The gonads regress during the inactive season. Most snakes, including corn snakes, are egg-layers. The normal gestation period (for eggs in the oviduct) in corn snakes is 30–45 days. Colubrid species can be induced to lay multiple clutches of eggs in a single year by manipulating their environment and diet. Young in captivity are initially raised on crickets before progressing to pinkies (newborn mice).

## AETIOPATHOGENESIS OF DYSTOCIA

Inappropriate husbandry conditions may predispose to reproductive disease. Animals not in peak body

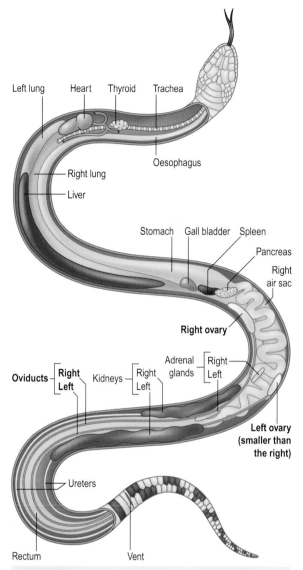

**Figure 19.2** Reproductive anatomy in a typical snake.

Labels on figure:
Left lung  Heart  Thyroid  Trachea
Oesophagus
Right lung
Liver
Stomach  Gall bladder  Spleen
Pancreas
Right air sac
**Right ovary**
Adrenal glands  Right Left
Oviducts Right Left  Kidneys  Right Left
**Left ovary (smaller than the right)**
Ureters
Rectum  Vent

Environmental cues such as lighting and temperature changes often stimulate reproductive activity – such as a reduction in day length and temperature over winter months in corn snakes. Animals with a history of dystocia are more likely to retain eggs in the future. This is likely to be due to the continued presence of factors resulting in the initial problem.

## TREATMENT

### Medical therapy

There was no evidence of obstructive dystocia from the investigations performed. Therefore in the first instance, supportive care was given to assist with passage of the eggs. The snake was hospitalized in a vivarium with supplemental heating to provide the POTR (preferred optimal temperature range) for the species. Fluids (warmed Hartmann's solution 30 ml/kg administered SC and intracoelomic [ICo]) and nutritional support (convalescent diet with easily digestible sugars, at 10 ml/kg) were administered. A warm water enema was administered to rehydrate cloacal material. Salpingitis commonly results in dystocia, and antibiosis was commenced (enrofloxacin at 10 mg/kg PO SID for a 3 week course).

> ### NURSING ASPECTS
>
> - Although it is tempting to provide nutrition daily to underweight snakes, there is a balance between providing support and causing undue stress due to excessive handling.
> - In larger snakes such as this corn snake, normal feeding is once a week. It is therefore acceptable to reduce assist-feeding to once or twice weekly.
> - Severely dehydrated animals are likely to require more intensive fluid therapy, sometimes requiring intravenous fluids via CRI (continuous rate infusion). Dehydration should be corrected before food is administered.

Calcium gluconate (20 mg/kg SC) was given prior to oxytocin (10 IU/kg IM, repeated three times with 90 minutes between injections).

A nesting area was advised, to encourage normal nesting behaviour and egg laying. The nest box was lined with moist sphagnum moss as substrate (an alternative is dampened vermiculite). Disturbance and handling should be minimized during the nesting time.

condition before hibernation or reproductive activity may have difficulty in sustaining egg development and parturition. Many gravid reptiles spend more time basking before laying their eggs. Lack of an appropriate oviposition site may result in dystocia. The incidence of dystocia increases with subsequent clutches produced in the same year.

## EPIDEMIOLOGY

Although social isolation prevents breeding, in many animals it does not stop reproductive activity.

## BOX 19.2   OXYTOCIN IN REPTILES

- For best results, oxytocin should be administered within the first 48 hours of dystocia.
- Although very effective (>90%) in chelonia, oxytocin in less effective in lizards, and even less so in snakes (<50% even in the early stages of dystocia).
- Reptile oviducts are more sensitive to arginine vasotocin, the natural oxytocin equivalent in reptiles. However, this hormone is usually unavailable.
- Oxytocin should not be used in cases of obstructive dystocia, as oviductal rupture, egg fracture, or haemorrhage may result (potentially fatally).
- Pre-treatment with propranolol (at 1 µg/kg) may increase the effectiveness of parturition-inducing drugs in reptiles.
- Calcium or reproductive steroids (such as oestrogen or progesterone) may be helpful.

## BOX 19.3   ANAESTHESIA OF THE CORN SNAKE

- Pre-medication was administered using butorphanol (2 mg/kg IM), also providing some analgesia, and ketamine (10 mg/kg IM).
- The snake was restrained manually. A gag was used to open the mouth and a 2 mm endotracheal tube (ETT) was inserted in the trachea of the mildly sedated snake.
- IPPV (intermittent positive pressure ventilation) was used to induce anaesthesia with isoflurane.
- After induction, a mechanical ventilator was used to maintain anaesthesia. Four breaths a minute at a pressure of 9.0 cmH$_2$O were sufficient to maintain a surgical depth of anaesthesia.
- The snake was placed on a heat pad to maintain body temperature during surgery, and warmed fluids were utilized for lavage.
- After surgery, the snake was disconnected from the anaesthetic circuit and returned to the vivarium. The ETT was left in place and IPPV performed using a small resuscitator device (Fig. 19.4). The ETT was removed once the patient was spontaneously breathing on a regular basis.

## FOLLOW-UP

Eight eggs were passed in the week following administration of oxytocin. However, the snake remained anorexic over the following month (despite continued supportive care with gavage-feeding every third day) and no further eggs were passed.

## FURTHER TREATMENT

### Exploratory coeliotomy

Prophylactic antibiosis was given (enrofloxacin, at 10 mg/kg IM at the time of surgery (see Box 19.3 for anaesthetic regime), continuing once daily PO for a week). A paramedian incision was made in the region of one of the masses located on ultrasound. The incision was ventro-lateral, between the first two rows of scales on the side (enabling closure without a suture line on the ventrum which contacts the substrate).

The oviducts were obvious on entry into the coelomic cavity, and found to contain several egg-shaped structures. There was no evidence of adhesions or coelomitis. After discussion with the owner, it was elected to perform a salpingectomy (Fig. 19.3) rather than a salpingotomy (i.e. caesarean section) due to the chronic

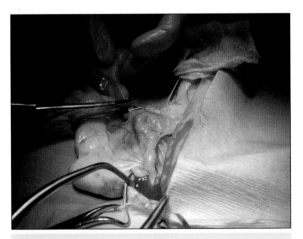

**Figure 19.3** Intraoperative view of the salpingectomy.

history of reproductive problems and as the animal was not required for future breeding. The oviducts were followed and removed to their cranial and caudal ends. Blood vessels supplying the oviducts are large and numerous, and must be ligated. The use of stainless steel vascular clips for rapid haemostasis reduced surgical time compared with ligatures with suture material (another rapid alternative is the use of lasers). Caudally, the oviducts were ligated close to their insertion into the cloaca before being removed. The procedure necessitated extension of the skin incision for approximately a third of the length of the snake.

When a salpingectomy is performed, it is preferable to perform an ovariectomy also (i.e. ovariosalpingectomy). Otherwise future folliculogenesis, ovulation and egg coelomitis will occur in some reptiles. The ovaries were not obvious during the coeliotomy of this case, and therefore a salpingectomy only was performed.

Closure of the coeliotomy incision was in two layers. The muscular wall of the coelomic cavity is thin, but can usually be closed with a simple continuous pattern using absorbable suture material. Horizontal mattress sutures of non-absorbable material (nylon) were used to close the skin, causing a deliberate eversion of the skin to prevent the edges rolling inwards.

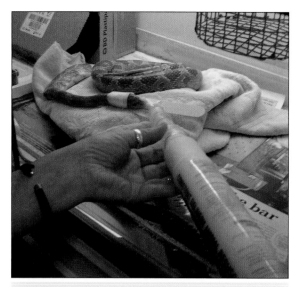

**Figure 19.4** Resuscitator devices; can be used to administer room air in IPPV.

### CLINICAL TIP

If a unilateral salpingectomy (with or without ipsilateral ovariectomy) is performed, reproduction is possible from the contralateral side of the reproductive tract.

### POSTOPERATIVE CARE

- The snake should be maintained in a vivarium within the species-specific POTR. Attention should be paid to other husbandry requirements such as optimizing ventilation, good hygiene, and nutritional support as required.
- Until the skin incision has healed, the snake should be maintained on a newspaper substrate. This prevents the possibility of substrate material abrading or entering the wound, and is also easily cleaned (replaced) daily.

### Laboratory investigations

It would have been useful to assess the excised oviductal material for evidence of infection (by culture) or other pathology (by histology). Further laboratory investigations were declined in this case.

## OTHER TREATMENT OPTIONS

### Medical

Other hormonal options for treatment of dystocia are described in Box 19.2.

### Manipulation of retained eggs

Under anaesthesia, retained eggs can sometimes be 'milked' caudally. Excess pressure may result in rupture or prolapse.

### Percutaneous ovocentesis

A sterile needle may be inserted through the ventrum of the snake to aspirate egg contents. This procedure carries a risk of coelomitis if egg contents contaminate the coelomic cavity. Once drained, the egg often collapses and the snake can expel it more easily. If not passed within 48 hours, the remainder of the egg should be surgically removed to reduce the risk of infection or coelomitis from residual yolk leakage. This technique is not useful in cases of prolonged dystocia, as the egg contents solidify with time and cannot be aspirated.

### Salpingotomy

If future breeding is required, a salpingotomy should be performed. The advantage of this technique is that eggs may be milked along the oviduct and fewer (and shorter) coeliotomy incisions will be necessary, although it may be less traumatic to make an incision over each egg. The oviduct is usually closed with a simple continuous pattern. The main disadvantage of this treatment is the risk of dystocia at future gestations.

## FOLLOW-UP AFTER SURGERY

The snake re-presented 4 weeks after surgery. After shedding, a small area of the wound had appeared inflamed. Antibiotic ointment (silver sulfadiazine) was applied to the lesion to reduce the risk of infection, and suture removal (normally performed approximately 6 weeks after surgery) was postponed. Skin sutures were removed 8 weeks after surgery. By this stage, the snake was active and her appetite was improving.

## PREVENTION

Attention to husbandry details such as appropriate temperature, humidity, and nest site provision are necessary to prevent egg retention in snakes. Prompt diagnosis of the problem and instigation of medical therapy may preclude the necessity for surgical intervention. Removal of reproductive tissue (bilateral ovariosalpingectomy) will prevent future reproductive disease.

## PROGNOSIS

Scarring of the skin after surgery is likely to result in dysecdysis – sometimes necessitating assistance from the owner to remove – although this problem should reduce with each shed. Although uncommon, the owner was also warned of the possibility of future follicles forming on the ovaries, being released into the coelomic cavity, and resulting in egg coelomitis.

In snakes where salpingotomy or unilateral (ovario-) salpingectomy have been performed to treat dystocia, future breeding is still likely. Many animals will breed within a year of medical or surgical treatment for dystocia, and some will produce clutches within 1–2 months.

# 20 Dysecdysis in a leopard gecko

## INITIAL PRESENTATION

Retained skin after shedding in a leopard gecko.

## INTRODUCTION

It is vital to assess the pet's husbandry in cases such as this. Frequently, chronic suboptimal conditions present with lesions that are not immediately life-threatening. However, they may indicate underlying problems that may predispose to stress, immunosuppression and potentially increased susceptibility to infectious agents. Alternatively, the individual may suffer from chronic metabolic problems.

### CASE PRESENTING SIGNS

A 3-year-old male leopard gecko (*Eublepharis macularius*) (Box 20.1) presented with retained skin after shedding (i.e. dysecdysis), which involved the digits, eyes and lips.

## HUSBANDRY

The leopard gecko was housed with a con-specific in a Perspex enclosure measuring approximately 60 cm long × 30 cm wide × 30 cm high, with a ventilated lid. The substrate – calcium sand – was spot-cleaned daily and completely replaced every 3 months, at which point the vivarium was disinfected with dilute bleach and rinsed with tap water. Supplemental heating was provided by a heat mat along the back wall on the outside of the tank and a small ceramic heat bulb at one end. The heat mat was switched on 24 hours per day, while the lamp was on for approximately 10 hours each day. A UV light was provided, but switched on for only 6 hours daily (Fig. 20.1). A plastic mould provided a hide area.

The temperature was monitored using an alcohol thermometer – positioned at the end with the heat bulb – and typically read 31°C during the day.

The geckos were fed on a selection of invertebrates, mainly small crickets and mealworms. The invertebrates were fed on various fruit and vegetables, and dusted with mineral supplement before feeding to the geckos.

## CASE HISTORY

The owner had noticed problems with the animal's skin over the previous week, since the last shed:
- Tags of skin around digits (Fig. 20.2)
- Eye lids appeared stuck together
- Previous skin sheds also resulted in some retained skin. Ecdysis approximately every 2 months
- No change in husbandry over previous year
- Appetite reduced over the past week, with the gecko appearing to have difficulty locating food
- Not known when last urine/faeces/urates were passed.

## CLINICAL EXAMINATION

The gecko was quite habituated to handling, but the small size of this species limits clinical examination to a degree. Findings included:
- Good body condition, evidenced by a substantial fat deposit at the base of the tail
- Alert demeanour. Mobility good and supporting weight well on all four limbs

## BOX 20.1   ECOLOGY OF LEOPARD GECKOS

- Range in the wild covers India, Pakistan and into Iran
- Terrestrial species. Crepuscular (primarily active at dawn and dusk)
- Normal habitat: rocky, dry grassland and desert regions. Spend daytime hidden under rocks or in dry burrows
- Require a hide area for security. This area should be moist to assist ecdysis. Rubbing against rough surfaces also helps to remove old skin
- Temperature range: 25–30°C
- Relative humidity: 30–40%, although humid microhabitats are required to assist shedding
- Average weight: 50–100 g
- Snout to tail tip length: <25 cm
- Free-ranging diet: mainly invertebrates, but will also take small vertebrates
- Reproduction: egg-laying. Pattern II temperature-dependent sex determination (i.e. females are produced at low and high temperatures, and males at intermediate temperatures)
- Longevity: up to 12 years in captivity.

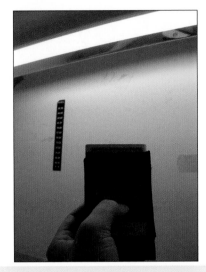

**Figure 20.1** Measuring the UV output from a light source using a meter.

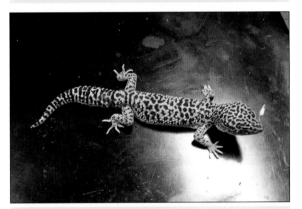

**Figure 20.2** Leopard gecko with dysecdysis, showing retained skin on digits.

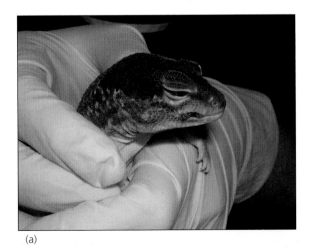

(a)

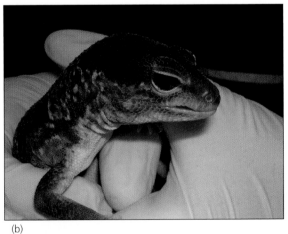

(b)

**Figure 20.3** (a) African fat-tailed gecko (*Hemitheconyx caudicinctus*) with retained shed in eye and at lip commissure. (b) Animal after retained skin removed.

- Bilateral eyes shut, with cream/brown material between the eyelids (similar to Fig. 20.3)
- Evidence of retained skin at commissures of jaw (similar to Fig. 20.3)
- Tags of skin covering all four feet ('glove' like) (Fig. 20.2). Missing distal tips of several digits
- Abdominal palpation revealed no obvious abnormalities
- No evidence of respiratory disease (e.g. open-mouth or noisy breathing, or nasal or oral discharges).

## DIFFERENTIAL DIAGNOSES

The differentials for *dysecdysis with retained skin* were:
- Poor husbandry, e.g. too hot, low relative humidity, lack of abrasive surfaces
- Malnutrition: hypoproteinaemia and hypovitaminosis A
- Dehydration
- Dermatitis
- Ectoparasites, e.g. mites and ticks
- Wounds or old scars: often result in dysecdysis for several cycles
- Seasonal influences, e.g. daylight length, temperature and/or relative humidity
- Systemic disease, septicaemia or hormonal conditions (hyperthyroidism has been reported in snakes, particularly older corn snakes).

## NURSING ASPECTS

### Condition assessment in leopard geckos
- Leopard geckos store fat reserves at the base of their tail.
- It is therefore relatively simple to ascertain body condition in these animals by assessing the width of the tail proximally.
- Underweight animals will have a thin tapering tail, and often the pelvic bones are prominent.
- Animals in good body condition will have a slightly rounded tail base.
- Overweight animals have an extremely round tail base.
- Muscle development can also be assessed by checking the amount of muscle in the limbs. The bones will be quite obvious and easily palpated in malnourished or unfit animals.

## CASE WORK-UP
### Husbandry
Assessment of the leopard gecko's husbandry suggested a lack of microclimate area with an elevated relative humidity – typically a hide area with moist substrate – which is necessary to assist ecdysis.

It was difficult to assess whether temperature problems were present. It is preferable to monitor the environmental temperature at both the cool and warm ends of the vivarium, using digital maximum–minimum thermometers. The cool end should be approximately 25°C, with a basking area of 32°C at the other end. Overnight, the temperature should not drop below 25°C.

The gecko's diet was good, with adequate supplementation. The water bowl in the enclosure was examined, finding no ectoparasites such as mites.

## OTHER POSSIBLE INVESTIGATIONS
### Skin
Microscopy on a Sellotape strip from the skin may identify ectoparasites more readily than using the naked eye. Cytology of impression smears – staining with Gram's stain to evaluate bacteria and/or Giemsa-style stain to assess cells present – may also be beneficial, particularly if an infection is suspected.

### Blood
It is sometimes useful to perform haematology, particularly if ectoparasites are present that may result in anaemia. Serum protein may be reduced if skin lesions result in exudates and fluid loss.

### Culture
Any discharges should undergo bacterial and fungal culture. Although superficial material may be contaminated from the environment it can still be useful to perform, as heavy growth of a micro-organism will be significant.

### Skin biopsy
Local anaesthesia – or preferably sedation or general anaesthesia – is required for this procedure. A sample may be sent for culture. Histology may identify bacterial or fungal conditions, such as mycobacteriosis or dermatophilosis, better than culture. Some skin lesions may be associated with viral infections such as poxviruses; diagnosis is based on virology on a biopsy sample.

## Imaging

Radiography and ultrasonography may identify systemic disease problems underlying or in association with the dysecdysis.

## DIAGNOSIS

Dysecdysis was diagnosed based on the clinical examination. The aetiology was not fully determined with the investigations performed, but husbandry deficits were suspected to be the most likely cause.

Dysecdysis is the abnormal shedding of skin in reptiles. While retained slough is the most common form encountered, dysecdysis may also present as excessive skin sloughing (e.g. with cases of thyroid dysfunction or hypo/hypervitaminosis A) or excessive sloughing of scutes in chelonia (e.g. in animals on diets high in protein and those with a low calcium to phosphorus ratio).

## ANATOMY AND PHYSIOLOGY REFRESHER

The skin of reptiles performs several functions. These include protection, water and electrolyte homeostasis, synthesis of hormone derivatives (e.g. production of vitamin D precursor) and camouflage. The epidermis and dermis make up the scales (and scutes in chelonia) (Fig. 20.4). The epidermis is composed primarily of three keratin layers, with an underlying layer for production. The dermis includes connective tissue, nerves, blood vessels and pigment cells.

Most lizards shed their skin piecemeal. However, normal ecdysis from the entire body should occur over a relatively short period of time and on a regular basis. The stratum germinativum generates new layers of

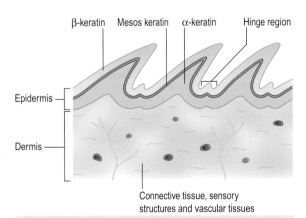

Epidermis —

Dermis —

β-keratin  Mesos keratin  α-keratin  Hinge region

Connective tissue, sensory structures and vascular tissues

**Figure 20.4** Normal reptile skin anatomy.

keratin underneath existing ones. Release of lymphatic fluids and proteolytic enzymes between the new and old layers creates a cleavage plane. The process usually occurs over about 2 weeks.

The eyelid geckos (Eublepharidae family) have movable eyelids rather than the transparent spectacles that most geckos possess. Eublepharidae also lack climbing pads on their feet.

## AETIOPATHOGENESIS OF DYSECDYSIS

The definition of dysecdysis is impaired shedding of the outer epidermal layers. Signs indicating dysecdysis in lizards include large areas of slough, multiple layers of keratin in slough, and/or retention of slough over extremities such as the digits and tail tip.

Retained skin around distal extremities may contract and result in tissue swelling, leading to gradual ischaemic necrosis. Leopard geckos and skinks are especially susceptible to this problem. The extremities are often lost. Periocular retained skin leads to conjunctivitis.

Reduced lymphatic output will reduce the efficacy of the cleavage plane. Low relative humidity in the environment therefore frequently causes dysecdysis through dehydration of the slough (in the short term) and the patient (long term, especially if water provision is inappropriate).

Snakes suffering from dysecdysis can be encouraged to move through a damp towel (i.e. moist abrasive surface) to aid shedding. Species such as snakes and species of gecko that do not possess eyelids – having spectacles instead – may suffer from retained spectacles when dysecdysis occurs.

## EPIDEMIOLOGY

As this condition is predominantly associated with husbandry problems, groups of animals housed in the same environment may present at the same time. Animals infested with ectoparasites or an enclosure containing ectoparasites will be a source of infection for other animals.

## TREATMENT

### Ocular

It was possible to remove some of the retained skin from the eyelids. The eyes were flushed with sterile saline using an intravenous catheter with the stylet removed to remove more of the debris.

## Rehydration

The leopard gecko was bathed in shallow warm water to aid rehydration, including of the retained skin. Gentle tension was then applied to the retained skin using forceps to remove it. Some areas were still quite firmly adhered to the underlying skin – these were left *in situ* at this time.

The animal was discharged with instructions for the owner to continue bathing for 15 minutes twice daily. Artificial tears were applied several times daily to soften the retained periocular skin.

## TREATMENT OPTIONS AND MANAGEMENT

### Husbandry

The owner was advised on improvements in husbandry conditions. The major requirement was provision of a hide area creating a humid microclimate. It is useful to monitor the relative humidity (aiming for 30–40% in the general enclosure). Digital hygrometers are available for this purpose.

In order to ensure an appropriate environmental temperature was provided, the owner was advised to use a digital maximum–minimum thermometer.

It is usually advisable to replace UV lights every 6–9 months, as UV output from bulbs will diminish over time. Some will produce UV for a longer period of time, but a UV meter is required to measure this.

It is advisable to increase relative humidity in cases of dysecdysis, for example by misting the vivarium, providing large shallow trays of water for evaporative loss into the environment and for bathing. Addition of a small hide enclosure with a microclimate of increased humidity – created by lining a plastic food container (with a doorway cut out) with moistened sphagnum moss or cotton wool – will assist normal shedding.

### Nutritional support

Since the gecko had not been feeding well, it was prudent to provide additional nutrition. Gavage-feeding was continued until the gecko was showing more interest in food.

## OTHER TREATMENT OPTIONS

### Diet

If the reptile is not eating, for example if vision is affected by periocular dysecdysis, assist-feeding may be required

> ### CLINICAL TIPS
>
> **Nutritional support**
>
> - Leopard geckos are predominantly insectivorous, and any nutritional aid administered should aim to replicate this.
> - For short-term use, baby food formulas may be used. A meat-containing dairy-free variety should be selected.
> - For longer term support, proprietary carnivore diets are available. Alternatively, invertebrates can be mashed and administered.
> - A volume of approximately 5 ml/kg may be administered at each gavage, and this may be repeated two or three times daily (depending on the animal's requirements). If dehydration is present, the food may be diluted to provide additional fluid.
> - A mouth gag, for example a wooden tongue depressor wrapped in bandage material, should be utilized to prevent damage to the animal's teeth or the gavage tube during the procedure.

for longer periods. In some cases, an oesophagostomy tube can be placed for this purpose.

### Ocular

On some occasions, ocular infections will develop. Topical antibiosis should be administered, preferably based on culture and sensitivity results.

## FOLLOW-UP

The gecko re-presented 1 week later. At this stage, it was possible to easily remove the remaining retained skin. The eyes were wide open and the gecko's appetite had improved.

## PREVENTION

Attention to appropriate husbandry requirements will avoid most aetiologies. Quarantine and good hygiene will reduce the risk of infectious agents.

## PROGNOSIS

With appropriate treatment, the prognosis for dysecdysis is good. However, lost extremities such as digits will not re-grow.

# 21 Aural abscesses in a map turtle

## INITIAL PRESENTATION

Head swellings on a map turtle.

## INTRODUCTION

Exotic pet – particularly reptilian – anatomy may vary significantly from commonly treated mammalian pets. This case discusses the anatomy of the reptilian ear, describing a common condition that is often associated with poor husbandry conditions. The veterinary clinician should be prepared to gain knowledge of differing anatomy and husbandry in order to best treat exotic pets.

## CASE PRESENTING SIGNS

A juvenile male map turtle (*Graptemys* species) (Box 21.1) presented with bilateral swellings on its head.

## HUSBANDRY

The client had owned the map turtle for 3 months, and housed it with a similar-sized con-specific. The enclosure was approximately 30 × 60 cm; it was constructed of a glass bottom and walls, and a plastic lid with ventilation slits. The water area had a gentle slope to permit easy access, and a maximum depth of 10 cm. An internal canister filter was present. A proportion of the water was changed weekly, equivalent to a complete water change approximately every 6 weeks. No routine water testing was carried out.

A basking area was provided, comprising a 'land' area with a substrate of soil and large pebbles. Some artificial plants were present, providing hiding places. A spot

bulb over this area produced a basking temperature of 32°C. A small underwater heater resulted in a water temperature (measured with a digital thermometer) of 24°C, dropping to 20°C overnight. A wire enclosure around the heater ensured that the turtles could not access it directly. A UV-B strip light was attached to the lid of the enclosure, sited approximately 30 cm above the surface of the substrate.

The map turtles' diet consisted of cat kibble (soaked in water), bloodworms and a small amount of spring greens. They were fed in their enclosure.

## CASE HISTORY

Two weeks prior to presentation, the owner had noticed swellings on the turtle's head. These had gradually increased in size. No other changes in behaviour, appetite or faecal output were noted. There had been no changes in husbandry since the turtle came into in the current owners' possession, although they did not have any details of the previous enclosure or diet.

## CLINICAL EXAMINATION

The map turtle was examined; findings included:
- Bright, alert and reactive
- Good body condition, weighing 100 g
- Moving around well, with no locomotor problems. Supporting body weight, standing up on all four limbs. No limb swellings or discomfort were detected
- Shell quality was firm. No skin lesions were present
- A firm swelling was present laterally on either side of the map turtle's head, caudal to the eyes. The

## BOX 21.1   ECOLOGY OF MAP TURTLES

- Range in the wild covers North America from Texas to Canada
- Normal habitat: semi-aquatic, freshwater (ponds, river-bottoms and lakes). Prefer large aquatic bodies, with areas of fallen trees or other debris for basking. Several animals may congregate to bask
- Average size: adult male = 10–25 cm in length, female = 18–27 cm in length, with weight 0.5–2.5 kg
- Sexual dimorphism: female much larger than male. Carapace more oval in males, who also have longer fore claws and a longer thicker tail (to contain the phallus)
- Reproduction: mating in deep waters, nesting (May–July) in unshaded sites with sandy soil. Clutch size = 6–20 eggs. Incubation = 50–70 days. Temperature-dependent sex determination
- Free-ranging diet: omnivorous, mainly feeding in water. Invertebrates such as aquatic insects, snails, crayfish and smaller crustaceans, also dead fish and plant material. The smaller male eats mainly insects, while the female consumes more molluscs and crustaceans. Older animals eat more plant material (<50% diet)
- Captive diet: animal material (70%) – rehydrated low-fat dried cat/dog/trout pellets, small raw fish, bloodworms, earthworms; fresh food (30%) – leafy green vegetables and aquatic plants
- Longevity: over 30 years
- Dormant: November–April.

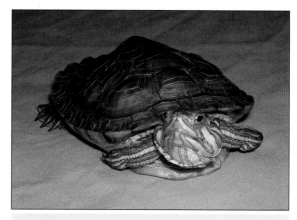

**Figure 21.1** Map turtle with bilateral cephalic swellings in the region of the tympanic membranes.

## DIFFERENTIAL DIAGNOSES

The differentials for *cephalic swelling(s)* were:
- Abscess of middle ear(s)
- Other infection: abscess, granuloma, fibriscess (granulomatous abscess); cellulitis; mycobacteria; viral (such as papillomas)
- Trauma: with haematoma formation, soft tissue damage or fractures
- Oedema
- Neoplasia (unlikely since bilateral)
- Foreign bodies (unlikely since bilateral)
- Parasites: cutaneous (such as ticks), subcutaneous (such as filarial worms, botfly)
- Sebaceous cysts.

swelling on the right protruded approximately 4 mm while that on the left extended approximately 3 mm (Fig. 21.1)
- No oral abnormalities were detected.

## CASE WORK-UP

### History and clinical examination

The most important aspects of investigation of this case were the above findings. Although some precautions were in place to address hygiene, they could be improved

upon (see below). The localization of the swellings on the lateral head just caudal to the eyes is the position of the ear in chelonia. Bilateral symmetrical lesions are most likely related to this anatomical structure.

### Other possible investigations that were not performed in this case

Imaging, such as radiography or ultrasound, would have been useful to rule out traumatic injuries or non-infectious fluid swellings. Computed tomography (CT) may also be useful to investigate head lesions in small animals.

A fine needle aspirate may have been useful to ascertain the contents of the swellings, with microscopic examination. This would have differentiated fluids, such as blood, serous exudates, or pus, and also help to rule out neoplasia as a differential.

## DIAGNOSIS

Bilateral aural abscessation: suspected on history and clinical examination, and proven on surgical exploration.

## ANATOMY AND PHYSIOLOGY REFRESHER

Chelonia, including terrapins such as the map turtle, do not have an external ear. The tympanic membrane is the outer limit of the middle ear. It lies level with the skin of the head and is covered by modified skin.

The eustachian tube is short and open. It leads to the pharynx from the middle ear, and thus the tube and middle ear are lined with mucous membrane. The entrance to the eustachian tube is visible in the pharynx, located just caudal to the mandible.

The middle ear contains one bone – the columella – that is rod-shaped. This connects to the tympanic membrane and the mandible (to the quadrate bone). Hearing relies on vibrations from the air or ground passing through this system – tympanic membrane to columella to perilymphatic fluid – to stimulate nerve impulses.

## AETIOPATHOGENESIS OF AURAL ABSCESSES IN CHELONIA

Abscesses in reptiles commonly involve Gram-negative bacteria (such as *Pseudomonas* or *Klebsiella*), although Gram-positive bacteria (such as *Staphylococcus* or *Streptococcus*) and anaerobes (such as *Bacteroides* or *Fusobacterium*) may be involved. Infective material generates an inflammatory response. This results in fibrin exudation, resulting in 'fibriscesses' (granulomatous abscesses). If pathogens are contained within the fibrin milieu a chronic infection may ensue. Thus reptilian abscesses are solid, and treatment is ideally by surgical excision (since lancing will not result in drainage as it does in mammals with liquid pus).

The columella and tympanic cavity are large. Aural abscesses are common at this site. Aquatic chelonia such as terrapins, including map turtles, are particularly susceptible to abscess/fibriscess formation in the middle ear. This infection may be associated with immunosuppression, which is often allied to poor husbandry conditions such as malnutrition or suboptimal environmental temperatures. Aural abscesses have also been associated with environmental pollutants in free-ranging chelonia.

## EPIDEMIOLOGY

Groups of animals housed in the same environment are likely to succumb to disease, due to the effects of inappropriate husbandry conditions on the immune system and the involvement of poor hygiene. Without improvements in husbandry, the condition may recur.

## TREATMENT

### General anaesthesia

Propofol (at 10 mg/kg) was injected into the sub-carapacial sinus to induce anaesthesia in the map turtle. The animal was then intubated using a 20-gauge intravenous cannula – with the stylet removed – attached to an endotracheal tube connector (Fig. 21.2). A short cannula is used to reduce the risk of intubating one bronchus (as the trachea bifurcates quite rostrally in chelonia). The tube and circuit were made rigid by attaching them to a wooden tongue depressor along the ventral surface of the patient's neck, thus preventing kinking and potential obstruction of the airway. Anaesthesia was maintained using isoflurane (at 2–3%), with intermittent positive pressure ventilation (IPPV) being performed.

> ### CLINICAL TIPS
>
> #### IPPV in chelonia
>
> - Many anaesthetic agents suppress respiration, often resulting in bradypnoea or apnoea. IPPV is useful to ensure adequate ventilation occurs, maintaining the supply of oxygen and anaesthetic gases.
> - IPPV may be performed by the anaesthetist or using a mechanical ventilator.
> - Tidal volume is larger in reptiles compared with mammals, but reptiles have a lower respiratory rate.
> - The airway pressure should peak at 8–10 cm $H_2O$ in chelonia. The patient should be observed, ensuring that body movements – i.e. small outward leg movements with the increase in intra-coelomic pressure during inspiration – are similar to those occurring in consciously breathing animals.
> - Inspiration should proceed over 1–2 seconds.
> - IPPV is usually administered at 4–8 breaths/minute.

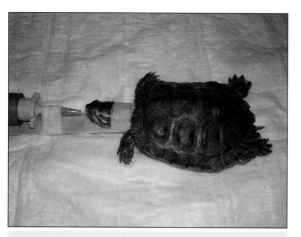

**Figure 21.2** Anaesthetized map turtle intubated with an intravenous cannula.

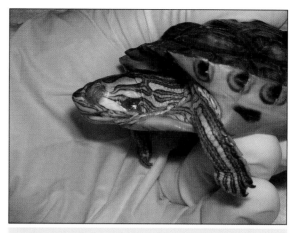

**Figure 21.3** Map turtle after surgery, showing semi-circular excision of tympanic membrane.

---

### NURSING ASPECTS

- Aquatic reptiles should not be permitted to return to their usual environment – with access to deep water – until fully recovered from anaesthesia.
- Until then they should be kept in a moist environment, e.g. on damp paper towels and sprayed with water.

### CLINICAL TIPS

**Injections in chelonia**

- When administering injections to chelonia, the skin should be thoroughly cleaned beforehand to reduce the risk of abscess formation.
- Intramuscular enrofloxacin injections are painful. Tissue necrosis and sterile abscesses may form. If administered subcutaneously, skin discolouration or necrosis may occur.

## Surgery

The map turtle was placed in sternal recumbency, permitting positioning of the head and neck laterally to allow access to each tympanic membrane in turn. The ventral portion of the tympanic membrane was removed by excising a semi-circular section of skin (Fig. 21.3). Abscessated material was removed using fine-tipped forceps and a small curette. The middle ear was then flushed with dilute povidone–iodine and sterile saline. A small catheter was passed into the eustachian tube, and flushed, to ensure patency.

## Medication

Fluids were given postoperatively (5 ml/kg of warmed Hartmann's solution administered intracoelomically). Analgesia was administered at the time of surgery (buprenorphine at 0.05 mg/kg and meloxicam at 0.1 mg/ kg IM). Systemic antibiosis was given in the form of enrofloxacin (at 5 mg/kg IM).

## TREATMENT OPTIONS AND MANAGEMENT

### Medication

Analgesia was continued postoperatively with meloxicam (at 0.1 mg/kg PO q24hr for a further 3 days). Enrofloxacin was continued for 2 weeks (at 5 mg/kg PO q48hr). The bilateral skin wounds were flushed with dilute povidone–iodine once daily for 1 week.

### Hygiene

The filtration system must be maintained. This will help ensure good hygiene in the water. The filter should be regularly cleaned, as well as performing regular water changes. Although internal canister filters usually suffice for smaller turtles, external ones are advisable for adult map turtles, due to the large amount of waste produced.

Water quality is improved if the turtles are fed in a separate tank, but this can be stressful for some individuals. Check water quality regularly using a test kit, assessing for toxic chemicals (such as nitrates and nitrites) and the pH. Water conditioning treatments can be used to neutralize toxic chemicals – such as chlorine and chloramine that are frequently used in public water supplies – in the water.

Most excreta are passed in the water, but the land area should also be kept clean. An animal safe disinfectant should be used in the enclosure.

## Husbandry

The environmental temperatures for this patient were adequate (with water temperature 24–26°C and a basking area of 32°C). The importance of monitoring – and recording – temperatures was impressed upon the owner.

Water quality should be checked regularly using a test kit. The filter should also be cleaned regularly.

---

### CLINICAL TIPS

#### Water quality

- A good quality test kit should be used to assess for nitrogenous waste products – ammonia, nitrite and nitrate – that are toxic.
- Other parameters that can be measured include temperature, pH and chlorine/chloramine (to ensure suitable water supply).
- Water should be routinely tested weekly (more frequently if a problem is present).
- Ammonia is oxidized by bacteria to nitrite, and thence to nitrate. The latter is the least toxic.
- Water temperature should be relatively constant.
- Ammonia and nitrite should not be detected if filtration is fully functional.
- Regular water changes should prevent significant accumulation of nitrate.

---

## Diet

The diet for this patient was satisfactory. However, growing reptiles should be supplemented with minerals such as calcium and phosphorus; this is usually accomplished by the addition of powdered supplements to feed, although for aquatic animals they should be trained to take this dusted food above water.

As the map turtles age, they should be offered a higher proportion of vegetable matter in their diet. The addition of aquatic plants to the environment may help; this will be easier in a larger enclosure (that will be required as the animals increase in size).

It is preferable to feed the map turtles in a separate enclosure, minimizing the presence of decomposing food that contributes to poor water quality.

## OTHER TREATMENT OPTIONS

### Surgery

In some cases, it may be possible to remove the abscess material without excising any overlying skin or tympanic membrane. In these cases, a semi-circular incision is made ventrally over the abscess and the material removed. In other instances with large abscesses, a complete circular area of skin and tympanic membrane needs to be excised to access and remove the abscess contents.

It is preferable to remove the abscess plug in one piece using a curette, as it can be difficult to ensure all infective material – particularly that within the eustachian tube – is removed if done piecemeal. If all such material has been removed, the skin may be sutured closed. However, it can be difficult to be certain that none remains and for most cases the middle ear is left open.

If the eustachian tube is not clear of infective material, the abscess will rapidly recur. The cavity should be flushed daily with antiseptic (such as chlorhexidine or povidone–iodine) until healing is progressing. Topical antibiotics may be useful in some cases.

### Supportive care

If the animal is not self-feeding, assist-feeding may be required. It can be difficult to maintain an oesophagostomy tube in aquatic species, as leakage at the skin incision commonly progresses to subcutaneous abscess formation.

If discomfort is noted – displayed, for example, by lethargy or other abnormal behaviour – further analgesia should be provided.

### Deterioration

If the animal becomes systemically unwell, a blood sample should be taken to assess haematological and biochemical parameters. If septicaemia is suspected, blood culture can be performed.

## FOLLOW-UP

The map turtle was reassessed at 1 week after surgery. It had been feeding well and behaving normally. The wounds had begun to dry. At 2 weeks after surgery, the skin had contracted significantly over the sites and granulation tissue was visible.

## PREVENTION

Optimal husbandry conditions – in particular good water hygiene, nutrition and sufficiently high environmental temperatures – are paramount to prevention of this condition. Ensuring aquatic animals are not exposed to toxins and pollutants is also advisable.

## PROGNOSIS

The prognosis for a full recovery in this case was good, providing the minor husbandry problems were addressed. In more debilitated animals, the prognosis may be poorer due to the likely presence of concomitant disease.

# Hypocalcaemia in a green iguana

## INITIAL PRESENTATION

Collapse and tremors in a green iguana.

## INTRODUCTION

Green iguanas are common reptile pets (Box 22.1). Destined to become large (<2 m in length) powerful animals, many owners struggle to provide an appropriate environment for them as they mature. This may lead to husbandry deficiencies as in this case and potentially fatal disease.

### CASE PRESENTING SIGNS

A 17-year-old female green iguana (*Iguana iguana*) presented with collapse and tremors.

## HUSBANDRY

The iguana's enclosure was a converted wooden cupboard measuring 1 m high × 1 m deep × 2 m wide; the front doors had been replaced by glass sliding doors. The substrate was newspaper. A hide box – made of cardboard – was present in the centre of the enclosure. Artificial plants were present. Several logs permitted the iguana to climb.

Supplemental heating was provided by two ceramic heat bulbs at one end of the enclosure. They were connected to a thermostat, set at 27–29°C. The owner did not measure the environmental temperature within the iguana's enclosure. A UV striplight was present at the top of the enclosure (approximately 30 cm above the highest branch), which had been replaced a few months previously.

The enclosure was spot-cleaned daily, with change of the newspaper substrate, and completely cleaned out and disinfected once every 3 months. A pet-safe disinfectant was used, and the enclosure and furniture (such as branches) rinsed well with water after cleaning.

The iguana was fed on a mixture of fresh and tinned vegetables and fruit. These included tinned mixed fruit, tinned mixed vegetables, fresh leafy greens, mixed salad leaves and spinach. A mineral supplement was added to the food once weekly. A shallow water bowl was provided for drinking and bathing.

Most of the time, the iguana was retained in the enclosure, but she was taken into the owner's living space occasionally for 1–2 hours at a time.

### CLINICAL TIPS

- It is important to use a safe substrate for lizards – either those that cannot be eaten or those that will not cause a gastrointestinal obstruction.
- Newspaper and Astroturf are safe to use.
- Wood chip-based substrates often result in blockages if eaten.

## CASE HISTORY

The owner had owned the green iguana for approximately 17 years, having purchased her from a local petshop. Several years previously, the iguana had been radiographed, showing the presence of poor bone density. The iguana did not have UV access for a prolonged period while still a growing juvenile. She had laid a clutch of eggs in the past; no problems were noted.

## BOX 22.1 ECOLOGY OF GREEN IGUANAS

- Range in the wild covers Central and South America, and the Caribbean. Introduced feral populations exist in the USA in south Florida, Hawaii and the Rio Grande Valley of Texas
- Tail: undergoes autotomy; re-grown tail will contain cartilaginous vertebrae. Will swim, using lateral tail movement for propulsion. Use tail to 'whip', protecting from predators; also use teeth and claws for protection
- Normal habitat: arboreal species – they are agile climbers using their long claws for grip. Rubbing against rough surfaces also helps to remove old skin during ecdysis. Diurnal
- Temperature range: 25°C (cool end) to 40°C (basking) during the daytime, and 20°C overnight
- Relative humidity: high
- Average adult weight: 5 kg (up to 10 kg)
- Snout to tail tip length: 1 m (maximum 2 m)
- Skin: scales are small and granular. Dorsal crest along full length of body and tail
- Free-ranging diet: herbivorous, feeding on leaves, flowers, fruit and growing shoots of many plant species. Occasionally consume invertebrates (usually as a by-product of eating plant material). Juveniles more likely to consume invertebrates
- Gender determination: sexual dimorphism. Males have well-developed dewlaps, used to regulate body temperature and for courtship and displays. Males also have prominent femoral pores on their ventral thighs. Hemipenal bulges present caudal to the cloaca in males. Adult males are highly territorial, particularly during the breeding season
- Reproduction: oviparous (egg-laying). Clutch of up to 40 eggs, laid in a nesting burrow. Temperature-dependent sex determination. Incubation 10–15 weeks. Young animals often remain in a group
- Parietal eye: present on dorsal skull, this is a photosensory organ
- Lateral nasal gland to excrete excess potassium and sodium chloride salts
- Popular pet. Also a food source – for both meat and eggs – in Latin America. Listed on CITES Appendix II.

Until 6 months previously, the iguana was housed with an adult male green iguana (which had died of unknown disease at that point).

The iguana was presented with an acute history of collapse, initially seen 2 hours prior to presentation. However, during the consultation it became clear that some other clinical signs had been present during the previous 48 hours.

- Previous 2 hours:
  - Collapse
  - Tremors/'shaking'
  - Intermittent stiffness of head and neck
- Previous 2 days:
  - Fell off log
  - Change in skin colouration, from brown to orange
  - Reduced appetite
  - Lethargy.

There was no history of access to potential toxins.

### CLINICAL EXAMINATION

A brief clinical assessment was performed to reduce the stress of restraint to the patient until a clearer picture of her health had been ascertained. Findings included:

- Body condition: thin. Animal small for her age. Weight = 1.31 kg
- Mucous membranes pink, but saliva quite viscous (suggested dehydration)
- Evidence of previous autotomy, with tail regrowth (obvious change to skin scales part-way down the tail, with smaller scales distal to the site of tail loss) (Fig. 22.1)

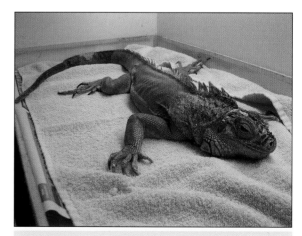

**Figure 22.1** Collapsed green iguana on presentation. Note the lack of body support by limbs, half-closed eyes, and re-grown distal tail after autotomy.

- No signs of respiratory disease
- Mandibular shortening and widening (likely associated with metabolic bone disease occurring as a growing individual)
- Unable to support body weight and limbs flaccid on presentation (Fig. 22.1). Paresis diagnosed (rather than ataxia)
- Both eyes half-shut (Fig. 22.1)
- Intermittent body tremors noted, also localized muscle fasciculations of the limbs
- Episode of rigid neck extension during clinical examination.

## DIFFERENTIAL DIAGNOSES

The differentials for *paresis, weakness and flaccidity* were:
- Hypocalcaemia
- Hypoglycaemia
- Central nervous system trauma
- Spinal trauma, often a sequel to secondary hyperparathyroidism (metabolic bone disease) if vertebral bodies collapse
- Other spinal pathology, such as spinal abscess
- Toxins, such as pesticides
- Septicaemia: usually with bacterial aetiology
- Renomegaly: resulting in pressure on the sciatic nerves
- Peripheral neuropathies, such as in hypothyroidism
- Central nervous system infection: bacterial, fungal, viral, parasitic (such as protozoa or visceral larva migrans)
- Cystic calculi.

The differentials for *lethargy* were:
- Husbandry inadequacies, such as inappropriate temperature, light pattern, relative humidity, or lack of UV lighting
- Nutritional disease, e.g. hypocalcaemia or hypovitaminosis A
- Musculoskeletal disease, e.g. poor mineralization
- Neurological disease, e.g. meningoencephalitis
- Hepatic disease, such as hepatic lipidosis
- Gastrointestinal disease, such as obstruction or endoparasitism
- Urogenital disease, e.g. follicular stasis or egg retention, or renal failure

- Psychological, e.g. with excessive noise or disruptive light patterns
- Respiratory disease, such as upper respiratory tract infection or pneumonia
- Sensual deprivation, such as loss of vision (e.g. with cataracts or other intraocular disease).

The differentials for *skin discolouration* were:
- Natural or behavioural changes: particularly in species such as anoles and chameleons, but many lizards can change colour to a degree
- Trauma, e.g. attack by another animal
- Ectoparasites, e.g. mites
- Septicaemia
- Burns
- Petechiae/ecchymoses.

The differentials for *loss of condition* were:
- Poor husbandry, e.g. inappropriate temperature and/or relative humidity
- Inappropriate diet or starvation
- Endoparasites
- Progressive dehydration, e.g. with a lack of fresh vegetables or fruit or accessible water, diarrhoea, or renal failure.

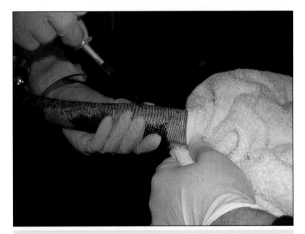

**Figure 22.2** Phlebotomy from the ventral coccygeal vein in a green iguana. The iguana is being restrained in dorsal recumbency.

## CASE WORK-UP

### Blood test

A blood sample was obtained from the ventral coccygeal vein (Fig. 22.2), and assessed using a portable blood analyser. Ionized calcium was low (0.6 mmol/l, normal

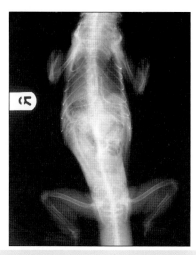

**Figure 22.3** Dorso-ventral radiograph showing gas distending the gastrointestinal tract.

range usually >1 mmol/l although species, gender and seasonal variations occur). Glucose and other electrolytes were within the normal reference range.

## Radiography

Conscious radiographs were taken. A vertical X-ray beam was used for the dorso-ventral view (Fig. 22.3) and a horizontal beam for the lateral view. Bone density was reasonably good, although some areas of the humeral and femoral cortices were irregular. The gastrointestinal tract was somewhat distended by gas, suggesting a degree of hypomotility. Some ingesta was present within the tract. No gastrointestinal obstruction or respiratory pathology was seen.

## DIAGNOSIS

Hypocalcaemia, resulting in muscular fasciculations and tetany, and gastrointestinal hypomotility.

## ANATOMY AND PHYSIOLOGY REFRESHER

Ionized calcium is the active portion of plasma calcium. Some 99% of the body's calcium store is in bone. If ionized calcium levels drop, parathyroid hormone (PTH) causes release of calcium and phosphorus from bone as well as further cholecalciferol (vitamin D3) absorption from the gastrointestinal tract. Cholecalciferol is a precursor to several steroid hormones, involved in PTH regulation, keratinocyte differentiation, immunity, insulin

secretion, muscle contractility and reproductive organ development.

Ultraviolet (UV) light on the skin results in the production of vitamin D. UV-B light, of a wavelength between 290 and 315 nm, is required for this photo-biosynthesis. An adequate skin temperature is also required. Reptiles vary in their ability to perform this synthesis, with some requiring much longer periods of UV exposure than other species.

## AETIOPATHOGENESIS OF NUTRITIONAL SECONDARY HYPERPARATHYROIDISM

Herbivore diets commonly contain low levels of both calcium and phosphorus. Animals not receiving appropriate supplementation will develop hypocalcaemia and increased PTH production (i.e. nutritional secondary hyperparathyroidism). The extra PTH will deplete bones of calcium, leaving osteopenia – that is readily detectable on radiographs. These osteopenic bones are weak and susceptible to pathological fractures.

Once bone reserves are depleted, serum hypocalcaemia may result. Clinical signs seen with hypocalcaemia include muscle tremors and fasciculation due to tetany. Digit twitching may progress to limb trembling and generalized tetanic spasms. Gastrointestinal hypomotility may occur. Death may be due to heart failure.

Other factors that may cause poor bone calcification include vitamin deficiencies (such as vitamin D (and/or its metabolites), A, C or K), minerals (such as calcium or phosphorus), hormone changes (including PTH or oestrogen) and/or inadequate exercise. Owing to the large number of functions of vitamin D, reptiles with a deficiency of this vitamin may also suffer from a broad range of problems such as obesity, heart disease and reduced immunocompetence.

## EPIDEMIOLOGY

Owing to the aetiology of this condition and the common presence of husbandry deficits in captivity, hypocalcaemia is frequently seen in herbivorous pet reptiles. (Carnivorous reptiles obtain minerals from bones in their diet of carcasses.) It is not unusual to see a group of conspecifics housed in similar conditions presenting together with clinical signs. It is important to note that such companion animals should be treated – with oral calcium supplementation and UV access – even if not showing clinical signs.

# TREATMENT

## Initial supportive care

As the iguana was extremely weak on presentation, supportive care was instigated with fluid administration (via an intraosseous catheter). The iguana was placed in a vivarium with supplemental heating (the environmental temperature was maintained at 25–30°C) and UV-B lighting. A small feed of convalescent diet – containing readily absorbable amino acids – was gavaged (5 ml/kg).

Excessive restraint appeared to trigger tetanic episodes. Handling was restricted to minimize any stress to the iguana. Medications were timed to reduce the frequency of handling.

---

### CLINICAL TIPS

Placement of an intraosseous (IO) catheter:
- IO catheters are usually contraindicated in reptiles with bone pathology such as severe metabolic bone disease, or those with infections in overlying soft tissues. In this case, the risk of an iatrogenic fracture was outweighed by the benefits of access to the circulation.
- The proximal tibia – in the tibial crest – is the commonest site for placement of an IO catheter or needle in lizards.

- Surgically prepare the skin over the stifle.
- In most cases, chemical restraint – such as a low dose of ketamine or propofol – is required to place the catheter. (This patient was extremely debilitated and did not require sedation or general anaesthesia for the procedure.)
- Inject local anaesthetic (0.01 ml of 2% lidocaine) into the periosteum.
- Use an intraosseous catheter, spinal needle or hypodermic needle. For the last, it can be helpful to use another needle or piece of sterile surgical wire as a stylet to prevent blocking with cortical bone. The needle should not measure more than half the length of the bone.
- Flex the stifle and insert the needle in a distal fashion while holding the tibia.
- The bone should move in the same direction as the needle when the needle hub is moved if positioning is correct. When a small amount of fluid is injected, there should be no resistance and no soft tissue swelling at the site. Radiographs can be used to assess positioning (Fig. 22.4).
- Continuous rate infusions are preferable to bolus injections IO in lizards owing to the small bone marrow space.

---

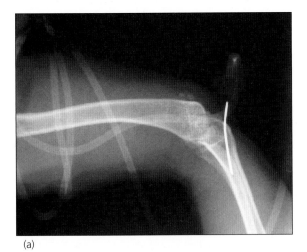

(a)

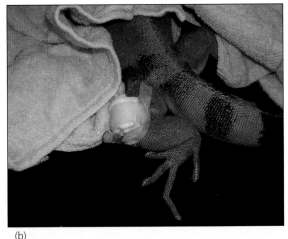

(b)

**Figure 22.4** Intraosseous needle placed in the tibia of a green iguana. (a) Radiographic confirmation of positioning within the medullary cavity. (b) Adhesive tape is used to hold the needle in place.

## Medication

Calcium gluconate was administered (100 mg/kg IM, repeating q8hr). Gastrointestinal motility was stimulated with metoclopramide (0.06 mg/kg PO q24hr). Analgesia was provided using buprenorphine (0.01 mg/kg IM q24hr).

## TREATMENT OPTIONS AND MANAGEMENT

### Nutritional support

Initially (for the first 2 days), fluids with additional amino acids and sugars were administered. Thereafter, a mix of herbivore convalescent diet was gavaged daily.

### Mineral supplementation

Once the patient was clinically stable, calcium supplementation was switched to daily oral administration using a liquid suspension containing calcium and phosphorus.

### Husbandry advice

The owner was advised to monitor the enclosure temperature using a maximum–minimum digital thermometer. The owner could adjust the supplemental heating as required, based on these readings.

Although some artificial lights may emit UV for prolonged periods, it is wise to either check their output with a UV meter or to renew them every 6–12 months.

The owner was advised to optimize the iguana's diet (see Nursing aspects, below), providing a variety of fresh vegetables and a small amount of fruit. Mineral supplementation should normally be given twice weekly, but in this case a daily addition was advised until blood levels stabilized.

### NURSING ASPECTS

Husbandry requirements of green iguanas:
- Environmental temperature: 25°C (cool end) to 40°C (basking area), with a minimum overnight of 21°C. Background heating is usually supplied by a tubular heater, heat mat (positioned on the back wall of the enclosure), ceramic bulb or heat plate – these can be attached to a thermostat. The heating should be covered, for example with a mesh grill, to prevent direct contact and burning of the pet.
- Provision of a branch or rock at the basking site will encourage its use.
- The use of a thermostat does not preclude the need for a thermometer to monitor temperature, as thermostats are often inaccurate.
- UV-B light, 30 cm above the iguana. This should be placed near the basking site.
- Mercury vapour lamps will provide heating and UV lighting. However, these cannot be attached to a thermostat and care should be taken that they do not overheat. Usually, these are switched on for 12 hours each day. Another source of background heating should be provided, particularly to maintain the temperature overnight.
- Relative humidity (RH): 80–90%. Regular spraying or misting the enclosure with a warm water spray will be required to maintain this high humidity. Placing the water bowl near the hot end of the enclosure will also elevate humidity. RH can be measured using a digital hygrometer.
- Diet: this should be 90% vegetable matter (e.g. parsley, cabbage, green beans, carrot tops, mustard, turnip, kale, spinach and broccoli) and 10% fruit (e.g. banana, pear, strawberries, grapes and apple).
- Supplementation: require 2:1 calcium to phosphorus ratio in the diet. A calcium and vitamin supplement should be added to the food twice weekly.
- If fed on animal protein, green iguanas develop pathologies, e.g. renal disease.

## OTHER TREATMENT OPTIONS

### Nutritional support

Where reptiles do not self-feed for prolonged periods, it can be useful to place an oesophagostomy tube. This will ease the administration of fluids, food and medication.

If a proprietary convalescent diet is not available, the clinician may use liquidized vegetables or vegetable baby food for assist-feeding.

### FOLLOW-UP

Muscle tone was improved within 30 minutes of administering calcium gluconate in the first instance.

The following day, the lizard was more alert and reactive. Although still unable to support her body weight, she was lifting her head and her eyes were fully open.

Faecal material was passed 4 days after admission. The iguana did not start to self-feed until 1 week after admission to the clinic. From that point on, muscular tone improved and she began moving around the vivarium. Calcium supplementation was switched to once daily oral administration at this point.

Blood calcium levels were repeated 48 hours after admission – at which point ionized calcium was 0.8 mmol/l – and 1 week later – by which time it had risen to 1.0 mmol/l. At the monthly re-check, the level was 1.2 mmol/l. A repeat blood test 6 months later showed ionized calcium to be 1.6 mmol/l, at which point the mineral supplementation was reduced to twice weekly.

## PREVENTION

This case had a long history of husbandry problems. Despite several veterinary clinicians stressing the importance of calcium, appropriate environmental temperatures and UV-B lighting, the owner failed to provide sufficient husbandry for prolonged periods. This resulted in a debilitated animal with a life-threatening illness. Good husbandry and diet would have prevented this problem.

## PROGNOSIS

The long-term prognosis for an animal with chronic metabolic disease is not favourable. Morbidity is likely to be present, although mortality is rare unless severe hypocalcaemia occurs. Reproduction should be avoided in females owing to the extra drain on calcium stores with egg production.

SECTION

4

# AMPHIBIANS

# 23 Amphibians – an introduction

## INTRODUCTION

There are over 4000 species in the three orders of the class Amphibia. Many are endangered in the wild, particularly due to worldwide spread of the fungal infection chytridiomycosis (*Batrachochytrium dendrobatidis*) that may also affect captive amphibians. Anurans (frogs and toads) are most commonly kept as pets, although members of the orders Caudata (salamanders and newts) or Gymnophiona (caecilians) may be seen from time to time.

## TAXONOMY

Taxonomic classification of amphibians commonly seen as pets is given in Table 23.1.

## BIOLOGY

The *thyroid* gland is predominantly responsible for controlling metamorphosis, and also ecdysis. Mexican axolotls (*Ambystoma mexicanum*) are obligate neotenic species, never metamorphosing in nature but doing so in captivity when thyroxine is administered. Tiger salamanders (*Ambystoma tigrinum*) are a facultative neotenic species, and metamorphose when TSH (thyroid-stimulating hormone) is produced in response to deteriorating environmental conditions.

As *ectotherms*, it is essential to house amphibians at an appropriate environmental temperature (both at the owner's home and at the veterinary clinic). Metabolic requirements vary depending on the environmental temperature and level of activity (increasing with illness or recovery from surgery). The preferred optimum temperature range (POTR) required may change according to species, age, season and current bodily functions (e.g. digestion or reproduction). Amphibians do not depend solely on the environmental temperature for thermoregulation. They can vary their body temperature by postural and locomotor changes, peripheral vasodilation and constriction, and changes in skin colour.

Anurans and caudates that hibernate have additional physiological adaptations to lower the freezing point of tissues, and permit ice formation in extracellular compartments. Although many species can survive at very broad temperature ranges, they adapt over a period of time. Rapid fluctuations in temperature should be avoided, as potentially fatal thermal shock may result.

*Moisture* is essential to amphibians. Physiology differs between terrestrial and aquatic amphibians. The former need to protect against water loss to the environment, while the latter need to cope with the threat of overhydration. Aquatic species thus excrete excess water and conserve plasma solutes.

These animals have various physiological means of preventing dehydration, such as secretion of waterproofing substances (e.g. South American tree frogs, *Phyllomedusa* spp), dried mucus on the skin, behavioural changes such as posture variation and limiting activity unless humidity is high. Some species, such as axolotls and mudpuppies, are completely aquatic. Some anurans have a 'drinking patch', an area of modified skin on their ventral pelvic region that is responsible for up to 80% of their water uptake.

Amphibian skin is relatively permeable, and is used for gas exchange. Desiccation may occur in excessively dry environments. Terrestrial animals require a relative environmental humidity of 60–80% for temperate species and 70–90% for tropical species. Water quality is extremely important to amphibian health, and parameters should be monitored. Water should be dechlorinated, and filtration or regular replacement of water is necessary for aquatic species or larval forms.

Amphibian *kidneys* cannot concentrate urine more than the concentration of plasma solutes. In aquatic anurans, ammonia is excreted via the kidneys as well as diffused across the skin. Most terrestrial anurans excrete urea.

**Table 23.1** Taxonomic classification of amphibians commonly seen as pets

| Order | Suborder | Family | Species |
|---|---|---|---|
| Gymnophiona | Caecilians | **6 families, e.g.**<br>Caeciliidae | **176 species** |
| Caudata | Salamanders and newts | **10 families, e.g.**<br>Sirenidae<br>Cryptobranchidae<br>Salamandridae<br><br>Proteidae<br>Ambystomatidae | **473 species, e.g.**<br>Sirens<br>Giant salamanders<br>Newts and European salamanders (e.g. fire salamander, *Salamandra salamandra*)<br>Olm, mudpuppies (*Necturus maculosus*) and waterdogs<br>Mole salamanders (e.g. tiger salamander, *Ambystoma tigrinum*, and axolotl, *Ambystoma mexicanum*) |
| Anura | Frogs and toads | **28 families, e.g.**<br>Pipidae<br><br>Bufonidae<br><br>Dendrobatidae<br>Ranidae<br>Hylidae<br><br>Bombinatoridae | **4750 species, e.g.**<br>Clawed frogs (e.g. African clawed frog, *Xenopus laevis*) and Surinam toads (*Pipa pipa*)<br>True toads, harlequin frogs and relatives (e.g. cane (marine) toad, *Bufo marinus*)<br>Poison frogs (e.g. poison dart frog, *Dendrobates* spp)<br>True frogs (e.g. leopard frog, *Rana pipiens*)<br>Tree frogs (e.g. green tree frog, *Hyla cinerea*, and White's tree frog, *Litoria caerulea*)<br>Fire-bellied toad (*Bombina* spp) |

Amphibian *hearts* are three-chambered, comprising two atria and one ventricle. The interatrial septum may be fenestrated, permitting mixing of oxygenated and deoxygenated blood. The lymphatic system is well developed, with lymph hearts (or lymph sacs) that return lymph (blood without erythrocytes) back to the heart.

The *haematolymphopoietic* system of amphibians differs from other taxonomic groups. Some species have bone marrow, although its function is not the same as in mammals. The spleen is the site of erythropoiesis and myelopoiesis. The thymus remains throughout life (although it may involute with chronic stress or malnutrition). The function of lymph nodes (which are absent in amphibians) is performed by gut-associated lymphoid tissue.

The *respiratory* system varies between orders and species, and intraspecies depending on life-stage and environment. Amphibians do not have a diaphragm. Most larval stages are aquatic, have external gills and rely on branchial respiration. Gills are often lost when amphibians metamorphose. Adult anuran respiration may be cutaneous, buccopharyngeal and/or pulmonic. In adult salamanders, branchial, cutaneous, buccopharyngeal or pulmonic respiration may occur. Neotenic species such as axolotls (*Ambystoma mexicanum*) have external gills. Sirens have lungs and gills. Adult caecilians have pulmonic (except for one lungless species), buccopharyngeal and cutaneous respiration.

Amphibian teeth are shed and replaced throughout life. Most anuran and salamander tongues can extend to capture prey. The *intestinal* tract is relatively short.

Gonads are paired in amphibians, with seasonal fluctuations in *reproductive* activity. Sexual dimorphism (e.g. nuptial pads developing in male White's tree frogs (*Pelodryas caerulea*) during the breeding season) is rarely present. Anurans are external fertilizers, most salamanders are internal fertilizers (via spermatophores), while all caecilians fertilize internally (copulating via a phallodeum). Many amphibians are seasonal breeders; visual and environmental cues are important for reproduction.

Anurans have well-developed *senses*. These include auditory structures, ocular structures (apart from caecilians), as well as taste, touch and olfaction. Amphibians have a Jacobson's organ for chemodetection.

## HUSBANDRY

Most species require a vivarium with a terrestrial area as well as shallow water. Good water quality should be maintained. Most species return to water to breed. Hide areas should be provided. Temperature and humidity gradients should be present. UV light is required by many species. Deep leaf litter is a good substrate for many amphibians. The vivarium should mimic the native environment for the species as closely as possible.

Many tadpoles are herbivorous (eating natural microflora on pond weed when small), converting to carnivores at metamorphosis. Adult amphibians are all carnivorous, mostly insectivores (being fed on earthworms, crickets, ants and mealworms in captivity), although larger species consume vertebrates (such as pinkies). Invertebrates should be supplemented with vitamins and calcium. Nutritional secondary hyperparathyroidism (NSHP) is common in captive amphibians if an inappropriate diet is consumed.

## Anura

Adult anurans do not possess a tail, nor do they have external gills (Fig. 23.1). The hindlimbs are usually longer than the forelimbs, and toes are often webbed. To improve jumping performance, the vertebrae are fused (including the pelvic girdle), with presacral, sacral and postsacral regions. There is no sacrum. Although tadpoles can regenerate lost limbs, generally adults cannot.

### White's tree frog ( Litoria caerulea)

A nocturnal species native to Australia and New Guinea, White's tree frog has been introduced to New Zealand and the USA. It may live 16 years in captivity. Obesity is common if animals are overfed. The environmental temperature should ideally be 26–28°C, but they are able to withstand lower temperatures. This arboreal species should be provided with branches for climbing.

### Poison arrow frogs ( Dendrobates spp)

These species come from tropical rainforests in Central and South America. They secrete toxins through their skin; as the chemicals are sequestered from prey items such as ants, captive animals do not have significant levels of toxins. They require a high environmental humidity (80–100%) and temperature (28–32°C).

### African clawed toads ( Xenopus laevis)

This totally aquatic species requires an aquarium, with water 10–20 cm deep at 20–26°C. They should be fed twice weekly on worms, fish or meat pieces.

## Caudata

Salamanders have an appearance similar to lizards. In most, the tail is flattened laterally. Most species have four limbs; however, sirens lack hindlimbs. Digits and limbs can be regenerated if lost. They will undergo autotomy. Some species have feather-like gills. Although mostly insectivorous, some will take small vertebrate prey (such as frogs or pinkies).

### Tiger salamander (Ambystoma tigrinum)

This species originates from North America, and requires a temperature of 15–25°C. Free-ranging individuals are generally terrestrial, returning to water to breed.

### Fire salamander (Salamandra salamandra)

These live in deciduous forests in southern and central Europe, hiding in fallen leaves and mossy tree trunks. Adults secrete the neurotoxic alkaloid samandarin. Most are ovoviviparous, but two subspecies are viviparous.

### Axolotl (Ambystoma mexicanum)

This is a neotenic species, with the adult an unmetamorphosed larval form. It is totally aquatic. Water temperature should be 10–25°C.

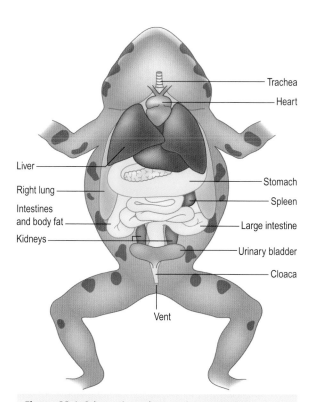

**Figure 23.1** Schematic to show major organs in an anuran (ventral view).

Trachea
Heart
Liver
Right lung
Intestines and body fat
Kidneys
Stomach
Spleen
Large intestine
Urinary bladder
Cloaca
Vent

## Gymnophiona

Caecilians are limbless, with a similar appearance to earthworms or snakes. The tail if present is very short. They do not possess pectoral and pelvic girdles, or a sacrum; locomotion is worm-like. Small olfactory and sensory tentacles are present just rostral to the eyes. Caecilians spend most of their time hidden underground. Their eyes are small and covered by skin for protection during burrowing. They originate from tropical regions of South-east Asia, Africa, the Seychelles islands and South America. Most species are viviparous, but some are oviparous.

## HISTORY

Husbandry is extremely important in the care of amphibians, with many diseases deriving from inappropriate conditions. Questioning of the owner will cover similar ground as that for reptiles (see Chapter 15), describing the vivarium and diet. Humidity and water quality are particularly important factors for amphibians.

## CLINICAL EXAMINATION

### Handling/restraint

Amphibians can be transported in containers with a damp substrate, except for aquatic species that require immersion in water. Ventilation should be provided.

Conscious examination may be possible in some amphibian species. However, conscious restraint can be very stressful for some smaller species. For example, the spot-legged poison frog (*Epipedobates pictus*) may die if manually restrained for a few minutes. Aggressive species such as horned frogs (*Ceratophrys* spp) may bite, and are best examined under sedation or anaesthesia.

If torn, skin defects permit entry of pathogens. Handlers should wear moistened powder-free examination gloves to reduce the risk of damage to the patient's skin. Some amphibians produce toxic (some potentially lethal) or irritating substances from their skin, and gloves will also protect the handler from contact with these.

Small animals can be cupped in the palm of the hand against the side of the enclosure. Larger species are restrained similarly but additionally holding the head between the first two fingers, with the thumb gently pressed against the neck. Fine nylon nets may be useful, but damage may occur during capture.

## Examination

The amphibian is initially observed in the enclosure or travel container, assessing body condition, locomotion, demeanour, skin secretions, and respiratory rate. Thereafter, the animal is restrained for a thorough physical examination. Areas of note include the head, skin and cloaca.

## INVESTIGATION

### Phlebotomy

The ventral coccygeal vein is accessed in salamanders. In larger anurans, the midline ventral abdominal vein or femoral vein may be used (Fig. 23.2). The lingual vein lies on the dorsal surface of the tongue when it is pulled forward (in the anaesthetized animal). General anaesthesia should be induced if cardiocentesis is to be performed.

### Imaging

Imaging techniques may be used for amphibians as in other species, although dental non-screen radiographic film is preferred in small animals to show finer detail. Radiography is useful to assess bone density in suspected cases of NSHP or for identification of radio-opaque foreign bodies. Contrast studies may be performed, usually with a 1:10 dilution of contrast medium.

Ultrasonography is easiest performed with the animal inside a water bath, precluding the obligation to apply coupling gel to the amphibian's skin (that may affect cutaneous respiration).

### Sampling

Skin lesions may be swabbed for microscopy or culture. Giemsa or Gram-staining is commonly performed, as well as dark-field microscopy for protozoa. The most sensitive test for chytridiomycosis is PCR performed on swabs taken from the skin (usually the ventral abdomen and inner thighs).

Faeces should be collected for wet microscopy, assessing for endoparasites. Tracheal swabs may be useful for investigation of respiratory disorders. It is preferable to perform this technique under general anaesthesia. Blood culture is useful for animals suspected to be septicaemic.

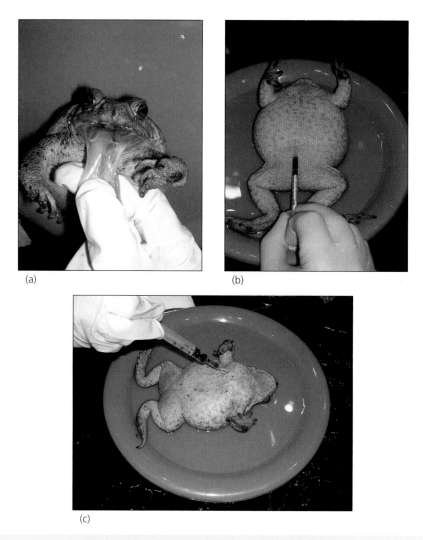

(a)

(b)

(c)

**Figure 23.2** Phlebotomy in anurans (anaesthetized cane toads, *Bufo marinus*). (a) The lingual venous plexus is located by flipping the tongue forward. (b) Midline ventral abdominal vein. (c) Cardiocentesis.

## TREATMENT

### Basic procedures

#### Drug administration

The easiest route of drug administration is *topical* application, due to the extremely permeable nature of amphibian skin. Irritant formulations or those that occlude the skin should be avoided. Medicated baths may also be used, taking into consideration that temperature and pH will affect absorption. With both these routes, the exact dose received is usually not known.

The *oral* route is preferred for accurate dosing. A small plastic gag is used to open the mouth before administration.

*Subcutaneous* injections are possible, although care should be taken not to tear the skin if performed in conscious animals. The *intramuscular* route is preferred for small volumes. *Intracoelomic* injections are possible. The *intravenous* route is possible in larger patients, usually the ventral abdominal vein, or alternatively the femoral vein (in larger species) or ventral tail vein (in salamanders). Some medications can be administered into the lymph sacs (e.g. the dorsal lymph sacs of anurans); this is equivalent to injecting into the circulation. *Intraosseous* injections are rarely required.

### Assist-feeding

Carnivore convalescent diets can be syringe-fed or administered by gavage to debilitated adult amphibians. Maintenance of water and electrolyte balance is vital, and ill animals are routinely bathed in shallow solutions of electrolytes.

## Anaesthesia

Sedation or anaesthesia may be required for the animal's safety (to reduce the stress of manual restraint), for the handler's safety (with aggressive species), or to perform certain procedures (such as internal transillumination, venepuncture, or surgery).

### Pre-anaesthesia

Aspiration after regurgitation is rare, but most species are fasted before elective procedures (for example <4 hours if <20 g body weight, 48 hours if >20 g, or 7 days if being fed vertebrates).

### Pre-medication

Pre-medicants are not usually administered to amphibians.

### Inhalation agents

Anaesthetics such as halothane and isoflurane may be administered to amphibians by mixing the liquid with a water-soluble gel and applying it to the skin. When a surgical plane of anaesthesia has been reached, the gel is wiped off. However, the dose administered is not known and prolonged maintenance of anaesthesia can be problematic.

---

### CLINICAL TIPS

- Large specimens may be intubated.
- However, cutaneous respiration means maintenance via pulmonic administration of anaesthetic gases is problematic.
- Cutaneous respiration is usually sufficient to maintain oxygenation.

---

### Injectable agents

In larger species, agents such as ketamine, propofol and tiletamine/zolazepam have been used, although results may be variable. Propofol has also been administered topically to small amphibians, resulting in sedation or anaesthesia.

### Immersion

This is the route of choice for anaesthesia of amphibians. Common agents include tricaine methanesulfonate (MS-222), benzocaine and clove oil (eugenol). For all of these agents, they are mixed with water from the animal's enclosure to minimize thermal or chemical shock. For prolonged procedures, air or oxygen should be bubbled into the bath to ensure sufficient oxygenation. The animal is induced with a higher concentration of anaesthetic agent, then removed completely from the bath for short procedures, or anaesthesia prolonged by applying a more dilute concentration of the agent over the skin. Recovery is speeded by washing off any residual anaesthetic with clean water.

MS-222 is buffered before use with sodium phosphate or sodium bicarbonate, aiming for pH 7–7.4. Higher concentrations are required for anaesthesia of larval forms. Induction in toads is slower than in frogs and salamanders.

### Monitoring anaesthesia

The cardiac impulse may be visible, or Doppler flow monitors can be used to assess the heart rate. The respiratory rate is counted by observation of buccopharyngeal or pulmonic movements.

### Peri-anaesthetic care

The patient should be maintained within its species POTR throughout the procedure and recovery periods. Hydration is aided by soaking the amphibian in a shallow water bath for 60 minutes prior to surgery. The patient is kept moist throughout the procedure.

## SURGERY

Many antiseptics are toxic to amphibians, including iodine products; 0.75% chlorhexidine may be used to prepare amphibian skin for surgery, rinsing with sterile saline at the end of the surgical preparation. The skin is closed using a simple interrupted or horizontal mattress pattern, ensuring skin edges do not roll inwards. Dehiscence is common, and interrupted patterns are preferred to continuous. Tissue glues may assist with waterproofing after surgery.

The most common surgery performed in amphibians is gastrotomy to remove gastric foreign bodies (often pieces of gravel used as substrate), in cases where endo-scopic retrieval is not possible. When performing a coeliotomy, a paramedian incision should be executed to avoid the ventral midline abdominal vein. Other surgeries such as limb amputations may also be performed.

Analgesia should be considered after painful procedures. Prophylactic antibiotics should be administered after surgery. Assist-feeding may be required postoperatively in some cases.

## EUTHANASIA

An overdose of barbiturates can be administered intravenously or intracoelomically. Alternatively an overdose of MS-222 or benzocaine in a water bath will result in euthanasia. Death is confirmed by a lack of heart beat (detected using a Doppler probe), or ensured by pithing.

## INITIAL PRESENTATION

Superficial wound in a marine toad.

## INTRODUCTION

Amphibians rarely present to veterinary clinics, but make interesting patients. Conditions are often related to husbandry issues, although infectious diseases such as chytridiomycosis are also prevalent. Care should be taken when handling and housing amphibians in the clinic.

## CASE PRESENTING SIGNS

An adult marine toad (*Bufo marinus*) (Box 24.1) presented with a superficial wound on the proximal ventral area of one hindlimb.

## HUSBANDRY

The toad was housed in a room with the owner's other pets, but within a separate enclosure. The terrarium was constructed of glass – measuring 30 × 45 cm – insulated on three sides and with a ventilation panel in the lid. It was positioned in an area of the owner's living room that was sheltered from direct sunlight. The substrate consisted of a moist layer of sphagnum moss overlying a layer of pea gravel, with bark chippings and a wooden branch at one end. A hide area of cork bark was also provided. The enclosure also contained some artificial plants.

A small freshwater pool – 2 cm in depth – was provided. The water was changed weekly. The enclosure was misted twice daily to increase the relative humidity. A UV light was positioned approximately 30 cm above the substrate, and had been new when the owner acquired the animal six months ago.

The enclosure temperature was 23–27°C and relative humidity 70–85%. These were monitored using a maximum–minimum digital thermometer and hygrometer.

The animal's diet comprised mealworms, crickets, locusts and pinkies (newborn mice). The invertebrates were gut-loaded during the 24 hours prior to feeding the toad, and dusted with a mineral supplement prior to feeding.

The owner kept several other amphibians, including a White's tree frog (*Litoria caerulea*), axolotls (*Ambystoma mexicanum*) and some fire salamanders (*Salamandra salamandra*). None of these animals had significant medical history. The marine toad had been quarantined for a period of 1 month on acquisition; it was housed in a separate room during this period and separate cleaning utensils were used.

## CASE HISTORY

The toad had been in the current owner's possession for 6 months. The problem had been noted 2 hours prior to presentation:

- A wound was seen on the right hind leg
- Demeanour, appetite and defaecation were normal
- A new plastic hide had been placed in the enclosure the previous day. No other husbandry changes had been made in the previous 6 months.

## CLINICAL EXAMINATION

A visual assessment was made of the toad while contained within the clear plastic transport container. This revealed:

## BOX 24.1 ECOLOGY OF MARINE TOADS

- Also known as cane, giant or Mexican toads
- Range in the wild: native to Central and South America, but introduced to many regions for agricultural pest control. Introduced into Australia in the 1930s to control pests in sugarcane plantations, but became a pest species
- Normal habitat: terrestrial. Require water to breed. Tropical/subtropical regions
- Average weight: females up to 2.5 kg (report of one individual measuring 38 cm and weighing 2.65 kg)
- Measure 10–15 cm from snout to vent (females <26 cm); tadpoles 1.0–2.5 cm in length
- Tongue strikes prey in 37 ms, taking about 143 ms to capture prey
- Free-ranging diet: mostly invertebrates such as ants, beetles, termites. Also anything that fits into the toad's mouth, such as small mammals (rodents), reptiles, birds and other amphibians
- Can project toxic fluid up to 1 m from their parotid glands. Human fatalities in Fiji and the Philippines have occurred after eating the toad, or even soup prepared from its eggs
- Reproduction: sexually mature at 9–10 cm in length; 8–25 000 small eggs per clutch, in rosary-like strings
- Life expectancy 10–15 years in the wild, <35 years in captivity
- Critical thermal maximum of 40–42°C and minimum around 10–15°C
- High tolerance of water loss.

- The toad was bright, alert and reactive
- A lesion was present on the ventral surface of the thigh on the right hind leg.

## CLINICAL TIPS

### Handling marine toads

- Care should be taken when handling marine toads owing to the risk of toxin ejection from their parotid glands.

- Examination gloves should be worn to reduce the risk to the handler, and they should be wetted with water to reduce the risk of trauma and transfer of infections to the toad. Eye goggles or a clear visor are useful to protect the face.
- Toads should be restrained by grasping around the abdomen (the 'waist' area), and supporting the cranial body (Fig. 24.1).

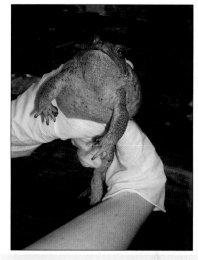

**Figure 24.1** Restraint of a marine toad.

Further clinical examination revealed:
- The toad was in good body condition – with good musculature but no excessive fat deposits – and weighed 1 kg
- Oral mucous membranes were pink
- No stomatitis, ocular lesions, or dysecdysis was present
- The owner had reported no lameness, and all four limbs appeared to be moving well. After the main clinical examination, the toad was released into a larger enclosure and its locomotion assessed further – and was found to be normal
- Minor haemorrhage was present from the wound, which was approximately 2 cm in length. The wound was relatively clean, although some moss was stuck to the skin edges.

The differentials for the *wound* were:
- Lacerations due to inappropriate handling, encounter with a sharp object within the enclosure, or injuries from live rodent prey (not legal in the UK)
- Attack from a con-specific (not possible in this case as housed in isolation)
- Pathology resulting in thin friable skin that is easily torn, e.g. bacterial or fungal infection (for example chytridiomycosis, Box 24.2), malnutrition, or neoplasia.

### BOX 24.2   CHYTRIDIOMYCOSIS

- This disease is caused by *Batrachochytrium dendrobatidis*.
- The fungus uses keratin as its substrate and, although infection usually causes only microscopic changes in tadpoles, overt disease is seen in adults.
- Osmotic regulation and other functions of the skin are disrupted. Clinical signs include excessive shedding of the skin, hyperaemia of pale skin, and sudden death. Secondary infections with other pathogens are possible.
- Owing to the extreme contagiousness of this infection, equipment should be sterilized between enclosures and between handling of amphibians. This is necessary, particularly in the veterinary clinic, if amphibians from more than one source are seen.
- Treatment of some cases is possible with itraconazole baths, but a complete cure is not guaranteed.

## CASE WORK-UP

### Cleaning

The wound was flushed with sterile saline to remove excessive debris and to enable closer examination of the lesion.

## OTHER OPTIONS FOR INVESTIGATION

### Culture

A swab from the lesion could have been submitted for bacterial and fungal culture. This is especially useful if the lesion is deep and suspected to be due to a bite. Although contaminants from the environment are likely to be present, a significant growth combined with the presence of obvious infection at a later date warrants sensitivity-based antibiosis.

### Imaging

If the toad was lame or had other signs of ill health, radiography would be useful to assess for fractures and also bone density (metabolic bone disease is relatively common in captive amphibians).

### Blood analysis

If the patient had been systemically unwell – or became so during treatment – phlebotomy would be advised to enable haematology and clinical chemistries to be performed.

## DIAGNOSIS

Owing to the history of a recent addition to the enclosure furniture with a sharp edge, a traumatic wound was suspected.

## ANATOMY AND PHYSIOLOGY REFRESHER

The skin of amphibians performs the roles of thermoregulation, homeostasis of hydration, sex recognition and reproduction. This layer also protects against entry of pathogens. The skin comprises the epidermal layer and the dermal layer. The stratum corneum layer of the epidermis is thin and easily damaged. The dermal layer comprises the stratum spongiosum and stratum compactum. The dermal layer also contains capillaries, nerves and smooth muscle. Respiration in anurans (frogs and toads) occurs partly via the skin.

## AETIOPATHOGENESIS OF SKIN LESIONS

Damage to the skin results in a break in the protective layer over the body. Fluids may be lost and pathogens may readily enter.

## EPIDEMIOLOGY

Skin lesions are not uncommon in amphibians because of the thin anatomy of the integument. However, they should be minimal if captive animals are maintained in an appropriate environment.

## TREATMENT

### Anaesthesia

MS-222 was used to induce anaesthesia in the toad, using a 0.3% (3 g/l) solution buffered with sodium

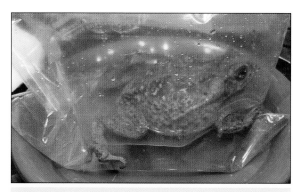

**Figure 24.2** Induction of anaesthesia in the marine toad, using MS-222 in a plastic zip-lock bag.

bicarbonate to produce a pH of around 7 (Fig. 24.2). Within 5 minutes, this resulted in surgical anaesthesia of 25 minutes' duration.

## Surgery

The wound was cleansed with 0.75% chlorhexidine and then rinsed with sterile saline. It was flushed with gentamicin solution. The skin edges were debrided and closed using poliglecaprone 25 (4/0 USP, 1.5 metric) in a horizontal mattress pattern. A small amount of tissue glue was applied to assist with waterproofing.

## Peri-anaesthetic care

Buprenorphine (0.075 mg/kg) was administered into the dorsal lymph sac to provide analgesia. The toad was bathed in normal saline for 20 minutes before induction of anaesthesia to ensure adequate hydration. (For obviously sick amphibians, recipes are available for other solutions that more closely mimic the animal's electrolyte status.)

The toad was hospitalized in a small plastic enclosure with damp kitchen roll as substrate until it had recovered from anaesthesia and was discharged. An upturned plastic box with cut-out doorway was provided as a shelter, along with a shallow water dish (added after recovery from anaesthesia). Dechlorinated water should be used for all water provision in the hospital. The patient took food the day after surgery, and assist-feeding was not required.

## TREATMENT OPTIONS AND MANAGEMENT

### Hygiene

It is important to maintain good hygiene in the enclosure during the healing period. It may be simpler to swap the moss substrate for moist kitchen paper as it is easier to

replace and keep clean. Water quality in the enclosure should also be the best possible, with checks made routinely.

### Husbandry

General husbandry should be optimal. This includes ensuring the correct environmental temperature and relative humidity. Prey items should be offered as appropriate.

The suspected source of the injury – the new hide box – was checked and found to have one sharp edge. This was filed to create a smooth surface.

> **NURSING ASPECTS**
>
> Medications may readily be administered within food providing the toad is eating.

## OTHER TREATMENT OPTIONS

### Medical management

In this case, the wound was relatively large and fresh and surgical closure deemed appropriate. However, in some cases, the wound may be small and/or contaminated, and healing by secondary intention may be preferred. The wound should be kept clean during this period, with daily flushing using sterile saline. Systemic antibiosis (e.g. enrofloxacin at 5–10 mg/kg PO/SC/IM q24hr or oxytetracycline at 25 mg/kg SC/IM q24hr) may be required for severe or problematic wounds. Analgesia and assist-feeding, e.g. by gavage, should be administered as deemed necessary.

## FOLLOW-UP

The toad was re-examined 1 week after the surgery and the wound was found to be healing well. The patient was eating as normal. The sutures were removed 2 weeks after surgery.

## PREVENTION

Care should be taken to ensure no sharp items are present within the enclosure of amphibians, and during handling.

## PROGNOSIS

The prognosis for this lesion was good, as it was fresh and minimally contaminated. For bite wounds, deep infections are common and do not always respond to therapy.

# FISH

# 25 Fish – an introduction

Many species of fish are kept in captivity, varying from small tropical species housed in indoor heated aquaria to larger temperate species in outdoor ponds. Enclosures are often expensive to build and maintain, and ornamental fish can themselves be expensive to purchase. Unlike some other captive animals, it is often imperative to treat the aquarium or pond inhabitants medically as a group, although there will be instances when individuals present for therapy.

## TAXONOMY

There are two superclasses of fish. Although some aquarists keep cartilaginous fishes such as small sharks and rays, most fish species kept as pets belong to the last class in Table 25.1, the ray-finned fishes (Actinopterygii). This group includes (among many others) carps, flatfishes, perch-like fishes and seahorses.

The most common captive cold freshwater fishes are the goldfish (*Carassius auratus*) and koi carp (*Cyprinus carpio*), both of which are *freshwater* fish and belong to the Cyprinidae family. Guppies (*Poecilia reticulata*) and tetras (such as the neon tetra, *Paracheirodon innesi*) are other freshwater fish popular with novice aquarists, although the latter species requires a tropical tank compared with cold water for the former. *Brackish-water* species such as the glassfish (*Chanda ranga*), mudskippers (*Periophthalmus* spp) and gobies (such as the spotted goby, *Stigmatogobius sadanundio*) are more difficult to maintain. Common *tropical marine* fish include angelfishes (such as the blue-ringed angelfish, *Pomacanthus annularis*), surgeons and tangs (such as the regal tang, *Paracanthurus hepatus*, and yellow tang, *Zebrasoma flavescens*), triggerfish (such as clown triggerfish, *Balistoides conspicillum*), wrasses (such as the cleaner wrasse, *Labroides dimidiatus*), and seahorses (such as the yellow seahorse, *Hippocampus kuda*). *Coldwater marine* fish include rainbow wrasse (*Coris julis*) and the tompot blenny (*Parablennius gattorugine*). Aquaria commonly hold a mixed collection (a 'community' tank) of fish species with the same environmental requirements, although some species can be kept only as single specimens.

Living plants are useful in aquaria for a number of reasons. They will provide shelter for the inhabitants, are a source of food, and improve water quality by absorbing nitrates.

## BIOLOGY

Most fish species have protective scales covered by a layer of mucus; damage to these leads to problems with osmotic balance. The main site for gaseous exchange is the gills; these are also involved in osmoregulation and excretion of nitrogenous waste. These delicate organs are often the site of pathology. Internal organs are similar to mammals, although there are no lungs or diaphragm, and the kidneys lie dorsally just beneath the spine. Some species have a swim-bladder to assist with buoyancy. Fish are poikilothermic, and thus water temperature is important for immune function and metabolism of drugs (Fig. 25.1).

Enclosures for fish in captivity vary enormously. Many small fish are maintained in little tanks, while bigger groups or larger fish require more substantial enclosures (often ponds). Whatever the size, water quality should be maintained (monitoring regularly to ensure it is optimal). Filtration is required to control levels of ammonia and nitrite (the main toxic products excreted from fish), usually involving mechanical, biological, chemical or ultraviolet components. Fish may require freshwater, brackish-water, or marine water. Tropical or marine species may require various salts to be added, and heating may be needed.

As a general rule, fish are fed commercial complete diets, sometimes supplemented with live foods.

**Table 25.1** Taxonomic classification of fish

| Superclass | Class | Order | Family | Species |
|---|---|---|---|---|
| Agnatha (jawless fishes) | Cephalaspidomorphi Myxini | Petromyzontiformes Myxiniformes | – | c.40 spp (lampreys) c.43–50 spp (hagfishes) |
| Gnathostomata (jawed fishes) | Chondrichthyes (cartilaginous fishes) | 14 orders | 34 families | c.915 spp (sharks, skates and rays, and chimaeras) |
| | Sarcopterygii (lobe-finned fishes) | 3 orders | 5 families | 8 spp (e.g. lungfishes) |
| | Actinopterygii (ray-finned fishes) | 39 orders | c.428 families | c.23600 spp |

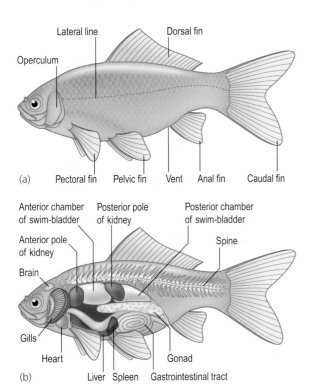

Figure 25.1 (a,b) External and internal anatomy of a fish, typified by the koi carp (*Cyprinus carpio*).

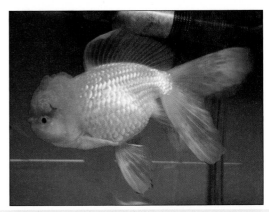

**Figure 25.2** The oranda is a variety of goldfish (*Carassius auratus*).

Thankfully, this means that nutritional deficiencies are infrequent.

## Goldfish (*Carassius auratus*)

Free-ranging goldfish originate from China (Fig. 25.2). They grow up to 25 cm in length. Captive breeding has produced many variations in colour, finnage and body form. This is a coldwater species (10–20°C), requiring a water pH of 6.5–7.5 and dH (hardness) to 15°. They produce a large amount of waste, necessitating efficient filtration and regular water changes (25% weekly). As with most fish, they are omnivorous; captive animals are usually fed on flake or pellet foods, but may also take vegetable matter and invertebrates. Eggs, when produced, are scattered in the tank.

## Guppy (*Poecilia reticulata*)

This live bearer comes from Central America, measuring 3–5 cm in length (although cultivated specimens are larger). Captive fish require a water temperature of 22–28°C. Their diet is similar to that of the goldfish. Many colour forms and fin varieties have been developed. Other *Poecilia* species are also popular, including the mollies.

## Neon tetra (*Paracheirodon innesi*)

These are the most popular aquarium fish. They originate from South America, grow to 4 cm, and can live over 10 years. They are omnivorous, being fed on small live foods (such as insect larvae) as well as frozen, flake, and pellet foods, and supplemented with green foods. Water temperature should be 22–26°C, with a pH of 5.0–7.0, and dH to 10°.

## Mudskippers (*Periophthalmus* spp)

These species originate in mangrove swamps, distributed from Africa through South-east Asia to Australia. They need a beach area to crawl out onto, along with rocks and roots for climbing out of the water. Air above the water should be warm and humid. Water temperature should be 25–30°C, with a pH of 8.0–8.5, dH to 15° and SG (salinity) 1.002–1.007. They feed on invertebrates (e.g. worms, crickets and flies), and may accept frozen and flake foods.

## Cleaner wrasse (*Labroides dimidiatus*)

These Indo-Pacific fish grow to 10 cm in the wild. They are carnivorous, and feed on finely chopped fish and shellfish in captivity, supplementing their natural diet of ectoparasites from other fish. Water should be 24–26°C, with a pH of 8.3–8.4 and SG 1.023–1.027.

## Tompot blenny (*Parablennius gattorugine*)

These originate from the eastern Atlantic coast from the Mediterranean to northern Scotland, and grow up to 20 cm in length. As a carnivorous species, they should be fed meaty foods (e.g. fish, shrimp and mussels). Water temperature should be 12–15°C, with a pH of 8.0–8.4 and SG 1.024–1.025.

## HISTORY

The environment of the fish is important in maintenance of health (Box 25.1). The veterinary clinician should obtain details of the aquarium or pond set-up, including monitoring protocols and records employed by the aquarist. For large or complicated enclosures, it is often easier to visit the owner's home to assess husbandry conditions visually.

Where water is analysed, a representative sample should be taken. This usually means a sample directly from the pond (rather than from the plastic bag within which the fish has been transported to the clinic), and preferably not just after a water change (when quality will be temporarily improved).

In community tanks, details should be obtained for all species of fish in the enclosure. The clinician should assess the suitability for co-habitation of the species (the reader is referred to other texts for further information on the various species).

> **BOX 25.1 SUGGESTED TOPICS TO COVER DURING HISTORY TAKING FOR FISH**
>
> - Animal:
>   - Species
>   - Gender (if known)
>   - Age
>   - Source
>   - Period in owner's possession
>   - In-contact species
>   - Previous medical problems (in individual, group, or aquarium)
>   - Current problem
> - Environment:
>   - Aquarium size, dimensions, substrate, furnishings, live plants
>   - Water: volume, source, pre-treatment(s) and routine treatments, changes, quality monitoring
>   - Filtration: type, cleaning, duration
>   - Heating and lighting: source, photoperiod, water temperature (day/night)
> - Cleaning and disinfection
> - Diet:
>   - Food (including source and storage)
>   - Frequency and amount of feeding
>   - Supplements
> - Recent weather conditions (outdoor ponds).

## CLINICAL EXAMINATION

Ideally, fish should be assessed within their normal enclosure. This will enable the veterinary clinician to assess the husbandry unit and any potential problems therein. If the fish is brought to the veterinary clinic, it should be transported in a sturdy container (e.g. a plastic bucket, or a water-tight plastic bag within a polystyrene box) filled with water from the aquarium. As anaesthesia is often necessary, request that the owner brings another container of water to mix with the anaesthetic agent. The fish should be kept in the dark during transport to reduce stress. Prior to long journeys, it can be useful to fast the fish for 24 hours to minimize excrement (and thence ammonia) production in transit.

### Handling/restraint

The stress of capture and restraint may result in collapse and death, and should therefore be performed deftly and with confidence. The period of restraint should be minimal. The best mode of capture is utilization of a net comprising fine mesh. The fish should be caught quickly to minimize damage and stress during the process. The fish should then either be moved to a smaller container of water for observation or held loosely in the net. Medium-sized fish in a small container may be gently restrained by hand. Wet examination gloves should be worn to reduce the risk of damaging the fish's integument during handling, and also to minimize transfer of potential zoonotic pathogens to the clinician (Box 25.2).

### BOX 25.2   ZOONOSES FROM FISH

- Fish tuberculosis (mycobacteriosis, e.g. *Mycobacterium marinum, M. fortuitum, M. chelonae*) may result in nodular skin disease in humans.
- *Nocardia* spp result in similar lesions to mycobacteriosis.
- *Vibrio* and *Aeromonas* spp may infect humans through ingestion or contamination of skin wounds.
- Other potential zoonotic diseases include *Pseudomonas* spp, protozoa and nematodes.
- Good personal hygiene will reduce the risk of disease transmission.

## Examination

If possible, the fish should first be visually assessed in their natural environment. If they have travelled to the veterinary clinic in a container, some assessment may still be made regarding locomotion and respiration.

Restraint is necessary for clinical examination. If this is done in the conscious individual, it should be extremely brief (and therefore often only cursory) to minimize stress. If anaesthetized, the period will be less brief, and a more meticulous examination can be conducted. In all cases, prepare sampling equipment (such as swabs, scalpel blade for skin scrape, scissors for a gill snip, and blood sampling tools) prior to handling.

If sedated or anaesthetized, a body weight is obtained (to assess body condition and enable accurate drug dosing). The skin and fins are thoroughly examined, and usually a skin scrape is taken. The head is assessed, including the oral cavity, eyes, opercula and gills (a gill snip is usually taken). The coelomic cavity may be palpated, but findings are often lacking unless a significant abnormality such as a large mass is present. The cloaca should be examined, and a faecal sample collected for microscopy.

### CLINICAL TIPS

**Gill snip**

- Anaesthetize the fish, using MS-222.
- Lift the operculum (gill cover).
- Cut a few small pieces of gill tissue (maximum 2 mm of primary gill lamellae) using fine scissors. Any haemorrhage should quickly cease.
- Prepare slides – using a drop of water from the fish's tank – and perform microscopy straight away.

## INVESTIGATION

### Water quality

Unless regularly performed by the owner using a good quality test kit, the clinician should analyse a water sample for nitrogenous waste products. Other parameters that may be measured as appropriate include temperature, pH, hardness and salinity.

### Phlebotomy

General anaesthesia (see below) is usually required to restrain fish sufficiently for phlebotomy. The caudal vein lies ventral to the vertebrae, and is accessed from ventrally in the midline or laterally. Larger koi carp have veins on the medial aspect of their operculae, which may be accessed (although these are preferred only for euthanasia, to avoid damaging the gills in a live animal). In teleost fish, the brachial arch may be useful.

### Imaging

Radiography is valuable in some cases. The fish should be anaesthetized for the procedure. The lateral view is easiest in most species that are laterally compressed, although it is ideal to take two orthogonal views to aid interpretation. The bony skeleton and swim-bladder (where present) are relatively easily visualized.

Ultrasound, CT, MRI and endoscopy are other imaging modalities that may prove useful. Interpretation of imaging results may be difficult unless a normal animal can be imaged for comparison.

### Sampling

As outlined above, routine samples taken during clinical examination include a skin scrape, gill snip and faecal sample. Microscopy is performed on wet preparations from all of these as soon as possible. Protozoa infections are common in fish, and samples should be fresh in order to visualize movement of these organisms.

Samples may also be submitted for culture, although culture from skin swabs typically grows contaminants from the environment. Biopsies from skin, fins, gills, and internal organs may be examined histologically.

## TREATMENT

### Basic procedures

#### Drug administration

Many medications can be administered by adding to the fish's water, such as those for treating ectoparasites and superficial infections. In some cases, the drug is added to the tank, while, in others, a separate medicated *bath* is prepared (although this necessitates the stress of handling the fish to move to and from the bath).

The *oral* route is commonly used, particularly for large groups of fish. Medication may be mixed with or coated onto feed. Uptake is often unreliable, particularly if the ill fish has a reduced appetite.

If possible, drugs should be administered by *injection* to ensure delivery (Fig. 25.3). However, this procedure requires restraint and is stressful to fish. The skin is irrigated with sterile saline before injection. Subcutaneous injections are avoided, as most of the injected material is expressed due to the lack of potential space. The epaxial muscles (approached either on the dorsal flank or alternatively from the dorsal midline), or sometimes under the pectoral fin from caudally, are used for intramuscular injections. Scale loss may occur at the site of injection. Intravenous injections may be given in anaesthetized animals (see Phlebotomy section above). Intracoelomic injections, given into the ventral midline between the vent and pelvic fins, should be administered with caution due to the proximity of internal organs.

### CLINICAL TIPS

- Drug metabolism will be affected by body temperature, and thence by environmental temperature. The fish should be maintained in an appropriate temperature range for the species.
- Any temperature alterations may necessitate recalculation of drug dosing (particularly the dosing interval).

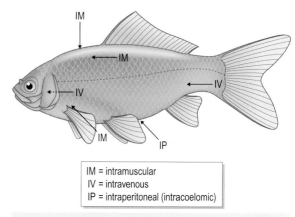

IM = intramuscular
IV = intravenous
IP = intraperitoneal (intracoelomic)

**Figure 25.3** Injection sites in fish.

#### Supportive care

It is not usually possible to assist-feed fish. However, changing the water composition of their environment will result in rehydration or solute supplementation. For example, placing a freshwater fish in a weak saline solution will result in a net water gain due to osmotic forces.

### Anaesthesia

#### Pre-anaesthesia

The fish should be fasted for a period prior to anaesthesia if possible. This is predominantly in order to maintain good water quality during travel to the clinic and during hospitalization.

#### Pre-medication

Pre-medicant sedatives are rarely utilized, as they necessitate additional handling (which is stressful) to administer. Eugenol may be used to sedate fish. Mild hypothermia will result in immobilization.

#### Injectable agents

These may be used in larger fish, but safety margins are often narrow and recovery prolonged. Ketamine combinations and propofol have been reported. Lidocaine may be used for local anaesthesia.

#### Immersion

Water-borne anaesthetic agents are most commonly used to anaesthetize fish. MS-222 (tricaine methanesulfonate) is the most frequently employed agent. This forms an acidic solution, and is therefore buffered before use. A concentration of 15–50 mg MS-222/l will usually result in sedation. Induction of anaesthesia is achieved

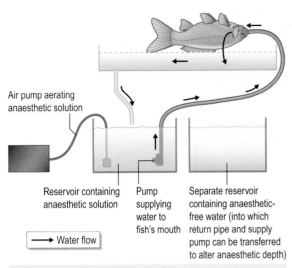

Air pump aerating
anaesthetic solution

Reservoir containing
anaesthetic solution

Pump
supplying
water to
fish's mouth

Separate reservoir
containing anaesthetic-
free water (into which
return pipe and supply
pump can be transferred
to alter anaesthetic depth)

→ Water flow

**Figure 25.4** A recirculating anaesthetic circuit for use with fish.

with a concentration of 100–200 mg/l, while mainte-nance usually requires 50–100 mg/l. Other water-borne agents that may be used include benzocaine, eugenol (clove oil), isoflurane (bubbled into the water) and ethanol.

A higher dose of anaesthetic agent is used to induce anaesthesia before maintenance with a lower dose. Medicated water is applied over the gills (via the oral cavity) using a pump with tubing or a syringe. Systems for maintenance may be non-recirculating (where 'spent' water is not re-used) or recirculating (where water is collected off the fish and re-cycled in the system) (Fig. 25.4).

The water should be oxygenated using an air-stone device, or by bubbling oxygen from an anaesthetic machine. Excessively high oxygen levels may damage the gills.

Recovery from anaesthesia is achieved by flushing fresh water over the gills. The fish is then held in the water and moved forwards until coordinated voluntary movement is present.

### Monitoring anaesthesia

As the fish becomes anaesthetized, it will lose its righting reflex as well as responses to tactile and surgical stimuli. Respiratory rate is monitored by visualizing opercular movement. The heart beat may be visible, or a Doppler flow monitor may be used to hear it. If desired, an ECG may be attached.

### Peri-anaesthetic care

Analgesia should be provided if a painful procedure is performed. During anaesthesia, the fish should be kept moist to prevent desiccation and skin damage.

---

**CLINICAL TIPS**

**Analgesics in fish**

- Butorphanol 0.1–0.4 mg/kg IM.
- Ketoprofen 2 mg/kg IM.

---

## Surgery

Suturing is usually not possible or practical in fish, either due to the lack of elastic skin to close over a defect (in which case healing occurs by secondary intention) and/or due to problems with waterproofing after closure. Super-ficial ulcers are common, and are treated by debridement and antiseptic application. Water-resistant ointments may be applied to dress wounds temporarily.

## Euthanasia

Overdosage of any of the anaesthetic agents will result in death. In some cases, anaesthesia is induced with water-borne agents before euthanasia is performed by injecting pentobarbitone intracoelomically.

# 26 Enucleation of an eye in a goldfish

## INITIAL PRESENTATION

Unilateral ocular swelling in a goldfish.

## INTRODUCTION

Goldfish are attractive fish, relatively hardy and long-lived (>20 years in optimum conditions). They are commonly kept as family pets and also as display fish in public ponds. External lesions are easily identified by owners, including ocular pathologies.

## CASE PRESENTING SIGNS

An adult goldfish (*Carassius auratus*) presented with unilateral ocular swelling of gradual onset.

## HUSBANDRY

The goldfish was housed in an indoor display pond, approximately 25 cm deep and 4.5 × 6.0 m in size. Water was changed continuously (from mains water), constituting a third of the water being changed every 6 weeks. Filtration was achieved using rapid sand and ultraviolet filters. The water was not routinely monitored for the presence of toxins such as nitrates and nitrites. Commercial goldfish food was offered once daily on 5 days each week. A relatively low stocking density was present, with several other goldfish in the pond. The other fish in the pond did not show any clinical signs of disease.

## CASE HISTORY

The goldfish's right eye had been noted to gradually increase in size over a period of 2 months. Otherwise the fish appeared unaffected by the ocular problem, but as it was in a display pond the facility's management were concerned about public perception and presented the animal to the veterinary clinic for assessment. The history presented was:
- No loss of appetite
- Activity normal
- Gradual development of right ocular swelling.

## CLINICAL TIPS

### Transport of fish to veterinary clinic
- A container large enough to permit some swimming is necessary. Usually this is a leak-proof plastic box or bucket, but may need to be a thick plastic bag within a firm container such as a polystyrene box.
- To avoid undue stress to the animal with water changes, the fish should be transported in water from its enclosure.
- It is advisable for the owner to bring another two containers of water also, which can be needed if anaesthesia is required.

## CLINICAL EXAMINATION

The patient was initially assessed in the presenting container:
- Swimming movements were normal (albeit in a small enclosure)
- There were no obvious lesions on the integument
- Respiration rate and depth were evidenced by opercular movement, and noted to be normal
- The right eye was distended, extending 2 cm out from the skull (Fig. 26.1).

It was decided to perform further investigations, and a 'hands on' examination was reserved for when the fish was anaesthetized.

## CLINICAL TIPS

### Clinical examination of fish

- Observation of the fish in water provides useful information, including assessment of the animal's mobility and respiratory movements.
- In some cases it is necessary to perform a brief conscious examination with the fish out of the water:
  - The fish can be gently grasped in the hands, or a net used to capture it.
  - Some of the examination may be performed with the fish in water, or it may be raised into the air for a brief period.
  - It is advisable to hold the fish above the water container in case a sudden movement by the animal releases it.
- A net should be used for larger fish before handling, or they should be anaesthetized.
- Handling is stressful for fish, and may result in physical damage. Although this may appear minor, for example with the loss of a few scales, this may provide an entry portal for infection that may progress to septicaemia and death. Great care should therefore be taken when handling specimens. Nets should be free of holes that may catch a fin, and of abrasive surfaces.

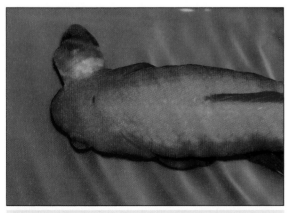

**Figure 26.1** Dorsal view of goldfish's head, showing distended right eye.

## DIFFERENTIAL DIAGNOSES

If possible, the practitioner should differentiate between buphthalmos (abnormal enlargement of the eye) and exophthalmos ('pop eye', abnormal protrusion of the eye, e.g. as a mass pushes it). Systemic disease usually results in bilateral exophthalmos, and other clinical signs or behaviour changes are often present concurrently.

The differentials for *ocular swelling* are:
- Infection: localized infection is often the cause of unilateral pathology
- Trauma: may cause ocular rupture
- Corneal damage: resulting in corneal oedema, may rapidly (within 24 hours) progress to cataract formation
- Retrobulbar oedema, e.g. due to gas in or behind the eye
- Retrobulbar mass, e.g. abscess, neoplasia
- Ocular neoplasia
- Gas supersaturation ('gas bubble disease')
- Ammonia toxicity
- Septicaemia
- Malnutrition, e.g. hypovitaminosis A (pitting of the cornea may lead to exophthalmos, uveitis and retinal degeneration).

## CASE WORK-UP

The goldfish was anaesthetized using tricaine methane-sulfonate (MS-222). Once induced, the fish was positioned in lateral recumbency on a wet incontinence pad. Water was dripped over the fish's body to keep the integument moist. Anaesthesia was maintained by slowly syringing a 100 mg/ml solution of buffered MS-222 into the oral cavity using a catheter-tip syringe (Fig. 26.2).

A full clinical examination was performed:
- Body weight was 250 g
- Right eye was enlarged. The cornea was opaque so intra-ophthalmic examination was not possible. No discharge was present
- The left eye did not have any apparent problems
- No other lesions were observed or palpated on the goldfish.

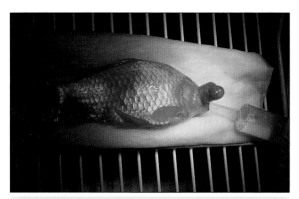

**Figure 26.2** Anaesthetized goldfish. MS-222 is being administered into the oral cavity using a syringe to maintain anaesthesia.

## Anaesthesia

Use water that has been de-toxified (see above). In preference, use water from the fish's own enclosure, as the animal will be accustomed to the chemical constituents and temperature. The aim is to buffer any changes such as thermal shock that may be stressful to the fish's physiology.

MS-222 is a sodium-channel blocking local anaesthetic agent that is absorbed across the gills in fish, resulting in sedation or general anaesthesia (depending on the concentration used and the time period the fish is in contact with the drug). Mixed with water, MS-222 produces a clear, colourless, acid solution. This solution should be buffered to pH 7.0–7.4 by adding phosphate buffer or sodium bicarbonate: either add sodium bicarbonate until the pH is measured at 7.0–7.4, or add sodium bicarbonate to saturation; this will result in a solution with a pH between 6.0 and 7.5. Human exposure to MS-222 should be avoided, as the powder or solutions may be irritant or corrosive.

Prepare three tanks of water: MS-222 at a concentration of 200 mg/l to induce anaesthesia, MS-222 at 100 mg/l for maintenance solution, and fresh stock water (i.e. from the fish's enclosure) for recovery. Place the fish in the induction tank and monitor closely. Once a surgical plane of anaesthesia is reached, the fish is removed from the induction tank.

The maintenance solution is administered into the oral cavity and flows out across the gills. It can be given either using a syringe or automatically using a pump to administer the solution. The system can be either non-recirculating (where the solution is not re-used after administration to the fish) or recirculating (where the solution is collected and recycled).

- The gills should be kept moist at all times to prevent damage. If anaesthetic solution is not required, water can be dripped onto the gills (bearing in mind that this may aid recovery from anaesthesia).

Recovery from anaesthesia is elicited by running fresh water over the gills. This is usually done by placing the fish in a tank of fresh water, and moving the fish in a forward motion through the water until conscious movements are present. The fish should be monitored for a period to ensure swimming movements are persistent and that opercular movements are regular.

## CLINICAL TIPS

### Stages of anaesthesia in fish

(0) Conscious: voluntary swimming, normal equilibrium and responsiveness.

(I) Sedation: decrease in reaction to stimuli, not swimming but normal equilibrium.

(II) Narcosis: further decreased response to tactile stimuli, decreased muscle tone and loss of response to postural changes.

(III) Surgical anaesthesia: weak (light anaesthesia) to no (surgical anaesthesia) response to strong tactile pressure, decreased respiratory rate (noted by opercular movement).

(IV) Medullary collapse: no response to tactile stimuli or postural changes, no respiration.

## CLINICAL TIPS

### Monitoring anaesthesia

- A Doppler probe can be used to assess heart rate.
- Opercular movements are equivalent to respiratory rate.

## FURTHER INVESTIGATIONS

### Husbandry

Investigations should include details of the aquarist's tank or pond set-up as well as water analysis.

## CLINICAL TIPS

### Water analysis

- Water should be sampled from the usual environment and tested as soon as possible.
- Parameters of interest include:
  - Temperature
  - Dissolved oxygen
  - Ammonia
  - Nitrite and nitrate
  - pH (e.g. this may be low if carbon dioxide supersaturation is present)
  - Hardness
  - Chlorine and chloramine (often present in mains water supply)
  - In marine systems, salinity and redox potential are also measured.

## Ophthalmoscopy

Ophthalmic examination can be performed as in other species. A slit lamp is useful for magnification to assess the cornea, anterior chamber, iris and lens (not possible in this case due to corneal opacity). Indirect ophthalmoscopy is used to examine the fundus. Fluorescein or rose bengal stains are used to assess corneal ulceration. Corneal scrapings may be collected for cytological examination. If intraocular pressure is raised, a transocular intraocular aspirate can be taken to relieve pressure (and provide a sample for culture and microscopy).

## Imaging

In order to further evaluate the lesion, it was suggested that imaging be performed. However, this was declined due to the financial implications. Ultrasound is the most useful modality to assess the globe and soft tissues in the periocular region.

Radiography may be useful if the pathology is more invasive. Soft tissue and fluid margins will be apparent, and if the ocular lesion had extended into the bony structures it is possible some changes may have been seen.

## Blood sampling

Since ocular signs may be associated with systemic disease, a complete physical examination should be performed. Blood sampling for haematology and biochemistry may be useful to assess for systemic disease. Blood culture and cytology will enable diagnosis of septicaemia.

## CLINICAL TIPS

### Venous access in fish

- Caudal vein: lies ventral to tail vertebrae, access via ventral midline or lateral approach.
- Medial aspect of operculae: accessible in larger koi for euthanasia.
- Brachial arch.

## DIAGNOSIS

Unilateral exophthalmos.

## ANATOMY AND PHYSIOLOGY REFRESHER

Ocular anatomy (Fig. 26.3) varies between species of fish, for example the shape of the pupil and colour of

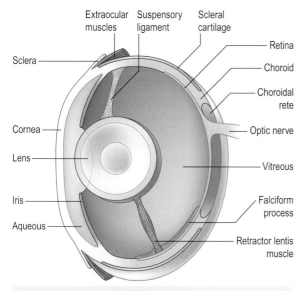

**Figure 26.3** Ocular anatomy in a fish.

the iris. Teleosts (bony fish including goldfish) do not have eyelids. Reaction to light relies on retraction of rods/cones into the retinal pigment epithelium or increasing pigment present in retinal epithelial processes. Both of these responses require time and therefore sudden exposure to intense light may result in retinal damage.

Extraocular muscles permit independent movement of each eye, although this movement is involuntary (following objects requires the fish to move its body within the water). The ocular globe is flattened and elliptical, and the cornea thickened. A cartilaginous ring is present within the sclera.

The choroid gland contains a vascular rete around the optic nerve. The iris attaches to the cornea, held in place by the annular ligament. The lens is large and spherical, suspended by the suspensory ligament assisted by the posterior retractor lentis muscle (this muscle moves the eye during accommodation).

## AETIOPATHOGENESIS OF EXOPHTHALMOS

Several aetiologies may result in this condition. Inadequate husbandry conditions may result in immune suppression and predispose to infection. Overstocking may result in intra- or inter-specific aggression and lesions that are susceptible to secondary infections. Examples of infectious agents that may affect the eye or periocular tissues include:

- Bacteria (e.g. *Streptococcus, Staphylococcus, Aeromonas, Pseudomonas,* or *Vibrio* spp; granulomatous lesions (e.g. *Mycobacteria, Nocardia* and *Flavobacterium*))
- Viruses (e.g. hepatic herpesvirus in salmon, lymphocystic disease)
- Parasites (e.g. the protozoan *Tetrahymena*)
- Fungi (e.g. secondary invasion of corneal ulcers with *Saprolegnia*, especially in poor water conditions).

Although primary neoplasia is rare, medulloepithelioma of the ciliary body has been reported in a goldfish.

Retrobulbar oedema and fluid retention commonly results in exophthalmos (unilateral or bilateral). The failure of osmoregulation is called 'dropsy', and is often due to infection or neoplasia. Fluid may also be retained elsewhere in the body, for example oedema of the vent, skin and bowel, or abdominal distension (where the scales become elevated to give a 'pinecone' appearance to the fish).

Gas supersaturation may produce exophthalmos. This may be associated with over-aeration from an air stone, or excessive oxygen production by algae and other plants. Supersaturation of the water results in gas bubbles in the circulation and/or skin and other tissues.

The optic nerve may become stretched in severe cases of exophthalmos, and blindness may ensue.

## EPIDEMIOLOGY

Exophthalmos is a relatively common presentation in ornamental fish.

## TREATMENT

This requires identification of the underlying cause of exophthalmos. Medical treatment, for example with antibiotics and local steroids, is rarely successful.

In this case, the eye was enucleated (Fig. 26.4), using a similar procedure to that used in other animals. Surgery involved dissection around the base of the mass, clamping the optic nerve and blood vessels (particularly the choroidal rete). Minor haemorrhage was present, and adrenaline on a cotton-bud was used to provide haemostasis. The orbit was packed with a waterproof ointment.

Antibiosis was provided by injections of amoxicillin (10 mg/kg IM) and enrofloxacin (5 mg/kg IM). Butorphanol (0.4 mg/kg IM) was administered to provide analgesia.

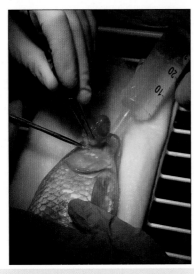

**Figure 26.4** Eye enucleation surgery in the goldfish.

## TREATMENT OPTIONS AND MANAGEMENT

In public displays, fish with an abnormal eye or missing an eye may be euthanized. However, many exophthalmos cases are associated with local pathology and may be readily treated by enucleation.

If infection is diagnosed, antimicrobials are best selected based on culture and sensitivity results. They are administered in-feed, or using baths or injections. Supportive treatment should be provided in cases with viral infections.

Neoplasia is best treated by surgical excision. Chemotherapy for ocular neoplasia is not reported in fish.

## OTHER TREATMENT OPTIONS

If the goldfish had presented earlier in the course of the disease, it may have been possible to consider medical treatment if trauma or an infection had been present. This may have enabled salvage of the eye, although it is not possible to say whether sight would have been retained.

Topical medication is likely to wash off under water. Antibiotics can be administered by injection or in-feed. Dosing a single animal in a group situation would be difficult, and isolation would be required during the treatment. External infections may be treated with baths, e.g. malachite green or formalin for fungal infections.

## FOLLOW-UP

The goldfish recovered well from anaesthesia and was discharged from the clinic the following day. The ointment did not remain in the orbit beyond a couple of days, but no problems were noted with healing. The animal continued to feed and swim well with only one eye.

## PREVENTION

Further investigations such as bacteriology and histology were not performed on this case, and an underlying aetiology was not diagnosed. The keeper was advised to optimize and monitor husbandry conditions (including diet and water quality) to reduce the risk of further disease due to immune suppression, infection or malnutrition.

## PROGNOSIS

Without a diagnosis, the prognosis given was guarded. However, case follow-up at 6 months showed the goldfish to be coping well with one eye.

# APPENDICES

# MCQs

## MAMMALS

**1. Degus belong to which taxonomic order?**
(a) Lagomorpha
(b) Chiroptera
(c) Rodentia
(d) Insectivora
(e) Diprotodontia

**2. What is the dental formula for rabbits (*Oryctolagus cuniculus*)?**
(a) I 2/1, C 0/0, PM 3/2, M 3/3
(b) I 1/1, C 0/0, PM 1/1, M 3/3
(c) I 1/1, C 1/1, PM 3/3, M 3/3
(d) I 1/0, C 0/0, PM 0/0, M 3/3
(e) I 1/1, C 1/1, PM 1/1, M 3/3

**3. Which of these species is NOT susceptible to heat stress?**
(a) African pygmy hedgehog (*Atelerix albiventris*)
(b) Chinchilla (*Chinchilla laniger*)
(c) Degu (*Octodon degus*)
(d) Guinea pig (*Cavia porcellus*)
(e) Rabbit (*Oryctolagus cuniculus*)

**4. Which of the following statements is TRUE for rabbits (*Oryctolagus cuniculus*)?**
(a) Acepromazine reduces tear production
(b) Alpha-2 agonists such as medetomidine produce peripheral vasodilation
(c) Atropine is an effective anticholinergic in most rabbits
(d) Ketamine is a good muscle relaxant
(e) Midazolam produces a longer period of sedation than diazepam

**5. Which of the following statements is TRUE? *Cheyletiella parasitivorax*:**
(a) May infest rabbits without clinical signs
(b) Is a common aetiological agent for dermatosis in chinchillas
(c) Is not zoonotic
(d) Is a burrowing mite
(e) Infestation is diagnosed by microscopy of a superficial skin scrape

**6. Which of the following statements about rabbit abscesses is TRUE?**
(a) For best results from culture, submit a sample from the abscess capsule
(b) The treatment of choice is lancing to allow drainage
(c) Oral penicillins are a good first-line antibiotic choice
(d) Abscesses rarely develop associated with dental disease
(e) Surgical excision of the abscess should not be attempted

**7. Which position is best for radiographic assessment of a chinchilla's (*Chinchilla laniger*) skull for potential otitis?**
(a) Laterals
(b) Oblique laterals
(c) Dorso-ventral
(d) Rostro-caudal
(e) Skyline

**8. Lack of appropriate analgesia in small mammals may:**
(a) Delay wound healing
(b) Impair immune function
(c) Increase the risk of sepsis after surgery
(d) Result in prolonged convalescence
(e) All of the above

9. Sugar gliders (*Petaurus breviceps*) are:
   (a) Insectivorous
   (b) Nectivorous
   (c) Omnivorous
   (d) Frugivorous
   (e) Insectivorous and sap-feeders

10. Which of the following is NOT usually associated with pain in rabbits?
   (a) Inappetence
   (b) Increased activity
   (c) Sitting very still
   (d) Tooth grinding
   (e) Unresponsive

11. Which statement about bacterial dermatoses in mice (*Mus musculus*) is FALSE?
   (a) *Staphylococcus aureus* may cause spontaneous ulcerative dermatitis
   (b) *Corynebacterium kutscheri* can cause furunculosis
   (c) Topical ointments are useful adjuncts to treatment
   (d) Many cases of bacterial dermatitis respond to penicillins or cephalosporins
   (e) Surgical excision may be necessary to treat some abscesses

12. Which of these CANNOT be used to monitor rabbit (*Oryctolagus cuniculus*) anaesthesia?
   (a) Ear pinch
   (b) Toe pinch
   (c) Palpebral reflex
   (d) Corneal reflex
   (e) Response to surgical stimuli

13. What are possible differential diagnoses for a Syrian hamster (*Mesocricetus auratus*) with haematuria?
   (a) Renal trauma with haemorrhage
   (b) Cystitis
   (c) Endometritis (females)
   (d) Uterine endometrial adenocarcinomas (females)
   (e) All of the above

14. Which of the following investigations are warranted in a ferret with vomiting?
   (a) Trial therapy with supportive treatment
   (b) Abdominal radiography
   (c) Abdominal ultrasound
   (d) Haematology and clinical chemistries
   (e) Any or all of the above

15. *Myobia musculi* infestation in mice (*Mus musculus*):
   (a) Usually results in lesions around the back and ventrum
   (b) Has a life cycle of 23 days
   (c) Is mostly transmitted by indirect contact, via fomites
   (d) Is usually treated with lime sulfur dip
   (e) Is usually non-pruritic

## BIRDS

16. A diet of seeds and nuts for a pet grey parrot (*Psittacus erithacus*) is:
   (a) A close approximation of the species' diet in the wild
   (b) Excessively high in fats
   (c) Deficient in vitamin A
   (d) Both **b** and **c**
   (e) **a**, **b** and **c**

17. Cream-coloured lesions in a raptor's oral cavity could be due to:
   (a) Trichomoniasis
   (b) Capillariasis
   (c) Bacterial infection
   (d) Avian pox virus
   (e) Any of the above

18. Which of the following antifungal medications will most rapidly reach therapeutic levels in the bloodstream of a parrot suffering from air sacculitis due to aspergillosis?
   (a) Amphotericin B, administered intravenously
   (b) Itraconazole, administered orally
   (c) Ketoconazole, administered orally
   (d) Nystatin, administered orally
   (e) Terbinafine, administered orally

19. *Knemidocoptes* spp infestation in budgerigars (*Melopsittacus undulatus*) results in which clinical signs?
   (a) Feather loss on the dorsal head
   (b) Feather picking over the abdomen
   (c) Paronychia (nailbed infection)
   (d) Scaly appearance of the beak and legs
   (e) Oculo-nasal discharge

**20. Air sacculitis in a cockatiel (*Nymphicus hollandicus*) commonly presents as:**
(a) Sneezing, with oculo-nasal discharge
(b) Coughing, with no discharges seen
(c) Gradual onset with vague signs of lethargy and inappetence
(d) Acute onset with vague signs of lethargy and inappetence
(e) No clinical signs seen until death

**21. Which of the following statements regarding avian anaesthesia is TRUE?**
(a) Induction in psittacine species is often achieved by mask induction with a gaseous anaesthetic agent
(b) Butorphanol administered as a pre-medicant never results in respiratory depression
(c) IPPV (intermittent positive pressure ventilation) should not routinely be used
(d) There is usually a long delay (minutes) between respiratory arrest and cardiac arrest in cases of anaesthetic overdose
(e) Halothane has a wide safety margin

**22. Which statement about egg binding in birds is FALSE?**
(a) Causes include malnutrition (e.g. hypocalcaemia), excessive egg production, abdominal wall herniation, hyperthermia, and oviduct infection
(b) Clinical signs may include lethargy and reduced respiratory rate
(c) Patient stabilization is important, with supportive care
(d) Diagnosis is usually by radiography
(e) Oxytocin is not recommended in birds

**23. Proventricular dilatation disease (PDD):**
(a) Is caused by a circovirus
(b) Has a short incubation period, usually less than a month
(c) Results in an increased gastrointestinal transit time
(d) Is usually diagnosed antemortem by biopsy of the proventriculus
(e) Is characterized histologically by degeneration of ganglia and lymphohistiocytic infiltrations

**24. Local anaesthetics in birds:**
(a) Have a wide safety margin
(b) Are often administered in topical ointments
(c) Should not be used for regional anaesthesia and analgesia
(d) May be administered intra-articularly
(e) Are best administered after a painful stimulus has occurred

**25. Which of the following bones is NOT part of the shoulder joint in birds?**
(a) Scapula
(b) Humerus
(c) Coracoid
(d) Sternum (keel)
(e) Clavicle

**26. Which statement about raptors is TRUE?**
(a) Owls do not have a crop
(b) In falconry equipment, the aylmeri connect the jesses to the swivel
(c) Harris' hawks (*Parabuteo unicinctus*) hunt best when solitary
(d) Bumblefoot usually develops on lame legs
(e) Working raptors are fed *ad libitum* to ensure sufficient energy reserves for flight

**27. Which of these would NOT be a common differential for a mass on the wing of a budgerigar (*Melopsittacus undulatus*)?**
(a) Feather cyst
(b) Xanthoma
(c) Fibrous osteodystrophy associated with nutritional secondary hyperparathyroidism (NSHP or metabolic bone disease, MBD)
(d) Haematoma associated with a fracture
(e) Articular gout

**28. A proven pair of zebra finches (*Taeniopygia guttata*) have recently had reduced reproductive success, with lower numbers of surviving chicks. Which of the following nutritional elements should be assessed in the investigation?**
(a) Vitamin A
(b) Vitamin D
(c) Vitamin E
(d) Calcium
(e) All of the above

29. A Moluccan cockatoo (*Cacatua moluccensis*) has fractured its tibiotarsus. You are going to use an external fixator and intramedullary pin for the repair, using a craniomedial approach to insert the pin in a retrograde fashion. Which of these structures will NOT be near the surgical field?
   (a) Digital flexor tendons
   (b) Cranial tibial muscle
   (c) Medial gastrocnemius muscle
   (d) Tibial artery and nerve
   (e) Deep fibular nerve

30. Which one of these statements about dyspnoea in a Eurasian eagle owl (*Bubo bubo*) is FALSE?
   (a) Non-respiratory tract disorders can result in signs of dyspnoea
   (b) Investigation should be as full as possible, including performance of faecal parasitology
   (c) Periocular swelling may be associated
   (d) Caudal air sac cannulation will always relieve dyspnoea
   (e) Open-mouth breathing may result

## REPTILES

31. Which of the following best describes a Hermann's tortoise (*Testudo hermanni*)?
   (a) No horny tip on tail, lack of thigh tubercles, grow up to 30 cm long (SCL, straight carapace length)
   (b) Horny tip on tail, lack of thigh tubercles, grow up to 30 cm SCL
   (c) No horny tip on tail, thigh tubercles, grow up to 35 cm SCL
   (d) Horny tip on tail, thigh tubercles, grow up to 35 cm SCL
   (e) No horny tip on tail, lack of thigh tubercles, grow up to 35 cm long

32. The most common antemortem test for OPMV (ophidian paramyxovirus) is:
   (a) Serology
   (b) Histology
   (c) Virus isolation from tissues
   (d) Virus isolation from an oral swab
   (e) Any of the above

33. What stimulates respiration in reptiles?
   (a) Low partial pressure of oxygen
   (b) High partial pressure of oxygen
   (c) Low partial pressure of carbon dioxide
   (d) High partial pressure of carbon dioxide
   (e) Presence of nitrous oxide in inspired gases

34. Which of the following species demonstrates autotomy?
   (a) Green iguana (*Iguana iguana*)
   (b) Leopard gecko (*Eublepharis macularius*)
   (c) Sheltopusik (glass lizard, *Ophisaurus apodus*)
   (d) Savannah monitor lizard (*Varanus exanthematicus*)
   (e) a + b + c

35. Which of the following is the best single test for diagnosis of metabolic bone disease?
   (a) Total serum calcium
   (b) Ionized serum calcium
   (c) Radiography
   (d) Vitamin D3 blood levels
   (e) History and clinical examination

36. Retained spectacles in snakes:
   (a) May be caused by excessive environmental humidity
   (b) May be associated with endoparasitism
   (c) Are always shed with the next shed
   (d) Should be managed conservatively
   (e) Should be managed surgically

37. A reason/reasons for castrating a green iguana (*Iguana iguana*) is/are:
   (a) Prevention of unwanted offspring
   (b) Treatment of testicular neoplasia
   (c) Reduced aggression towards women during their menstrual period
   (d) a + b
   (e) a + b+ c

38. Which species do NOT have eyelids?
   (a) Royal python (*Python regius*)
   (b) Bearded dragon (*Pogona vitticeps*)
   (c) Leopard gecko (*Eublepharis macularius*)
   (d) a + b
   (e) a + c

**39. The surgical approach of choice for ovariectomy in a bearded dragon (*Pogona vitticeps*) is:**
(a) Trans-plastron
(b) Paramedian
(c) Inguinal
(d) Midline
(e) Flank

**40. Clinical signs of respiratory disease in snakes may include:**
(a) Coughing up discharges
(b) Stomatitis
(c) Seeking cooler areas of the enclosure
(d) Altered posture, with head and cranial body raised vertically
(e) All of the above

**41. Which ONE of the following statements about spiny-tailed lizards (*Uromastyx acanthinurus*) is FALSE?**
(a) They are herbivorous
(b) They belong to the Agamidae family of lizards, and thus have acrodont dentition (with teeth fixed to the maxillary and mandibular bones)
(c) Their body shape is dorso-ventrally flattened to enable them to burrow and hide under rocks
(d) They should be kept in a vivarium with a moderately high humidity
(e) They are sexually dimorphic

**42. A rescue centre presents a Horsfield's tortoise (*Testudo horsfieldi*) at your clinic to 'do a health check and test for infectious disease' before mixing with the centre's resident population. Which of the following would you NOT perform routinely?**
(a) Faecal parasitology and bacteriology
(b) Oro-pharyngeal swabs for herpesvirus and mycoplasma PCR
(c) Full-body radiographs to assess bone density
(d) Haematology and clinical chemistry
(e) Blood culture

**43. Which of the following statements about dysecdysis in a Burmese python (*Python molurus*) is FALSE?**
(a) It may be a result of excessive humidity in the environment during shedding
(b) Ectoparasite infestation may result in the condition
(c) A lack of bathing area or rubbing stones may predispose the condition
(d) Pieces of retained skin can be gently removed
(e) It is best treated by placing the snake in wet towels to move through and remove retained skin

**44. Cryptosporidiosis in snakes:**
(a) Results in constipation as the primary clinical sign
(b) Is readily detected on faecal microscopy
(c) Is diagnosed on histology using a silver stain
(d) Results in gastric wall hypertrophy
(e) Is treated with fenbendazole

**45. Which of the following statements about shell trauma in chelonia is FALSE?**
(a) The chelonian should be radiographed to assess the extent of bony damage
(b) Analgesia is not required as reptiles do not possess nociceptive receptors
(c) Contaminated wounds should be managed as open wounds, with lavage and dressing changes until infection (or potential infection) is under control
(d) Wires or screws may be used to hold fragments of shell in apposition
(e) Epoxy resin or hoof acrylic are commonly used to repair shell defects

## AMPHIBIANS

**46. Respiration in amphibians may be:**
(a) Branchial (via external gills)
(b) Buccopharyngeal (across oral mucous membranes)
(c) Pulmonic (via lungs)
(d) Cutaneous (across the skin)
(e) All of the above

47. **Which of the following statements about the cardiovascular system in amphibians is INCORRECT?**
    (a) Venepuncture is possible in the midline ventral abdominal vein in some species such as larger toads
    (b) The lingual plexus in anurans lies ventral to the tongue
    (c) The amphibian heart lies midline, dorsal to the pectoral girdle and sternum, and is located by visualization, palpation or Doppler flow
    (d) Phlebotomy in salamanders is usually performed via the ventral tail vein
    (e) Amphibian hearts are three-chambered (right atrium, left atrium, and a single ventricle)

48. **Cloacal prolapse in a frog:**
    (a) May be due to gastrointestinal foreign body
    (b) Is often associated with tenesmus
    (c) May resolve spontaneously if small
    (d) Treatment should include elimination of the underlying cause
    (e) All of the above

## FISH

49. **Which of the following is NOT a useful indicator of anaesthetic depth in a fish?**
    (a) Eye position
    (b) Opercular movements
    (c) Response to pinching at the tail-base
    (d) Swimming movements
    (e) Doppler probe over heart

50. **Which of the following may cause low oxygen levels in water?**
    (a) Reduced surface area of pond or tank, e.g. by surface plants
    (b) Algal bloom
    (c) Hot weather and low atmospheric pressure
    (d) Decomposition of excess food in aquarium
    (e) All of the above

# MCQs – Answers

1. **(c)** Degus (*Octodon degus*) are rodents. They belong to the Hystricognathi, the cavy-like rodents. There are 118 families in this suborder, which includes pets in the Caviidae (e.g. guinea pig), Chinchillidae (e.g. chinchilla) and Octodontidae (e.g. degu) families. Although little is published about degus, medicine can be extrapolated from the other hystricognaths.

2. **(a)** Rabbits have two upper incisors, with the smaller 'peg' teeth caudal to the other upper set. Incisors grow at approximately 3 mm per week, and cheek teeth (premolars and molars) 3 mm per month.

3. **(a)** African pygmy hedgehogs (*Atelerix albiventris*) are used to an environmental temperature range of 23–32°C, usually requiring supplemental heating when captive in temperate zones. The other species originate from cooler climes; although supplemental heating may be required for debilitated animals or during anaesthesia, they will suffer if excessively heated.

4. **(a)** Sedated or anaesthetized rabbits should always have ocular lubricant applied to prevent the eyes drying out and to reduce potential trauma from substrate. Medetomidine causes peripheral vasoconstriction. Most rabbits possess anticholinesterase, so glycopyrrolate is the anticholinergic drug of choice.

5. **(a)** Similar to other companion animals, *Cheyletiella* may be found on some rabbits without clinical signs. In other individuals, a scaling dermatosis with partial alopecia may be seen. Pruritus may be present. Some rabbits appear to develop a hypersensitivity reaction, and more severe signs are seen.

6. **(a)** Although a useful culture may be obtained from some samples of purulent material, this is often sterile and the clinician has an increased chance of success with a sample from the abscess capsule.

7. **(c)** The dorso-ventral view permits assessment of both the external ear canals and tympanic bullae. The tympanic bullae are very large in the chinchilla, and this species is used in auditory research.

8. **(e)** Pain may also result in an increase in metabolic demands, tissue catabolism, anorexia, and cardiovascular stress. Herbivores such as rabbits are also susceptible to gastrointestinal hypomotility.

9. **(e)** Free-ranging sugar gliders feed on gum and sap from eucalyptus and acacia trees during the winter. They are mainly insectivorous during the rest of the year. Captive diets are usually a mix of fruit, insectivore or carnivore diet, and artificial nectar; several 'recipes' exist.

10. **(b)** Any abnormal behaviour in rabbits may be due to pain, but usually activity is reduced. Abdominal or spinal pain may be demonstrated by a hunched or crouched posture.

11. **(c)** Fastidious grooming by mice will remove most ointments, and toxicity may be seen associated with parenteral intake. Topical antiseptics (e.g. chlorhexidine 0.5–1.0%) are often beneficial.

12. **(c)** The palpebral reflex is an unreliable indicator of anaesthetic depth in the rabbit. The corneal reflex should normally be retained at a surgical plane of anaesthesia, but is lost if medetomidine is used.

13. **(e)** Urinary tract disease may result in true haematuria. There are separate urethral and vaginal openings in female hamsters, but blood from the reproductive tract may contaminate urine samples. Endometritis and reproductive tract disease are relatively common. It should be noted that a white discharge is normal at the end of the oestrous cycle in hamsters.

14. **(e)** Depending on the severity of clinical signs, all of these would be useful investigations. Common differentials include gastritis with ulceration, gastroenteritis, oesphageal/gastrointestinal obstruction (often a foreign body, but neoplasia such as lymphoma is also common), insulinoma, or other metabolic disease. Megaoesophagus will result in regurgitation.

15. **(b)** Owing to the life cycle of 23 days, the treatment is repeated to kill newly hatched mites (usually ivermectin at 0.2–0.4 mg/kg SC/PO/topically, repeated every 7–14 days for three doses). Parent mice usually pass the mite to offspring, but lesions often do not develop until the animal reaches maturity. Pruritus varies, with some animals being asymptomatic and others intensely so due to an allergic response. Lesions of alopecia and ulceration are typically around the head, neck, lateral thorax and flanks.

16. **(e)** Free-living African grey parrots feed mostly on seeds and nuts. However, they are more active and have a higher energy demand than more sedentary captive birds. This results in consumption of a greater quantity of food in free-living birds, including appropriate energy and sufficient nutrients. A pet bird fed a similar diet will suffer from malnutrition, and should be fed a proprietary pelleted food supplemented with fresh fruit and vegetables.

17. **(e)** Further investigation of the lesions are warranted to make a diagnosis before treatment can be started. Samples should be examined microscopically in the first instance; microbiology or histology may be appropriate.

18. **(a)** Amphotericin B is fungicidal, and rapidly effective. Fluids should be administered simultaneously as the drug is potentially nephrotoxic. The azole family take several days before they are effective. These drugs are variably hepatotoxic, and itraconazole appears to be toxic in grey parrots.

19. **(d)** The burrowing knemidocoptic mange mite is relatively common in budgerigars and can affect other species. Most frequently the cere becomes grey, scabby and crusting. Burrowing tracts may be seen in the beak. Leg lesions, on the scaled part of the limb, are less common in budgerigars but cause 'tassle foot' in canaries. Diagnosis is by skin scrape. Ivermectin is the treatment of choice.

20. **(d)** Birds hide signs of illness until severely ill. Clinical signs of disease are usually vague. Birds do not have a diaphragm and therefore cannot cough, although increased respiratory effort may be seen in the form of tail-bobbing or open-mouth breathing. Sneezing and oculo-nasal discharge may be seen with upper respiratory tract disease.

21. **(a)** The facemask should be closely-fitting to reduce environmental contamination by anaesthetic gases. After induction, most species can be intubated for maintenance.

22. **(b)** Tachypnoea is commonly seen. Other clinical signs may include a wide-based non-perching stance, or hindlimb paresis or paralysis, dypnoea, swollen cloaca, and straining. Supportive care includes fluids and housing in a warm quiet area. A comprehensive history and blood analysis are useful to ascertain predisposing factors. Oxytocin results in profound cardiovascular effects, and smooth muscle contractions of the oviduct are usually ineffective.

23. **(e)** PDD is caused by a bornavirus. The incubation period is variable, and may be years. Gastrointestinal transit time is slowed, and many secondary infections occur associated with this stasis. Although the proventriculus usually has histopathological changes, surgery on this organ carries a high risk of rupture; the crop is more commonly biopsied. Histological lesions are mainly detected in the autonomic nerve plexus of the proventriculus and other parts of the gastrointestinal tract, or in the central nervous system in neurological cases.

24. **(d)** Bupivacaine has been injected intra-articularly in birds with experimentally induced arthritis. Systemic uptake of local anaesthetics is rapid in birds, and overdosage is easy in small patients. Toxicity results in tremors, ataxia, recumbency, seizures, stupor and cardiovascular effects (including cardiac arrest and death). Accurate dose calculation and dilution of drugs will reduce the risk of toxicity. Ointments are not commonly used, as dose calculation is difficult, plumage may be damaged, and oral ingestion after preening is likely. As with other analgesics, pre-emptive administration is preferable.

25. **(d)** The left and right clavicles are fused to form the furcula in most birds. The sternum supports the thoracic girdle, which also includes the scapulae and coracoid.

26. **(a)** The crop is a dilation of the oesophagus. It is present in most birds and serves as a storage area for food *en route* to the stomach (proventriculus). Owls (Strigiformes) do not have a crop. Their casting material will include bone as well as fur and feathers, whereas, in Falconiformes, bone is absorbed due to the longer time ingested material remains in the gastrointestinal tract before the pellet is regurgitated.

27. **(c)** NSHP occurs in animals with calcium and vitamin D deficiencies. Reptiles often respond to NSHP by replacing decalcified bone with fibrous connective tissue, with gross thickening of the bone cortex visible as firm swellings of long bones (commonly femurs). Clinical signs in birds with NSHP include muscle fasciculation and seizures associated with the hypocalcaemia, osteodystrophy (e.g. bowing of the tibiotarsus) and pathological fractures, and poor reproductive performance (e.g. abnormally shaped and thin-shelled eggs, and weak chicks with poor bony calcification). Neurological signs are treated with injections and oral administration of calcium. Bone deformities are common in young growing animals. Radiographic lesions are often seen in the spine, tibiotarsi, radii and humeri. Surgery may be required to correct bone deformities, or euthanasia considered in severe cases. Prevention, and long-term treatment, includes provision of UV-B radiation as well as an appropriate diet containing calcium and vitamin D.

28. **(e)** Many elements are involved in good reproductive performance. Birds that are used repeatedly for breeding have a much greater metabolic demand, particularly the females, and are more likely to show clinical signs of chronic nutritional deficiencies than non-breeding birds. Marginal deficiencies of adults may first be highlighted by clinical signs in their offspring.

29. **(a)** The digital flexor tendons are ventral to the phalanges of the digits. Access both laterally and medially is required to place the external fixator pins. The craniomedial incision to allow access to insert the intramedullary pin is between the cranial tibial and medial gastrocnemius muscles. The tibial artery and nerve run caudally over the stifle joint. The deep fibular nerve runs from caudally at the stifle across the tibiotarsus, and lies medially at the hock (intertarsal) joint.

30. **(d)** Space-occupying masses in the coelomic cavity (e.g. egg binding or organomegaly) commonly compress the air sacs and result in dyspnoea. Faecal parasitology is necessary to check for eggs from respiratory parasites such as *Serratospiculum* spp and *Syngamus trachea*. Periocular swelling may be seen with an upper respiratory tract infection if sinusitis is present; differentials for the swelling include trauma resulting in subcutaneous haemorrhage or emphysema, or neoplasia. Clinical signs of respiratory tract disease in birds are varied, including exercise intolerance, coughing, sneezing, tachypnoea, dyspnoea, change in vocalization, and nasal discharge. Dypnoea will only be relieved by placement of an air sac cannula in a caudal air sac if the respiratory pathology is in the upper respiratory tract. The cannula permits access to the air sacs and thence the lungs, bypassing the upper airways.

31. **(b)** Identification of tortoise species is important, to permit appropriate husbandry conditions to be selected. Hermann's tortoises originate from France, Italy, Spain and various Mediterranean islands. They require a daytime temperature range of 20–30°C with a basking spot of 40°C. They eat mainly weeds such as dandelions, sow thistle, clover and plantains. As with other chelonia, they require supplemental UV-B when housed indoors or when exposed to reduced sun outside.

32. **(a)** Serological tests detect antibodies against OPMVs. The most commonly used are haem-agglutination inhibition (HI) tests. Seroconversion may take 6–8 weeks, so false negatives may occur in acutely ill animals. Postmortem diagnosis is often based on histology of lung and CNS tissue. The virus may be isolated in cell culture, usually from lung, but also from kidney, intestine and liver. Virus can also be isolated from oral and cloacal swabs.

33. **(a)** This is important during recovery from anaesthesia, when 100% oxygen should not routinely be administered to reptiles. Similarly, provision of high levels of oxygen may be contraindicated in patients with respiratory disease, as it may actually reduce respiratory rate and depth.

34. **(e)** Autotomy is the self-amputation of a part of the body, such as the tail in some species of lizards. It is a mechanism of self-defence, where the animal hopes a predator will follow the tail after separation – permitting the animal to escape. Caution should be exercised when handling these species, particularly if phlebotomy is to be performed from the ventral coccygeal vein. Tail re-growth does not include bony vertebrae (they are cartilaginous), and scales may have a slightly different appearance.

35. **(c)** The other tests are also useful, but radiography is most valuable for assessment of bone mineralization. Ionized calcium is the active fraction of calcium in the bloodstream, and therefore a more useful parameter than total blood calcium (which is often within the normal range in cases with metabolic bone disease).

36. **(d)** Whenever possible, conservative treatment should be utilized. Over-zealous removal of the retained spectacle may damage the normal basal spectacle. It is preferable to correct predisposing husbandry and nutritional problems. Increasing environmental humidity should ensure hydration. Synthetic artificial tears may be used to provide local hydration; mucolytics such as acetylcysteine may aid loosening of the spectacle. If surgery is required, it should be delicate and microscopy should be used.

37. **(e)** Mature intact green iguanas can be very aggressive during the breeding season. Castration of mature iguanas is less likely to successfully reduce aggression than castration of immature animals as a preventative measure. The testes are intra-abdominal, and the surgical procedure is quite technically demanding.

38. **(e)** Most geckos have eyelids, and can blink. Leopard geckos have fused eyelids (i.e. spectacles), as in snakes.

39. **(b)** In order to avoid the ventral midline abdominal vein, the coeliotomy incision is made slightly off midline. A similar procedure in a laterally compressed chameleon would be performed via a lateral (flank) incision.

40. **(e)** Signs may relate directly to the respiratory tract, including coughing, dyspnoea, tachpnoea, or open-mouth breathing. Increased respiratory noise or cyanosis of mucous membranes may be seen. General signs may include weight loss, lethargy and dehydration. Animals may spend more time in cooler areas to lower their metabolic rate, as a coping mechanism for hypoxia.

41. **(d)** The species originates from North Africa, living in rocky outcrops in desert areas of low humidity.

42. **(e)** Although blood culture may be indicated in chelonia with signs suggestive of septicaemia (e.g. plastron flushing, severe lethargy, or heterophilia with toxic changes), it is not routinely performed in a baseline health check.

43. **(a)** Dysecdysis is more common if humidity is too low during shedding. Burmese (or Indian) pythons require a relative humidity of 30–70%, and a daytime temperature range of 25–30°C (5–10°C higher at the 'hot spot', and 5–10°C lower at night).

44. **(d)** The coccidian organism (*Cryptosporidium serpentis*) causes an intense inflammatory reaction within the gastric crypts. Diagnosis without biopsy is difficult; the oocysts may be seen on gastric washes or using a fluorescent antibody test on faeces. The oocysts stain red with acid-fast reagents (e.g. Ziehl–Neelsen). Paromomycin may be useful to reduce shedding of oocysts, but does not eradicate the organism.

45. **(b)** All vertebrate species experience pain, but nociceptive pathways have not been fully elucidated in all reptile species. An endogenous opioid system has been demonstrated in reptiles. Assessment of pain is difficult in chelonia, as subtle behavioural changes may be the only clinical signs. If bone or soft tissues have been damaged, analgesia should be provided.

46. **(e)** The amphibian respiratory system varies between orders and individual species, as well as intraspecies depending on life-stage. Most larvae stages are aquatic and rely on branchial respiration. Anurans (frogs and toads) possess lungs, and in adults respiration may be cutaneous, buccopharyngeal and/or pulmonic. Neotenic species of Caudata such as the axolotl rely heavily on branchial respiration.

47. **(b)** The lingual plexus lies dorsally at the base of the tongue, and is readily accessed by pulling the tongue rostrally.

48. **(e)** Other causes of cloacal prolapse include local irritation, endoparasitism, gastroenteritis, and cloacal masses. The frog should be kept in water to prevent dessication of the prolapsed tissue. Larger prolapses require reduction and replacement, often under general anaesthesia.

49. **(a)** Eye position will not alter during fish anaesthesia. Of the other parameters, swimming movements are lost before reaction to tactile stimuli (pinching the tail-base) as anaesthesia deepens. Opercular movements are equivalent to respiratory rate, and a Doppler probe can be used to measure heart rate.

50. **(e)** Low oxygen levels in water may result in severe effects in fish. Respiratory distress is seen, with fish gasping at the surface of the water; this may be fatal. Gill damage, anaemia and methaemoglobinaemia may ensue, resulting in clinical hypoxia.

# APPENDIX 1
# Critical care

Good exotic patient assessment and preparation before procedures will reduce the development of critical problems. However, despite optimizing care of animals, there may be times when an animal requires emergency intervention to resuscitate it.

## PREPARATION

It is important to have supplies of drugs and equipment readily to hand in case an emergency occurs. The author recommends having a 'crash kit' (Fig. A1.1) that is portable enough to be carried between rooms in the clinic. In smaller establishments, it may be feasible to have a stock of materials in one central location. Emergency situations often arise when the patient is undergoing a procedure, particularly if anaesthesia is required. In practice, it is useful to keep basic equipment – such as that required for anaesthetic, drug and fluid administration – in this kit (Box A1.1) along with emergency drugs.

Other facilities that are useful include:

- Resuscitators (Fig. A1.2), e.g. Ambu®-bags
- Microscope: to perform rapid cytology on blood or other aspirated samples
- Blood analysers: those that can produce results with a small aliquot of blood are ideal for small animals (e.g. iStat® portable analyser)
- Imaging: radiography and ultrasonography in particular, e.g. to identify fluid in a coelomic cavity
- Blood pressure monitoring equipment – usually Doppler probe and sphygmomanometer for indirect method
- Digital thermometer – along with sources of supplemental heating (such as heat pads or a forced warm air blanket) and cooling (such as fluids at room temperature or ice packs).

## PRINCIPLES OF CCPR

Cardiocerebral pulmonary resuscitation (CCPR) is an emergency procedure performed in patients with cardiac or respiratory arrest. The inclusion of 'cerebral' indicates the need to preserve brain function.

In line with other pets, some basic principles (**ABCDEF**, see below) should be followed when treating a collapsed animal. If the animal undergoes respiratory or cardiac arrest while anaesthetized, switch off anaesthetic gases and administer reversal agents for injectable anaesthetics. CCPR is frequently unsuccessful. It is not usually performed in animals with end-stage disease.

- **A**irway
  - Ensure the airway is patent.
  - Intubate the patient. A tracheostomy (or air sac cannulation in birds) can be performed if orotracheal intubation is not possible.
- **B**reathing
  - Provide IPPV (intermittent positive pressure ventilation) with 100% oxygen (or atmospheric air via an Ambu-bag). Ideally, this is done via an endotracheal tube, but a close-fitting facemask will also create a seal and enable thoracic inflation (although there is a risk of air entering the gastrointestinal tract).
  - Chest wall compressions are an alternative method of deflating and inflating the lungs.
- **C**ardiovascular
  - Obtain venous access. If this is not possible, the intraosseous route may be used to access the circulation. If the patient is hypovolaemic, administer fluids (see below).
  - Perform external cardiac compression. (Internal cardiac compression is more effective but not usually feasible in small patients.)
- **D**rugs
  - At certain times, drugs are required to aid resuscitation (see below).
- **E**lectrical defibrillation
  - Not usually applicable to small exotic pets.
- **F**ollow-up
  - Assess the animal's history and perform a clinical examination to identify any underlying

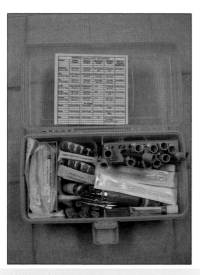

**Figure A1.1** Typical 'crash kit'.

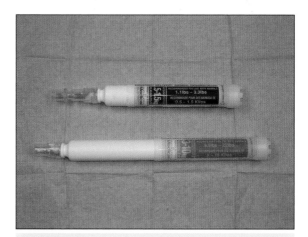

**Figure A1.2** Small animal resuscitators.

---

### BOX A1.1    CONTENTS OF A 'CRASH KIT'

- Drugs
  - Adrenaline
  - Atropine (glycopyrrolate for rabbits and rats that possess atropinesterase)
  - Doxapram
  - Diazepam
  - Local anaesthetic spray
  - Local anaesthetic ointment (e.g. lidocaine/prilocaine, EMLA®)
- Intubation equipment
  - Endotracheal tubes (uncuffed, 1–6 mm diameter)
  - Laryngoscope, with size 0–1 Wisconsin blade
- Intravenous catheters (20–26 gauge)
- Needles (18–24 gauge) and syringes (1–5 ml)
- Ocular lubricant
- Adhesive tape.

---

pathological conditions. Treatments will depend on the condition present, for example if the patient is hypothermic, provide supplementary heating.

- Continue support with fluids, monitor urine output, IPPV until spontaneous breathing resumes, oxygen (via nasal catheter or oxygen-enriched cage) until animal is stable, restore body temperature with active warming.

## DRUGS FOR USE IN EMERGENCIES
(TABLE A1.1)

- **Adrenaline** for cardiac arrest (fibrillating or asystole).
- **Anticholinergics** (atropine and glycopyrrolate) for bradycardia, or where excess oral or respiratory secretions are present. Note that anticholinergics will reduce the volume of secretions but they will be more viscous, and potentially more likely to result in obstruction of small airways. Glycopyrrolate should be used in animals that possess atropinesterase, including most rabbits and some rats.
- **Dexamethasone** and prednisolone sodium succinate for shock. May be ineffective, and may cause severe immune suppression (particularly in rabbits and birds) and gastrointestinal ulceration.
- **Diazepam** for seizures.
- **Doxapram**, a respiratory stimulant. Use in cases of respiratory depression or arrest. It has a short duration of effect and therefore may require repeated dosing. Mechanical ventilation should not be administered with doxapram. (Some adverse effects have been noted with this drug: improved cardiac output results in a pressor response. This effect may lead to a fall in arterial $pO_2$ due to a worsening of ventilation–perfusion matching in the lungs. Hyperventilation results in a lowered $pCO_2$, and thence cerebral vasoconstriction and slowing of the cerebral circulation. Doxapram also results in an increased release of catecholamines. Stimulation of the central nervous system may result in seizures. Cardiovascular effects may cause dysrhythmias.)

**Table A1.1** Emergency drug doses

| Drug | Species | Dose (mg/kg) | Route | Comment |
|---|---|---|---|---|
| Adrenaline | Rabbit | 0.2 | IV/IT | Combine with cardiac (usually external) compressions if asystole occurs |
| | Guinea pig | 0.003 | IV | |
| | Ferret | 0.02 | IV/IM/SC/IT | |
| | Non-human primates | 0.2–0.4 (diluted in 5 ml sterile water) | IT | |
| | | 0.5–1.0 ml/kg (of 1:10 000 dilution) | IV | |
| | Birds | 0.5–1.0 ml/kg (of 1:1000 dilution) | IV/IM/IO/IT | |
| | Fish | 0.2–0.5 ml/kg (1:1000) | IP/IM/IV/IC | |
| Atropine | Rodents | 0.05–0.1 | SC/IM | – |
| | Ferret | 0.02–0.04 | SC/IM | |
| | Non-human primates | 0.02–0.05 | IM | |
| | Birds | 0.2–0.5 | IV/IM/IO/IT | |
| | Reptiles | 0.2 | SC/IM/IV | |
| | Amphibians | 0.03 | IM/SC | |
| | Fish | 0.1 | IM/ICe/IV | |
| Dexamethasone | Rabbit | 2 | IM/IV | – |
| | Rodents | 0.5–2.0 | SC/IM/IV/PO | |
| | Ferret | 4–8 | IM/IV | |
| | Non-human primates | 0.25–1.00 | PO/IM/IV | |
| | Birds | 2–6 | IM/IV | |
| | Amphibians | 1–5 | SC/IM | |
| | Fish | 1–2 | IM/ICe | |
| Diazepam | Rabbit | 1 | IM/IV | Can repeat boluses as required |
| | Rodents | 1–5 | IM/IV | |
| | Ferret | 1 | IM/IV | |
| | | 0.5–1.0 mg/kg/h | CRI (IV) | |
| | Non-human primates | 0.25–5.0 | IM/IV | |
| | Birds | 0.5–1.0 | IM/IV | |
| | Reptiles | 2.5 | IM/IV | |
| Doxapram | Rabbit | 2–5 | IV/SC | Repeat every 10–15 min if required |
| | Chinchilla, gerbil, guinea pig, hamster, mouse, rat | 2–10 | IV/IP | |
| | Ferret | 1–11 | IV | |
| | Non-human primates | 2 | IV | |
| | Birds | 5–20 | IV/IM/IO/IT | |
| | Reptiles, amphibians | 5 | IM/IV | |
| | Fish | 5 | IV/ICe | Been used in sharks (prn) to treat respiratory depression |
| Frusemide | Rabbit | 0.3–5.0 | SC/IM/IV/PO | Duration 6–12 hr |
| | Rodents | 1–10 | SC/IM/PO | |
| | Ferret | 1–4 | SC/IM/IV/PO | |
| | Non-human primates | 1–2 | IV/PO | |
| | Reptiles | 5 | PO/IM/IV | Effects of loop diuretic are questionable as reptile kidneys lack a loop of Henle |
| | Fish | 2–5 | IM | |

**Table A1.1** Emergency drug doses *continued*

| Drug | Species | Dose (mg/kg) | Route | Comment |
|------|---------|--------------|-------|---------|
| Glycopyrrolate | Rabbit, rodents | 0.01–0.02 | SC | – |
| | Ferret | 0.01 | IM | |
| | Non-human primates | 0.005–0.010 | IM | |
| | Birds | 0.01 | IM/IV | |
| | Reptiles | 0.01 | SC/IM/IV | Not effective at these doses in the green iguana (*Iguana iguana*) |
| Lidocaine (lignocaine) | Rabbit | 2 | IV/IT | – |
| | Non-human primates | 1–2 | IV | |
| | | 0.01–0.05 mg/kg/min | IV CRI | |
| Prednisolone sodium succinate | Non-human primates | 1–15 | IV | – |
| | Birds | 10–20 | IM/IV | |
| | Amphibians | 5–10 | IM/IV | |
| Naloxone | Non-human primates | 0.01–0.05 | IM/IV | – |

CRI, continuous rate infusion; IC, intracardiac; ICo, intracoelomic; IM, intramuscular; IO, intraosseous; IP, intraperitoneal; IT, intratracheal; IV, intravenous; prn *(pro re nata)*, 'as the situation arises'; SC, subcutaneous; Top, topically. Note: Where a drug dose has neither been licensed nor published for a specific species, in an emergency situation the author would use the dose reported for a closely related species.

- **Frusemide**, a diuretic. Use in cases of heart failure, pulmonary congestion or oedema.
- **Lidocaine** (lignocaine) for cardiac arrhythmia.
- **Reversal agents** for anaesthetic drugs, e.g. atipamezole against $\alpha_2$-agonists, or partial opioid agonists (such as buprenorphine or butorphanol) or full opioid antagonists (such as naloxone) against opioids such as fentanyl or morphine.

## FLUID ADMINISTRATION

Many exotic pets are dehydrated when presented to the veterinary clinician (Table A1.2). Some may become dehydrated, or suffer significant blood loss during procedures. Fluids are often necessary to treat hypovolaemic shock; blood pressure should be monitored when administering fluids. The use of fluids is discussed further in the introductory chapters.

## OTHER ASPECTS OF CRITICAL CARE

- **Environment**
  - As discussed in the introductory chapters, it is important to ensure the animal is housed in an appropriate environment during hospitalization.

Provision of the animal's usual temperature, humidity, hide and substrate will help optimize the patient's metabolic functions. A UV light should be present for those species requiring one (i.e. most reptiles, amphibians and some birds).
- It is also vital to offer appropriate food and water. If you do not routinely stock certain foods, ask the client to supply some for a short hospital stay (or go shopping).
- **Heating**
  - Many small animals are susceptible to hypothermia and supplemental heating should be provided, particularly after anaesthesia.
  - Species from tropical climates – particularly reptiles – will require additional heating to provide their preferred optimal temperature range (POTR).
- **Oxygen**
  - Bubble through water in the aquarium for aquatic species such as fish.
  - Increase ambient oxygen levels for other species.
  - An intranasal catheter can be placed to provide oxygen.
  - Care should be taken when supplementing oxygen in reptiles, as a low oxygen saturation is

**Table A1.2** Principles of fluid administration

| Fluid | Species | Route | Dose | Frequency | Comment |
|---|---|---|---|---|---|
| Isotonic crystalloids, lactated Ringer's, dextrose (4%)/ normal saline (0.18%) | Rabbit | IP/IO/IV/SC | Maintenance = 100–150 ml/kg/day | CRI, or divide and administer a bolus q6–12hr | Use lactated Ringer's for fluid and electrolyte deficits, dextrose/saline for primary water deficit to support intravascular fluid volume; chipmunk IV/IO doses are for shock therapy. Only small boluses possible via reptile IO route due to small marrow space |
| | Chinchilla | IV/SC | 30–60 ml/day | | |
| | Chipmunk | SC; IP; IV/IO | 2–5 ml; 3–5 ml; 5–7 ml | | |
| | Gerbil | IP; SC | 3–4 ml; 2–3 ml | | |
| | Mouse | IP; SC | 1–3 ml; 1–2 ml | | |
| | Rat | IP; SC | 10–15 ml; 5–10 ml | | |
| | Ferret | IV/SC | 60–70 ml/kg/day | | |
| | Birds | IV/IO/SC | 50 ml/kg/day <10 ml/kg/hr | | Can administer 10 ml/kg IV/IO as a bolus in birds, one or two times |
| | Reptiles | IV/IO/SC/ICo | 5–10 ml/kg/hr | | |
| | Fish | IV/IP | 20–60 ml/kg/day (lactated Ringer's); 18 ml/kg prn (Ringer's) | Usually administered in divided doses | |
| Glucose 5% | Rabbit | IV/SC | 10 ml/kg | – | Anorexia |
| | Rodents | SC | | | Use routinely in small rodents pre-anaesthesia, and for pregnancy toxaemic in guinea pigs |
| | Birds | IV | | | – |
| | Amphibians | Shallow bath | | | For treating hydrocoelom and SC oedema |
| | Fish | IV/ICo | 40–60 ml/kg/day | | Severe dehydration |
| Colloids, e.g. hetastarch | Rabbit | IV/IO | 5 ml/kg | Repeat if still hypotensive | Hypovolaemic shock, hypoproteinaemia. Administer over 5–10 minutes and re-assess blood pressure. Caution in patients with congestive heart failure or renal failure. Can administer with crystalloids, reducing crystalloid volume by 33–50% |
| | Chipmunk | | 5–7 ml | | |
| | Gerbil | | 0.1 ml | | |
| | Ferret | | 5 ml/kg, maximum total 10–20 ml/kg/day | | |
| | Birds | | 10–15 ml/kg (or 5 ml/kg + 15 ml/kg lactated Ringer's) | q8hr, <4 treatments | |
| Liquidized diet, e.g. proprietary nutritional support diets, baby food, liquidized pellets | Rabbit, rodents | PO | 50 ml/kg/day in total | Divide and give bolus q8hr | Anorexia. Warm food first. Use organic, lactose-free baby foods; use vegetarian types for herbivores and carnivorous types for carnivores. Dilute carnivore convalescent diet in chlorine-free fresh water for amphibians |
| | Ferret | | 5–10 ml/animal | q8hr | |
| | Birds | | <50 ml/kg | q6–24hr | |
| | Reptiles | | 10–30 ml/kg | q24hr | |
| | Amphibians | | 10–20 ml/kg | q24hr | |

**Table A1.2** Principles of fluid administration *continued*

| Fluid | Species | Route | Dose | Frequency | Comment |
|---|---|---|---|---|---|
| Blood | Rabbit | IV | 10–20 ml/kg, maximum rate 22 ml/kg/h | Can repeat, advise cross-match | Anaemia. Monitor for transfusion reactions. Maximum volume from donor 1% of body weight; 6 ml blood into 1 ml anticoagulant (e.g. acid–citrate–dextrose) |
| | Ferret | IV/IO | 6–12 ml/animal | No need to cross-match | |
| | Birds | IV | 10–20% blood volume (5–26 ml/kg) | Homologous donor preferred; heterogeneous species donor acceptable for single transfusion | |
| Haemoglobin solutions | Ferret | IV | 6–15 ml/kg | Infusion over 4 hours, once or twice in 24 hour period | Anaemia. Administer slowly |
| | Birds | IV/IO | 5 ml/kg | One or two boluses | Alternative in birds with hypovolaemia and shock is hypertonic saline 7.5% (5 ml/kg bolus over 10 min) |

CRI, continuous rate infusion; ICo, intracoelomically; IM, intramuscularly; IO, intraosseously; IV, intravenously; PO, orally; prn, 'as the situation arises'; q8hr, every 8 hours; SC, subcutaneously.

required to stimulate breathing, and provision of an elevated oxygen environment will reduce the animal's respiratory drive.

- **Fluids**
  - Reptiles: Bathing reptiles in shallow warm water often encourages them to drink (and also to pass urine, faeces and urates). This is usually performed once or twice daily for 10–15 minutes.
  - Amphibians: Normal (0.5–0.8%) saline may be used as an electrolyte bath for ill terrestrial amphibians. Provide access to a bath of untreated fresh water in the enclosure simultaneously. Other electrolyte solutions may be used for longer term fluid therapy, such as 'amphibian Ringer's solution' (6.6 g NaCl, 0.15 g KCl, 0.15 g $CaCl_2$ and 0.2 g $NaHCO_3$ in 1 litre water).
  - Fish: 1–3 g sodium chloride (non-iodinized)/l tank water is a supportive measure against stress-induced mortality in freshwater fish.
- **Nutritional support**
  - Often necessary with ill exotic pets (further details in introductory chapters).
- **Medication**
  - Drugs such as analgesics and prokinetics are often required to aid recovery from illness.
  - Antimicrobial agents may be required for certain infectious diseases.

# APPENDIX 2
# Zoonoses

A zoonosis is a disease of animals transmissible to man. In some cases, this disease transmission is difficult and hence rarely occurs; in other cases, extreme caution should be taken when dealing with animals, as transmission is relatively easy. Some diseases may be subclinical in man while others can be fatal. In certain instances, individuals – such as those who are immunocompromised – will be more susceptible to disease and the disease may be much more severe in them than in the general population.

Appropriate precautions should be taken to reduce risks to owners and staff when dealing with exotic pets. This may be a simple case of good hygiene – such as washing hands after handling the animal – or wearing personal protective equipment (PPE) – such as examination gloves and a facemask. For some conditions, it is advisable to humanely euthanize the animal and dispose of the body safely (e.g. by cremation) to avoid any further risk to humans. Separate equipment for different enclosures will help reduce the spread of diseases. Immunosuppressed individuals should avoid handling potentially infected animals or materials.

Infections are often more common in free-ranging animals, so veterinary clinicians dealing with wildlife are more likely to be exposed to disease. However, exotic pets may have an unknown origin, and poor biosecurity or lack of quarantine after addition of a new animal to a collection may permit the spread of pathogens.

Some zoonotic diseases are listed in legislation to safeguard human health, e.g. the Psittacosis or Ornithosis Order 1953 in the UK. Legislation will vary between countries.

## MAMMALS

### Bacterial

- **Bordetella bronchiseptica:** Usually associated with respiratory disease. Other bacterial respiratory infections that may be zoonotic are *Klebsiella pneumoniae* and *Pasteurella* spp.
- **Campylobacter spp:** Causes enteric disease.
- **Chlamydophila psittaci:** May cause conjunctivitis in guinea pigs; the infection is usually self-limiting (see Birds section below for further details).
- **Escherichia coli:** Transmission is usually via the faeco-oral route. Certain strains will cause serious illness (potentially fatally) in humans.
- **Leptospira:** Most mammal species can become infected with pathogenic *Leptospira*. Maintenance host species (usually wildlife) such as mice, rats, opossums and skunks shed the organisms in their urine for a prolonged time period. *Leptospira ballum* in hamsters (from contaminated mice) results in nephritis and hepatitis. Disease in humans may include pulmonary haemorrhage, renal failure and jaundice.
- **Listeria monocytogenes:** Symptoms in humans include fever, nausea and diarrhoea. It can be fatal.
- **Salmonella:** Causes disease in many mammals, although some individuals may be asymptomatic, e.g. *Salmonella typhimurium* and *S. enteritidis* in rodents. They cause food poisoning in humans which may become systemic. As an example, *Salmonella* serotype Tilene in pygmy hedgehogs has caused illness in humans. As animals may become asymptomatic carriers after infection, those diagnosed with salmonellosis should be euthanized.
- **Shigella spp:** Cause enteric disease.
- **Streptobacillus moniliformis:** Causes polyarthritis in mice and rats, and 'rat bite fever' in humans (with fever, rigors, and migratory polyarthralgias).
- **Tuberculosis** (*Mycobacterium tuberculosis*): Most commonly from non-human primates. Tuberculosis causes gastrointestinal disease with granulomas and lymphadenopathy in ferrets. Transmission is usually

by inhalation, especially aerosolized fluids from coughing. It is of concern in humans due to the spread of strains with drug resistance.

- **Wild-caught** animals such as rabbits or prairie dogs can transmit tularaemia (*Francisella tularensis*) and plague (*Yersinia pestis*), listeriosis.
- **Yersiniosis** (*Yersinia pseudotuberculosis*). The source of infection is often contamination of food by wild birds or rodents. Many species are asymptomatic carriers. The infection causes gradual loss of weight and body condition with diarrhoea in guinea pigs. In callitrichids and other primates, sudden death may be the first sign of an outbreak. Treatment in pets is not advised.

## Fungal

- **Dermatophytosis** (ringworm, e.g. *Microsporum* spp and *Trichophyton* spp) may be asymptomatic.

## Viral

- **Hantavirus** is transmitted to humans via inhalation of aerosolized virus in urine, saliva or faeces of infected rodents. Disease in humans may be haemorrhagic fever with renal syndrome (in Asia and Europe) or pulmonary syndrome (in the Americas). It is very rare in the UK and rare in North America, but often fatal in humans.
- **Hepatitis** can be transmitted from primate body fluids. It results in fever, anorexia and jaundice in humans.
- **Lymphocytic choriomeningitis virus** (LCMV) is a potential zoonosis from rodents.
- **Monkey pox** causes a smallpox-like disease. Direct contact will transmit infection from primates and rodents (e.g. prairie dogs in an outbreak in the USA in 2003) to humans. Symptoms in humans include a febrile rash. The disease can be fatal.
- **Rabies:** The disease results in neurological signs. All mammals are prone to infection, but susceptibility varies. Reservoir hosts commonly include bats and terrestrial carnivores. An endemic cycle of one distinct phylogenetic clade has been demonstrated in common marmosets. Human exposure is usually after being bitten or scratched by an infected animal. Pre-exposure vaccination provides some protection, but post-exposure treatment is recommended if exposure is thought to have occurred. Untreated human cases are fatal.
- Mouse **rotavirus** and rat rotavirus-like agent may be zoonotic.

## Parasites

- Rodent **cestodes:** Dwarf tapeworm (*Rodentolepis* (previously *Hymenolepis*) *nana*) and rat tapeworm (*Hymenolepis diminuta*) are a threat particularly to children.
- *Cheyletiella parasitivorax:* Causes erythematous pruritic lesions in humans, particularly on the arms (often due to direct contact when holding a pet rabbit).
- **Fleas:** Usually cat or dog flea (*Ctenocephalides felis* or *canis*) from other pets may be found on pet rabbits (not usually the rabbit flea, *Spilopsyllus cuniculi*).
- Various **helminths** affecting non-human primates are zoonotic. The raccoon ascarid *Baylisascaris procyonis* is also zoonotic.
- **Sarcoptic mange:** *Sarcoptes scabiei*. *Trixacarus caviae* may result in dermatitis in infected humans.
- **Protozoal**
  - **Cryptosporidiosis** is potentially zoonotic.
  - *Encephalitozoon cuniculi:* Causes illness mainly in immunocompromised humans (such as those with AIDS).
  - *Entamoeba histolytica:* Can cause diarrhoea in primates and amoebic dysentery in humans.
  - *Toxoplasma gondii* is transmitted by eating undercooked rabbit meat. Animals usually become infected through food contamination by cat faeces containing oocytes. It may cause abortion or still-birth if contracted during pregnancy.

## Other infections

- Mammals carry many **other infections**, especially bacterial and fungal – that are zoonotic. Particular caution should be taken when dealing with non-human primates, as many diseases – including viruses – will transfer between them and humans (as well as *vice versa*).
- Some infections are found in both animals and humans but cross-species transmission does not appear to occur, e.g. *Giardia* in rabbits.

## REPTILES

### Bacterial

- *Escherichia coli.*
- **Mycobacteria.** Mycobacteriosis has been identified in reptiles (typically *Mycobacterium avium* complex (MAC), *M. marinum*, *M. chelonae*, *M. fortuitum*, *M. smegmatis*, *M. phamnopheos* and *M. phlei*), with

lesions mainly affecting the integument, gastrointestinal and respiratory tracts. Infection usually originates from soil or stagnant water. Disease in humans is commonly cutaneous granulomas. The organism enters via skin lesions.

- *Pseudomonas.*
- Tick-borne **rickettsiae** such as Q fever.
- *Salmonella.* Many healthy reptiles harbour *Salmonellae* asymptomatically in their gastrointestinal tract, shedding bacteria intermittently. This is a potential risk for handlers, which can be protected against by wearing gloves while handling reptiles or by washing hands afterwards. Immunosuppressed individuals – such as the elderly, infants or those with impaired immune systems – are more at risk.
- *Yersinia* (see above for detail).

## Parasites
- **Pentastomids.**

# BIRDS

## Bacterial

- *Campylobacter* **spp:** Bacteria are usually waterborne. Human disease is a severe form of food poisoning.
- *Erysipelothrix rhusiopathiae.* Rodents act as reservoirs. Disease is common in turkeys and is also reported in raptors.
- *Escherichia coli.*
- *Pasteurella multocida* (avian cholera).
- **Psittacosis** (*Chlamydophila psittaci*). Host species include psittacines (parrots), pigeons, poultry and waterfowl. Clinical signs often involve the respiratory system but may be vague in a sick bird, and so this disease should therefore be considered with most sick cage birds. Conjunctivitis and rhinitis are common clinical signs in pigeons. Adult raptors commonly have chronic disease with non-specific respiratory signs, weight loss and diarrhoea; young raptors usually succumb to acute disease. Owners should always be warned of the risk of this zoonotic disease, and euthanasia should be considered in animals shown to be positive. Transmission is via inhalation of dust from faeces or feathers, or via direct contact. Symptoms in humans are 'flu-like', including fever, headache, non-productive cough, lymphadenopathy, confusion, and myalgia. Immunocompromised individuals – such as those with HIV or on immunosuppressive drug therapies – are most at risk. Care should be taken when performing avian necropsies, which should preferably be carried out inside a fume-hood. It is advisable to perform microscopic examination using a modified Ziehl–Neelsen stain on an impression of spleen or air sac at the start of the necropsy before proceeding further. If a suspect case is hospitalized, staff should wear PPE (gloves, facemasks, plastic aprons and hats).
- *Salmonella* **spp:** Pigeons are known carriers of *Salmonella*, especially *S. typhimurium*. Disease in humans varies, but is often gastrointestinal; a fever may be present.
- **Tuberculosis:** Difficult to cure so advise euthanasia of infected birds to reduce the human risk. The environment should also be decontaminated. Disease in humans varies from local – particularly *Mycobacterium tuberculosis* – to systemic – particularly *M. avium* – disease.
- *Yersinia pseudotuberculosis* (pseudotuberculosis).

## Fungal
- *Aspergillus* **spp.**

## Viral
- **Avian influenza:** Close contact with infected birds – currently poultry or wild birds – may result in human disease. Outbreaks of the H5N1 strain resulted in human fatalities in 1997 (Hong Kong) and 2003–2004 (throughout Asia).
- **Newcastle disease** (PMV-1 infection). In most countries this is a notifiable disease in poultry. In humans, a brief conjunctivitis or flu-like symptoms are seen.
- **West Nile virus.** Originating in Uganda in 1937, this virus has since spread widely. An outbreak in the USA in 1999 resulted in deaths in humans, horses and many wild birds (predominantly corvids). Disease typically causes encephalitis and fever, although some species may be asymptomatic. Vectors include mosquitoes and ticks.

## Parasites
- **Red mites** (*Dermanyssus gallinae*). These may infect passerines, and can bite humans. Pruritus and skin lesions are seen in humans.

# AMPHIBIANS

## Bacterial

- **Mycobacteria** are not very infective to other in-contact amphibians, but can result in persistent granuloma formation in humans ('aquarist's nodule'). Infected animals should be euthanized.

- Other **aquatic bacteria** as listed in the Fish section.

## FISH

### Bacterial (in aquatic environments)

- *Aeromonas hydrophila.* Bacteria are ubiquitous in aquatic environments. Humans are infected by ingesting contaminated water or via direct contact with a wound. Usually symptoms are of gastroenteritis and localized wound infection.
- *Campylobacter* spp.
- *Edwardsiella tarda.*
- *Escherichia coli* (enterotoxic and enteropathogenic types).
- *Erysipelothrix* spp.
- *Legionella pneumophila.*
- **Mycobacteria** (*Mycobacterium fortuitum*, *M. marinum*, *M. chelonia*): Also called fish tank granuloma, fish fancier's finger or fish handler's disease. Granulomatous nodules – usually on hands or fingers – often heal without treatment in several months. Sometimes localized infection spreads to local lymph nodes – particularly with *M. marinum* – or deep into adjacent tissues – resulting in arthritis, osteomyelitis and tenosynovitis. Owing to unresponsive T-cells, immunosuppressed individuals are most at risk.
- **Nocardia** (*N. asteroids, N. kampachi*) cause similar clinical signs to mycobacteria.
- *Pseudomonas* **spp** (*Pseudomonas fluorescens*). Common in freshwater and marine aquarium fish.
- *Vibrio* (*Vibrio fluvialis, V. parahaemolyticus, V. vulnificus*). These organisms can be present in marine and estuarine environments. Infection, occasionally fatal, in humans is usually via eating infected marine fish or through contamination of skin wounds.
- *Yersinia enterocolitica.*

### Parasites

- *Cryptosporidium* may infect both fish and humans. No reported zoonotic cases.

- **Nematodes** can be transmitted via ingestion of food fish and therefore are no risk to humans working in aquaria.

## OTHER POTENTIALLY INJURIOUS FACTORS (NOT ZOONOSES) TO CONSIDER WHEN DEALING WITH EXOTIC PETS

- **Allergy:** For example to rabbit or rodent dander or urine. Acute respiratory compromise may occur in humans with allergies in response to aerosolized rat urine.
- **Constriction** by large snakes.
- **Drowning:** This is particularly a risk in large public aquaria where divers are required for tank maintenance.
- **Electrocution:** From electric fish such as the electric eel, electric catfish and several genera of rays. Wear arm-length rubber gloves to reduce the risk to the handler.
- **Toxins**, such as those from the fangs of venomous snakes or Heloderm lizards, from the parotid glands in marine toads, or the skin of poison arrow frogs (*Dendrobates* spp). Several fish species possess spines – some of which are venomous – such as lionfish, stingrays, some catfish, and surgeonfish.
- **Trauma:** From bites, scratches, pecks and tail whipping. These may become infected.

## HUMAN INFECTIONS CAUSING DISEASE IN ANIMALS (i.e. REVERSE ZOONOSES)

- **Human herpes Epstein–Barr virus** (human herpesvirus 4) may induce lymphoproliferative conditions in callitrichids.
- **Human herpes simplex I.** This virus causes chronic hepatitis in African pygmy hedgehogs (*Atelerix albiventris*). *Herpes simplex* has also been implicated in callitrichid (marmosets and tamarins) fatalities with disseminated disease associated with open lip or mouth ulcers on owners or keepers.
- **Measles** may be asymptomatic in non-human primates or may be fatal (particularly in New World primates).

# APPENDIX 3
## Suppliers

- Easily-digestible formulae for other species e.g. Carnivore Care®, and Critical Care® or Critical Care Fine Grind® for herbivores from Oxbow Animal Health, Murdock, NE 68407 USA.
- Warm air blanket, e.g. Bair Hugger®, Arizant Healthcare Inc., Eden Prairie, MN 55344, USA.
- Portable blood analysis, e.g. i-STAT®, Abbott Laboratories, Abbott Park, IL, USA.
- Local anaesthetic cream, e.g. EMLA®, AstraZeneca, Macclesfield, Cheshire UK.
- Easily digestible avian formula, e.g. Harrison's Recovery Formula, Harrison's Bird Foods, Loughborough, UK.
- Brooder, e.g. Brinsea TLC (Thermal Life-support Cabinet) 4M Intensive Care Unit (see Fig. 10.1a), Brinsea Products Ltd, North Somerset, UK.
- Incubator, e.g. Animal Intensive Care Unit (see Fig. 10.1b), Animal Care Products, various suppliers.
- Resuscitator, e.g. Constant Delivery Animal Resuscitator (see Fig. A1.1), McCulloch Medical, McCulloch Products Ltd, Auckland, New Zealand.
- Fentanyl/fluanisone, e.g. Hypnorm, VetPharma Ltd, Leeds, UK.
- Romanovsky stain, e.g. Diff Quick, Andwin Scientific, Thermo Fisher Scientific Ltd, various suppliers.

# Further reading

## SECTION 1    MAMMALS

### CHAPTER 2    Mammals – an introduction

Carpenter JW (2005): Exotic Animal Formulary. 3rd edn. Elsevier/Saunders.

Harcourt-Brown F (2002): Textbook of Rabbit Medicine. Butterworth-Heinemann, Oxford.

Johnson-Delaney CA (2008): Exotic Companion Medicine Handbook for Veterinarians. Zoological Education Network, Lake Worth, Florida.

Keeble E, Meredith A (2009): Manual of Rodents and Ferrets. British Small Animal Veterinary Association, Quedgeley, Gloucester.

Longley LA (2008): Anaesthesia of Exotic Pets. Elsevier/Saunders, Edinburgh.

MacDonald D, Norris S (2004): The New Encyclopedia of Mammals. Oxford University Press, Oxford.

Meredith A, Redrobe S (2002): Manual of Exotic Pets, 4th edn. British Small Animal Veterinary Association, Quedgeley, Gloucester.

O'Malley B (2005): Clinical Anatomy and Physiology of Exotic Species: Structure and Function of Mammals, Birds, Reptiles and Amphibians. Elsevier/Saunders, Edinburgh.

Quesenberry KE, Carpenter JW (2004): Ferrets, Rabbits and Rodents: Clinical Medicine and Surgery, 2nd edn. Saunders, St Louis, pp. 135–230.

### CHAPTER 3    Post-spay complications in a rabbit

Carpenter JW (2005): Rabbits. Exotic Animal Formulary, 3rd edn. Elsevier/Saunders, St Louis, pp. 409–444.

Harcourt-Brown F (2002): Textbook of Rabbit Medicine. Butterworth-Heinemann, Oxford.

Keeble E, Meredith A (2006): Self-Assessment Colour Review of Rabbit Medicine & Surgery. Manson Publishing, London.

Quesenberry KE, Carpenter JW (2004): Ferrets, Rabbits and Rodents: Clinical Medicine and Surgery, 2nd edn. Saunders, St Louis, pp. 135–230.

### CHAPTER 4    Spinal fracture in a rabbit

Girling SJ (2006): Diagnostic imaging. In: Meredith A, Flecknell P (eds) Manual of Rabbit Medicine and Surgery, 2nd edn. British Small Animal Veterinary Association, Quedgeley, Gloucester, pp. 52–61.

Harcourt-Brown F (2002): Textbook of Rabbit Medicine. Butterworth-Heinemann, Oxford.

Keeble E (2006): Nervous and musculoskeletal disorders. In: Meredith A, Flecknell P (eds) Manual of Rabbit Medicine and Surgery, 2nd edn. British Small Animal Veterinary Association, Quedgeley, Gloucester, pp. 103–116.

O'Malley B (2005): Rabbits. Clinical Anatomy and Physiology of Exotic Species: Structure and Function of Mammals, Birds, Reptiles and Amphibians. Elsevier/Saunders, Edinburgh, pp. 173–195.

Ward ML (2006): Physical examination and clinical techniques. In: Meredith A, Flecknell P (eds) Manual of Rabbit Medicine and Surgery, 2nd edn. British Small Animal Veterinary Association, Quedgeley, Gloucester, pp. 18–36.

### CHAPTER 5    Ferret with abdominal mass

Johnson-Delaney CA (2008): Ferrets. In: Johnson-Delaney CA (ed.) Exotic Companion Medicine Handbook. Zoological Education Network, Lake Worth, Florida, Vol 1: pp. 1–42.

Lewington J (2005): Ferrets. Clinical Anatomy and Physiology of Exotic Species: Structure and Function of Mammals, Birds, Reptiles and Amphibians. Elsevier/Saunders, Edinburgh, pp. 237–261.

Lewington J (2007): Ferret Husbandry, Medicine and Surgery, 2nd edn. Saunders/Elsevier, Edinburgh.

Quesenberry KE, Carpenter JW (2004): Ferrets, Rabbits and Rodents: Clinical Medicine and Surgery, 2nd edn. Saunders, St Louis, pp. 135–230.

### CHAPTER 6    Urolithiasis in a chinchilla

Hoefer H, Latney La'T (2009): Rodents: urogenital and reproductive system disorders. In: Keeble E, Meredith A (eds) Manual of Rodents and Ferrets. British Small Animal Veterinary Association, Quedgeley, Gloucester, pp. 150–160.

Quesenberry KE, Donnelly TM, Hillyer EV (2004): Biology, husbandry, and clinical techniques of guinea pigs and chinchillas. In: Quesenberry KE, Carpenter JW (eds) Ferrets, Rabbits and Rodents: Clinical Medicine and Surgery, 2nd edn. Saunders, St Louis, pp. 232–244.

### CHAPTER 7    Cheilitis in a guinea pig

Hollamby S (2009): Rodents: neurological and musculoskeletal disorders. In: Keeble E, Meredith A (eds) Manual of Rodents and Ferrets. British Small Animal Veterinary Association, Quedgeley, Gloucester, pp. 161–168.

Longley L (2009): Rodents: dermatoses. In: Keeble E, Meredith A (eds) Manual of Rodents and Ferrets. British Small Animal Veterinary Association, Quedgeley, Gloucester, pp. 107–122.

Quesenberry KE, Carpenter JW (2004): Ferrets, Rabbits and Rodents: Clinical Medicine and Surgery, 2nd edn. Saunders, St Louis, pp. 135–230.

## CHAPTER 8    Skin neoplasia in a hamster

Bennett RA (2009): Rodents: soft tissue surgery. In: Keeble E, Meredith A (eds) Manual of Rodents and Ferrets. British Small Animal Veterinary Association, Quedgeley, Gloucester, pp. 73–85.

Burnie D (2001): Animal. Dorling Kindersley, London.

Longley LA (2008): Rodent anaesthesia. Anaesthesia of Exotic Pets. Elsevier/Saunders, Edinburgh, pp. 59–84.

Longley L (2009): Rodents: dermatoses. In: Keeble E, Meredith A (eds) Manual of Rodents and Ferrets. British Small Animal Veterinary Association, Quedgeley, Gloucester, pp. 107–122.

MacDonald D, Norris S (2004): The New Encyclopedia of Mammals. Oxford University Press, Oxford.

O'Malley B (2005): Hamsters. Clinical Anatomy and Physiology of Exotic Species: Structure and Function of Mammals, Birds, Reptiles and Amphibians. Elsevier/Saunders, Edinburgh, pp. 227–236.

# SECTION 2    BIRDS

## CHAPTER 9    Birds – an introduction

Chitty J, Lierz M (2008): Manual of Raptors, Pigeons and Passerine Birds. British Small Animal Veterinary Association, Quedgeley, Gloucester.

Harcourt-Brown N, Chitty J (2005): Manual of Psittacine Birds, 2nd edn. British Small Animal Veterinary Association, Quedgeley, Gloucester.

Harrison GJ, Lightfoot TL (2006): Clinical Avian Medicine. Spix Publishing, Palm Beach, Florida.

Lennox AM (2009): Avian advanced anaesthesia, monitoring and critical care. BSAVA Annual Congress. British Small Animal Veterinary Association, Birmingham, pp. 54–57.

Longley LA (2008): Anaesthesia of Exotic Pets. Elsevier/Saunders, Edinburgh.

## CHAPTER 10    Regurgitation in a cockatoo

Garner MM (2006): Overview of tumors: Section II A retrospective study of case submissions to a specialty diagnostic service. In: Harrison GJ, Lightfoot TL (eds) Clinical Avian Medicine. Spix Publishing, Palm Beach, Florida, pp. 566–571.

Hadley T (2005): Disorders of the psittacine gastrointestinal tract. Veterinary Clinics of North America: Exotic Animal Practice 8 (2), 329–349.

Harcourt-Brown NH (2005): Diagnostic imaging. In: Harcourt-Brown NH, Chitty J (eds) Manual of Psittacine Birds, 2nd edn. British Small Animal Veterinary Association, Quedgeley, Gloucester, pp. 97–106.

Harrison GJ, Lightfoot TL (2006): Emergency and critical care: Section 1. In: Harrison GJ, Lightfoot TL (eds) Clinical Avian Medicine. Spix Publishing, Palm Beach, Florida, pp. 213–232.

Lawrie A (2005): Systemic non-infectious disease. In: Harcourt-Brown NH, Chitty J. (eds) Manual of Psittacine Birds, 2nd edn. British Small Animal Veterinary Association, Quedgeley, Gloucester, pp. 245–265.

Lightfoot TL (2006): Overview of tumors: Section 1. Clinical avian neoplasia and oncology. In: Harrison GJ, Lightfoot TL (eds) Clinical Avian Medicine. Spix Publishing, Palm Beach, Florida, pp. 560–565.

Longley LA (2008): Avian anaesthesia. In: Longley LA (ed.) Anaesthesia of Exotic Pets. Saunders/Elsevier, Edinburgh, pp. 127–182.

O'Malley B (2005): Avian anatomy and physiology. Clinical Anatomy and Physiology of Exotic Species: Structure and Function of Mammals, Birds, Reptiles and Amphibians. Elsevier/Saunders, Edinburgh, pp. 97–161.

## CHAPTER 11    Harris' hawk with bumblefoot

Bailey T, Lloyd C (2008): Raptors: disorders of the feet. In: Chitty J, Lierz M (eds) Manual of Raptors, Pigeons and Passerine Birds. British Small Animal Veterinary Association, Quedgeley, Gloucester, pp. 176–189.

Hirschberg RM (2008): Anatomy and physiology. In: Chitty J, Lierz M (eds) Manual of Raptors, Pigeons and Passerine Birds. British Small Animal Veterinary Association, Quedgeley, Gloucester, pp 25–41.

Kemp A, Newton I (2003): Hawks, eagles, and Old World vultures. In: Perrins C (ed.) The New Encyclopedia of Birds. Oxford University Press, Oxford, pp.162–173.

O'Malley B (2005): Avian anatomy and physiology. Clinical Anatomy and Physiology of Exotic Species: Structure and Function of Mammals, Birds, Reptiles and Amphibians. Elsevier/Saunders, Edinburgh, pp. 97–161.

Schmidt RE, Lightfoot TL (2006): Integument. In: Harrison GJ, Lightfoot TL (eds) Clinical Avian Medicine. Spix Publishing, Palm Beach, Florida, Vol 1: pp. 395–409.

## CHAPTER 12    Tibiotarsal fracture in a dove

Harcourt-Brown N, Chitty J (2005): Manual of Psittacine Birds, 2nd edn. British Small Animal Veterinary Association, Quedgeley, Gloucester.

Harcourt-Brown NH (2005): Orthopaedic and beak surgery. In: Harcourt-Brown NH, Chitty J (eds) Manual of Psittacine Birds, 2nd edn. British Small Animal Veterinary Association, Quedgeley, Gloucester, pp. 120–135.

Orosz SE (2003) Long bone fracture repair and bandaging: clinical anatomy of the humerus, femur, and tibiotarsus. AAV Annual Conference, Pittsburgh, Pennsylvania, pp. 277–283.

Redig PT (2003) Orthopedic principles and methods for the humerus, antebrachium, femur, and tibiotarsus of birds. AAV Annual Conference, Pittsburgh, Pennsylvania, pp. 285–295.

## CHAPTER 13    Feather plucking in a parrot

Chitty J (2005): Feather and skin disorders. In: Harcourt-Brown NH, Chitty J (eds) Manual of Psittacine Birds, 2nd edn. British Small Animal Veterinary Association, Quedgeley, Gloucester, pp. 191–204.

Coles BH (1997): Avian Medicine and Surgery, 2nd edn. Blackwell Science, Oxford.

Glendell G (2007): Breaking Bad Habits in Parrots. Interpet Publishing, Surrey.

Harrison GJ, Lightfoot TL (2006): Clinical Avian Medicine. Spix Publishing, Palm Beach, Florida.

O'Malley B (2005): Avian anatomy and physiology. Clinical Anatomy and Physiology of Exotic Species: Structure and Function of Mammals, Birds, Reptiles and Amphibians. Elsevier/Saunders, Edinburgh, pp. 97–161.

Raftery A (2005): The initial presentation: triage and critical care. In: Harcourt-Brown NH, Chitty J (eds) Manual of Psittacine Birds, 2nd edn. British Small Animal Veterinary Association, Quedgeley, Gloucester, pp. 35–49.

## CHAPTER 14    Stomatitis in a Harris' hawk

Dalhausen RD (2006): Implications of mycoses in clinical disorders. In: Harrison GJ, Lightfoot TL (eds) Clinical Avian Medicine. Spix Publishing, Palm Beach, Florida, Vol 2: pp. II: 691–704.

O'Malley B (2005): Avian anatomy and physiology. Clinical Anatomy and Physiology of Exotic Species: Structure and Function of Mammals, Birds, Reptiles and Amphibians. Elsevier/Saunders, Edinburgh, pp. 97–161.

Stanford M (2008): Raptors: infectious diseases. In: Chitty J, Lierz M (eds) Manual of Raptors, Pigeons and Passerine Birds. British Small Animal Veterinary Association, Quedgeley, Gloucester, pp. 212–222.

# SECTION 3    REPTILES

## CHAPTER 15    Reptiles – an introduction

Fudge AM (1999): Laboratory Medicine: Avian and Exotic Pets. Saunders, London.

Girling SJ, Raiti P (2004): Manual of Reptiles, 2nd edn. British Small Animal Veterinary Association, Quedgeley, Gloucester.

Halliday T, Adler K (2002): The New Encyclopedia of Reptiles & Amphibians. Oxford University Press, Oxford.

Highfield AC (1996): Practical Encyclopedia of Keeping and Breeding Tortoises and Freshwater Turtles. Carapace Press, London.

Jackson OF (1980): Weigh and measurement data on tortoises (Testudo graeca and Testudo hermanni) and their relationship to health. Journal of Small Animal Practice 21, 409.

## CHAPTER 16    Gastrointestinal foreign body in a tortoise

Benson KB (1999): Reptilian gastrointestinal diseases. Seminars in Avian and Exotic Pet Medicine 8, 90–97.

Calvert I (2004): Nutrition. In: Girling SJ, Raiti P (eds) Manual of Reptiles, 2nd edn. British Small Animal Veterinary Association, Quedgeley, Gloucester, pp. 18–39.

Carpenter JW, Mashima TY, Rupiper DJ (2005): Miscellaneous agents used in reptiles. Exotic Animal Formulary, 3rd edn. WB Saunders, Philadelphia, pp. 90–93.

Diaz-Figueroa O, Mitchell MA (2006): Gastrointestinal anatomy and physiology. In: Mader DR (ed.) Reptile Medicine and Surgery, 2nd edn. Saunders/Elsevier, St Louis, pp. 145–162.

Esque TC, Peters EL (1994): Ingestion of bones, stones and soil by desert tortoises. In: Bury RB, Germano DJ (eds) Biology of North American Tortoises. Fish and Wildlife Research, US Department of the Interior, Washington DC, pp. 105–111.

Hailey A, Coulson IM (1996): Differential scaling of home-range area to daily movement distance in two African tortoises. Canadian Journal of Zoology 74, 97–102.

Hasbun C, Samour J, Al-Ghais S (1998): Duodenal volvulus in free-living green turtles from coastal United Arab Emirates. Journal of Wildlife Disease 34, 797–800.

Hernandez-Divers SJ (2004): Surgery: principles and techniques. In: Girling SJ, Raiti P (eds) Manual of Reptiles, 2nd edn. British Small Animal Veterinary Association, Quedgeley, Gloucester, pp. 147–167.

Jacobson ER (1994): Causes of mortality and disease in tortoises: a review. Journal of Zoo and Wildlife Medicine 25, 2–17.

Marlow RW, Tollestrup K (1982): Mining and exploitation of natural mineral deposits by the desert tortoise Gopherus agassizii. Animal Behaviour 30, 475–478.

McArthur S, Barrows M (2004): Nutrition. In: McArthur S, Wilkinson R, Meyer J (eds) Medicine and Surgery of Tortoises and Turtles. Blackwell Publishing, Oxford, pp. 73–85.

McArthur S, Hernandez-Divers S (2004): Surgery. In: McArthur S, Wilkinson R, Meyer J (eds) Medicine and Surgery of Tortoises and Turtles. Blackwell Publishing, Oxford, pp. 403–464.

O'Malley B (2005): Tortoises and turtles. Clinical Anatomy and Physiology of Exotic Species: Structure and Function of Mammals, Birds, Reptiles, and Amphibians. Elsevier/Saunders, Edinburgh, pp. 41–56.

Schumacker J, Papendick R, Herbst L, et al. (1996): Volvulus of the proximal colon in a Hawksbill turtle (Eretmochelys imbricata). Journal of Zoo and Wildlife Medicine 27, 386–391.

## CHAPTER 17    Bearded dragon with hepatic disease

Barten SL (2006): Differential diagnoses by symptoms, Section VI: Lizards. In: Mader DR (ed.) Reptile Medicine and Surgery, 2nd edn. Saunders/Elsevier, St Louis, pp. 683–695.

Funk RS (2006): Specific diseases and clinical conditions, Section VII: Anorexia. In: Mader DR (ed.) Reptile Medicine and Surgery, 2nd edn. Saunders/Elsevier, St Louis, pp. 739–741.

Girling SJ, Raiti P (2004): Manual of Reptiles, 2nd edn. British Small Animal Veterinary Association, Quedgeley, Gloucester.

Hernandez-Divers SJ, Cooper JE (2006): Specific diseases and clinical conditions, Section VII: Hepatic lipidosis. In: Mader

DR (ed.) Reptile Medicine and Surgery, 2nd edn. Saunders/Elsevier, St Louis, pp. 806–813.

O'Malley B (2005): Lizards. Clinical Anatomy and Physiology of Exotic Species: Structure and Function of Mammals, Birds, Reptiles and Amphibians. Elsevier/Saunders, Edinburgh, pp. 57–75.

### CHAPTER 18    Osteomyelitis in a Hermann's tortoise

Done L (2006): Neurologic disorders. In: Mader DR (ed.) Reptile Medicine and Surgery, 2nd edn. Saunders/Elsevier, St Louis, pp. 852–857.

Fitzgerald KT, Vera R (2006): Spinal osteopathy. In: Mader DR (ed.) Reptile Medicine and Surgery, 2nd edn. Saunders/Elsevier, St Louis, pp. 906–912.

Longley LA (2008): Chelonian (tortoise, terrapin and turtle) anaesthesia. Anaesthesia of Exotic Pets. Elsevier/Saunders, Edinburgh. pp. 228–237.

Mader DR (2006): Abscesses. In: Mader DR (ed.) Reptile Medicine and Surgery, 2nd edn. Saunders/Elsevier, St Louis, pp. 715–719.

Mader DR, Bennett RA, Funk RS, et al. (2006): Surgery. In: Mader DR (ed.) Reptile Medicine and Surgery, 2nd edn. Saunders/Elsevier, St Louis, pp. 581–630.

McArthur S, Hernandez-Divers S (2004): Surgery. In: McArthur S, Wilkinson R, Meyer J (eds) Medicine and Surgery of Tortoises and Turtles. Blackwell Publishing, Oxford, pp. 403–464.

McArthur S, Meyer J, Innis C (2004): Anatomy and physiology. In: McArthur S, Wilkinson R, Meyer J (eds) Medicine and Surgery of Tortoises and Turtles. Blackwell Publishing, Oxford, pp. 35–72.

Rees Davies R, Klingenbery RJ (2004): Therapeutics and medication. In: Girling SJ, Raiti P (eds) Manual of Reptiles, 2nd edn. British Small Animal Veterinary Association, Quedgeley, Gloucester, pp. 115–130.

Wilkinson R, Hernandez-Divers S, Lafortune M, et al. (2004): Diagnostic imaging techniques. In: McArthur S, Wilkinson R, Meyer J (eds) Medicine and Surgery of Tortoises and Turtles. Blackwell Publishing, Oxford, pp. 187–238.

### CHAPTER 19    Dystocia in a snake

DeNardo D (2006): Dystocias. In: Mader DR (ed.) Reptile Medicine and Surgery, 2nd edn. Saunders/Elsevier, St Louis, pp. 787–792.

Hernandez-Divers SJ (2004): Surgery: principles and techniques. In: Girling SJ, Raiti P (eds) Manual of Reptiles, 2nd edn. British Small Animal Veterinary Association, Quedgeley, Gloucester, pp. 147–167.

Obst FJ, Richter K, Jacob U (1988): The Completely Illustrated Atlas of Reptiles and Amphibians for the Terrarium. T.F.H, Neptune City, New Jersey.

### CHAPTER 20    Dysecdysis in a leopard gecko

Blood DC, Studdert VP (1988): Baillière's Comprehensive Veterinary Dictionary. Baillière Tindall, London.

Fraser MA, Girling S (2004): Dermatology. In: Girling SJ, Raiti P (eds) Manual of Reptiles, 2nd edn. British Small Animal Veterinary Association, Quedgeley, Gloucester, pp. 184–198.

Halliday T, Adler K (2002): The New Encyclopedia of Reptiles & Amphibians. Oxford University Press, Oxford.

Varga M (2004): Captive maintenance and welfare. In: Girling SJ, Raiti P (eds) Manual of Reptiles, 2nd edn. British Small Animal Veterinary Association, Quedgeley, Gloucester, pp. 6–17.

### CHAPTER 21    Aural abscesses in a map turtle

Fraser MA, Girling S (2004): Dermatology. In: Girling SJ, Raiti P (eds) Manual of Reptiles, 2nd edn. British Small Animal Veterinary Association, Quedgeley, Gloucester, pp. 184–198.

Halliday T, Adler K (2002): The New Encyclopedia of Reptiles & Amphibians. Oxford University Press, Oxford.

Hernandez-Divers SJ (2004): Surgery: principles and techniques. In: Girling SJ, Raiti P (eds) Manual of Reptiles, 2nd edn. British Small Animal Veterinary Association, Quedgeley, Gloucester, pp. 147–167.

O'Malley B (2005): General anatomy and physiology of reptiles. Clinical Anatomy and Physiology of Exotic Species: Structure and Function of Mammals, Birds, Reptiles and Amphibians. Elsevier/Saunders, Edinburgh, pp. 7–39.

O'Malley B (2005): Tortoises and turtles. Clinical Anatomy and Physiology of Exotic Species: Structure and Function of Mammals, Birds, Reptiles, and Amphibians. Elsevier/Saunders, Edinburgh, pp. 41–56.

### CHAPTER 22    Hypocalcaemia in a green iguana

Burnie D (2001): Animal. Dorling Kindersley, London.

Calvert I (2004): Nutritional problems. In: Girling SJ, Raiti P (eds) Manual of Reptiles, 2nd edn. British Small Animal Veterinary Association, Quedgeley, Gloucester, pp. 289–308.

Eatwell K (2009): Variations in the concentration of ionised calcium in the plasma of captive tortoises (Testudo species). The Veterinary Record 163 (3), 82–84.

Fraser MA, Girling S (2004): Dermatology. In: Girling SJ, Raiti P (eds) Manual of Reptiles, 2nd edn. British Small Animal Veterinary Association, Quedgeley, Gloucester, pp. 184–198

Halliday T, Adler K (2002): The New Encyclopedia of Reptiles & Amphibians. Oxford University Press, Oxford.

O'Malley B (2005): General anatomy and physiology of reptiles. Clinical Anatomy and Physiology of Exotic Species: Structure and Function of Mammals, Birds, Reptiles and Amphibians. Elsevier/Saunders, Edinburgh, pp. 7–39.

O'Malley B (2005): Tortoises and turtles. Clinical Anatomy and Physiology of Exotic Species: Structure and Function of Mammals, Birds, Reptiles, and Amphibians. Elsevier/Saunders, Edinburgh, pp. 41–56.

## SECTION 4    AMPHIBIANS

### CHAPTER 23    Amphibians – an introduction

Halliday T, Adler K (2002): The New Encyclopedia of Reptiles & Amphibians. Oxford University Press, Oxford.

Helmer PJ, Whiteside DP (2005): Amphibian anatomy and physiology. In: O'Malley B (ed.) Clinical Anatomy and Physiology of Exotic Species: Structure and Function of Mammals,

Birds, Reptiles and Amphibians. Elsevier/Saunders, Edinburgh, pp. 3–14.

Longley LA (2008): Amphibian anaesthesia. In: Longley LA (ed.) Anaesthesia of Exotic Pets. Saunders/Elsevier, Edinburgh, pp. 245–260.

Williams DL (2002): Amphibians. In: Meredith A, Redrobe S (eds) Manual of Exotic Pets, 4th edn. British Small Animal Veterinary Association, Quedgeley, Gloucester, pp. 257–266.

Wright KM, Whitaker BR (2001): Amphibian Medicine and Captive Husbandry. Krieger Publishing, Malabar, Florida.

## CHAPTER 24   Trauma in an amphibian

Barnett SL, Cover JF, Wright KM (2001): Amphibian husbandry and housing. In: Wright KM, Whitaker BR (eds) Amphibian Medicine and Captive Husbandry. Krieger Publishing, Malabar, Florida, pp. 35–61.

Halliday T, Adler K (2002): The New Encyclopedia of Reptiles & Amphibians. Oxford University Press, Oxford.

Helmer PJ, Whiteside DP (2005): Amphibian anatomy and physiology. In: O'Malley B (ed.) Clinical Anatomy and Physiology of Exotic Species: Structure and Function of Mammals, Birds, Reptiles and Amphibians. Elsevier/Saunders, Edinburgh, pp. 3–14.

Wright KM (2001): Trauma. In: Wright KM, Whitaker BR (eds) Amphibian Medicine and Captive Husbandry. Krieger Publishing, Malabar, Florida, pp. 233–238.

# SECTION 5   FISH

## CHAPTER 25   Fish – an introduction

Fiddes M (2008): Fish anaesthesia. In: Longley LA (ed.) Anaesthesia of Exotic Pets. Saunders/Elsevier, Edinburgh, pp. 261–278.

Maclean B (2002): Ornamental fish. In: Meredith A, Redrobe S (eds) Manual of Exotic Pets, 4th edn. British Small Animal Veterinary Association, Quedgeley, Gloucester, pp. 267–279.

Sandford G (1999): Aquarium: An Owner's Manual: The Complete Illustrated Guide to the Home Aquarium. Dorling Kindersley, London.

Wildgoose WH (2001): Manual of Ornamental Fish, 2nd edn. British Small Animal Veterinary Association, Quedgeley, Gloucester.

## CHAPTER 26   Enucleation of an eye in a goldfish

Fiddes M (2008): Fish anaesthesia. In: Longley LA (ed.) Anaesthesia of Exotic Pets. Saunders/Elsevier, Edinburgh, pp. 261–278.

Harms CA (2003): Fish. In: Fowler ME, Miller RE (eds) Zoo and Wild Animal Medicine, 5th edn. Saunders/Elsevier, St Louis, pp. 2–20.

Lawton MPC (2002): Exotic species. In: Petersen-Jones S, Crispin S (eds) Manual of Small Animal Ophthalmology, 2nd edn. British Small Animal Veterinary Association, Quedgeley, Gloucester, pp. 285–295.

Lewbart GA (1998): Self-Assessment Colour Review of Ornamental Fish. Manson Publishing, London.

Wildgoose WH (2001): Manual of Ornamental Fish, 2nd edn. British Small Animal Veterinary Association, Quedgeley, Gloucester.

# APPENDICES

## Appendix 1   Critical care

Carpenter JW (2005): Exotic Animal Formulary. Elsevier, St Louis.

Lennox AM (2009): Avian advanced anaesthesia, monitoring and critical care. BSAVA Annual Congress. British Small Animal Veterinary Association, Birmingham, pp. 54–57.

Longley LA (2008): Anaesthesia of Exotic Pets. Elsevier/ Saunders, Edinburgh.

Wright KM, Whitaker BR (2001): Amphibian Medicine and Captive Husbandry. Krieger Publishing, Malabar, Florida.

## Appendix 2   Zoonoses

Chitty J, Lierz M (2008): Manual of Raptors, Pigeons and Passerine Birds. British Small Animal Veterinary Association, Quedgeley, Gloucester.

Fowler ME, Miller RE (2003): Zoo and Wild Animal Medicine, 5th edn. Saunders, St Louis.

Girling SJ, Raiti P (2004): Manual of Reptiles, 2nd edn. British Small Animal Veterinary Association, Quedgeley, Gloucester.

Harcourt-Brown F (2002): Textbook of Rabbit Medicine. Butterworth-Heinemann, Oxford.

Harcourt-Brown N, Chitty J (2005): Manual of Psittacine Birds, 2nd edn. British Small Animal Veterinary Association, Quedgeley, Gloucester.

Hosey G, Melfi V, Pankhurst S (2009): Zoo Animals: Behaviour, Management, and Welfare. Oxford University Press, Oxford.

Keeble E, Meredith A (2009): Manual of Rodents and Ferrets. British Small Animal Veterinary Association, Quedgeley, Gloucester.

Meredith A, Redrobe S (2002): Manual of Exotic Pets, 4th edn. British Small Animal Veterinary Association, Quedgeley, Gloucester.

Wildgoose WH (2001): Manual of Ornamental Fish, 2nd edn. British Small Animal Veterinary Association, Quedgeley, Gloucester.

# Index

NB: Page numbers followed by *f* indicate figures; *t* indicate tables; *b* indicate boxes